AF556840

An Atlas of Investigation and Treatment

HEMORRHAGIC STROKE

For the Stroke Center team at Hartford Hospital

IES

For the Stroke Team at Saint Luke's Hospital, Kansas City

MMR

An Atlas of Investigation and Treatment

HEMORRHAGIC STROKE

Isaac E Silverman, MD
Vascular Neurology
Co-Medical Director
The Stroke Center at Hartford Hospital
Hartford, Connecticut
USA

Marilyn M Rymer, MD
Saint Luke's Brain and Stroke Institute
Saint Luke's Hospital
UMKC School of Medicine
Kansas City, Missouri
USA

Foreword by

Joseph P Broderick, MD
Professor and Chair
Department of Neurology
University of Cincinnati Neuroscience Institute
Cincinnati, Ohio
USA

Special contributions by

Gary R Spiegel, MDCM (Neuroimaging)
Jefferson Radiology
Director of Neurointervention
Co-Medical Director
The Stroke Center at Hartford Hospital
Hartford, Connecticut
USA

Robert E Schmidt, MD, PHD (Neuropathology)
Professor, Pathology and Immunology
Washington University School of Medicine
St Louis, Missouri
USA

CLINICAL PUBLISHING

OXFORD

Clinical Publishing
an imprint of Atlas Medical Publishing Ltd
Oxford Centre for Innovation
Mill Street, Oxford OX2 0JX, UK

Tel: +44 1865 811116
Fax: +44 1865 251550
Email: info@clinicalpublishing.co.uk
Web: www.clinicalpublishing.co.uk

Distributed in USA and Canada by:
Clinical Publishing
30 Amberwood Parkway
Ashland OH 44805, USA

Tel: 800-247-6553 (toll free within US and Canada)
Fax: 419-281-6883
Email: order@bookmasters.com

Distributed in UK and Rest of World by:
Marston Book Services Ltd
PO Box 269
Abingdon
Oxon OX14 4YN, UK

Tel: +44 1235 465500
Fax: +44 1235 465555
Email: trade.orders@marston.co.uk

First published 2010

A catalogue record of this book is available from the British Library

ISBN-13 978 1 84692 039 4
ISBN e-book 978 1 84692 616 7

Project manager: Gavin Smith, GPS Publishing Solutions, Herts, UK
Illustrations by Graeme Chambers, BA(Hons)
Typeset by Phoenix Photosetting, Chatham, Kent, UK
Printed by Marston Book Services Ltd, Abingdon, Oxon, UK

Contents

Foreword

A picture is worth a thousand words but in a stroke patient, a picture also provides the definitive answer as to whether there is bleeding in or around the brain. The introduction of CT imaging of the brain in 1972 revolutionized the field of the epidemiology, pathophysiology, and treatment of stroke – particularly that of intracerebral and subarachnoid hemorrhage. For example, prior to CT and MR brain imaging, intracerebral hemorrhage (ICH) was thought to be uncommon, mostly fatal, and due to hypertension in most instances. We know now that intracerebral hemorrhage is a common cause of stroke and in many instances cannot be differentiated from ischemic stroke by clinical features alone. We have also learned that imaging of the location of bleeding, as well as associated structural changes, provides critical clues as to the probable cause.

Thus, an atlas that uses pictures to teach the epidemiology, pathophysiology and treatment of hemorrhagic stroke is a marvelous way to teach and to learn about these devastating stroke subtypes which have much higher mortality and morbidity than ischemic stroke. For example, the pattern of multiple cortical old microhemorrhages on gradient echo imaging, combined with a new lobar ICH, speaks very strongly to the likely diagnosis of amyloid-associated ICH whereas a pattern of old microhemorrhages in the deep basal ganglia and white matter structures with a new subcortical hemorrhage speaks very strongly to the likelihood of hypertensive hemorrhage. Only brain imaging can make this probable diagnosis without autopsy, and only a pictorial atlas showing the appropriate brain imaging, illustrations and pathology can allow physicians to recognize this pattern and make the likely diagnosis in their patients with hemorrhagic stroke. Imaging of ongoing bleeding in patients with intracerebral hemorrhage during the first hours after onset conveys better than any words the urgency required to slow and halt the process. Brain imaging in patients continues to evolve, with radiopharmaceutical agents using PET imaging that can image amyloid deposition in the brain and associated blood vessels in patients with lobar intracerebral hemorrhage.

A host of technologic advances to treat structural causes of ruptured intracranial vessels such as clips, coils, stents, balloons, embolization and focused radiation therapy have evolved over the past 40 years. Surgical techniques to remove hemorrhage in the brain and ventricles have unfortunately not demonstrated clear benefit for patients but are frequently used. Again, imaging, as shown in an atlas, provides the best way to highlight these therapeutic technologies.

The brain imaging, illustrated figures and pathologic images in this atlas are superb and the accompanying text is clear and straightforward. This book is a great way for students, resident physicians, stroke fellows and neurologic physicians to learn about hemorrhagic stroke. These powerful images will remain with the reader long after they close the book.

Joseph P. Broderick, MD
February, 2010

Preface

Hemorrhagic stroke has always been the poor sibling to its ischemic counterpart. Not only is hemorrhage much less common, but it also has significantly worse clinical outcomes, and relatively fewer emergent therapies. The reality that only about 20% of patients with a primary intracerebral hemorrhage (ICH, the most common type of major bleeding in the brain) survive to make an independent recovery should be a call to focus upon this important disease.

Hemorrhagic stroke is grabbing the attention of neurovascular clinicians for several reasons. First, an aging population facilitates the development of the most common forms of hemorrhagic stroke, primary ICH (due to hypertension and cerebral amyloid angiopathy), and subarachnoid hemorrhage (due to the development of intracranial aneurysms, with its chief risk factors of hypertension and tobacco use). Second, advancing neuroimaging is better at detecting not only acute hemorrhagic stroke but also at identifying subclinical hemorrhage, such as the gradient-echo magnetic resonance imaging (MRI) detection of microhemorrhage and cavernous malformations, and computed tomography (CT) and MR angiography's definition of unruptured intracranial aneurysms and vascular malformations. There is still a role for old-school conventional cerebral angiography in the management of many patients with hemorrhagic stroke.

An era of increased awareness of hemorrhagic stroke may soon translate into a wider proliferation of treatments. The success of recombinant factor VIIa in preventing the expansion of ICH was an important first step from a large international clinical trial evaluating an emergent drug therapy. Efforts to reduce the delayed impact of toxic by-products of free blood upon brain parenchyma may conceivably hold clinical benefit at much wider time windows than have proven helpful for therapies of acute ischemic stroke. In addition, although earlier efforts of neurosurgical evacuation of hemorrhage within the brain have been unsuccessful, ongoing studies are looking at less invasive means; e.g. endoscopic aspiration and thrombolytic agents delivered via external ventricular devices, in order to reduce clot burden; or are focusing upon subgroups of patients; e.g. those patients with lobar lesions. For complex neurovascular disorders, large comparative trials have either been completed (i.e. in intracranial aneurysms, comparing neurosurgical clipping versus endovascular coiling) or are under way (i.e. in unruptured vascular malformations, comparing conservative medical therapy versus aggressive interventions).

Finally, hemorrhagic stroke is bringing together neurovascular clinicians with distinct training backgrounds. Its in-hospital management gathers together vascular neurology, interventional neuroradiology, vascular neurosurgery, and neurocritical care medicine. For example, during the past 15–20 years, endovascular approaches have been developed to complement open neurosurgery in the management of intracranial aneurysms. In addition, radiation treatment is a viable option for some arteriovenous malformations.

Continuing from where our previous volume left off (*Ischemic Stroke: An Atlas of Investigation and Treatment*), we again intend to introduce clinicians, residents in training, and medical and nursing students to the breadth of the 'dark side' – hemorrhagic stroke – of neurovascular disorders. In addition to this survey of neuroimaging and neuropathology, case studies demonstrate the clinical management considerations surrounding various types of hemorrhagic stroke. The result is a broader range of clinical pathology than found in our earlier volume. We conclude this volume with a survey of *'Extreme'* Neurovascular Disorders, as a means to convey the wide array of interesting and challenging disorders we encounter as clinicians.

We hope that you find this volume on hemorrhagic stroke a useful companion to *Ischemic Stroke: An Atlas of Investigation and Treatment*.

Isaac E. Silverman, MD
Marilyn M. Rymer, MD
December 2009

Abbreviations

ACA	anterior cerebral artery
ACE	angiotensin-converting enzyme
A-Comm	anterior communicating artery
ADC	apparent diffusion coefficient
AICA	anterior inferior cerebellar artery
AIS	acute ischemic stroke
AP	anteroposterior
AV	arteriovenous
AVF	arteriovenous fistula
AVM	arteriovenous malformation
BA	basilar artery
CA	conventional angiography
CAA	cerebral amyloid angiopathy
CADASIL	cerebral autosomal dominant arteriopathy with subcortical infarcts and leukoencephalopathy
CCA	common carotid artery
CM	cavernous malformation
CNS	central nervous system
CS	cavernous sinus
CSF	cerebrospinal fluid
CT	computed tomography
CTA	CT angiography
CVP	central venous pressure
DM	diabetes mellitus
DVA	developmental venous anomaly
DWI	diffusion-weighted imaging
DW-MRI	diffusion-weighted magnetic resonance imaging
ECA	external carotid artery
ECASS	European Cooperative Acute Stroke Study
FLAIR	fluid attenuated inversion recovery
GCS	Glasgow Coma Scale
GE	gradient-echo
H&E	hematoxylin and eosin (stain)
HELPP	hemolysis, elevated liver enzymes, low platelets
HI	hemorrhagic infarction
HTN	hypertension
IA	intracranial aneurysms
ICA	internal carotid artery
ICH	intracerebral hemorrhage
ICP	intracranial pressure
ISAT	International Subarachnoid Aneurysm Trial
IV	intravenous
JNC-7	The Seventh Report of the Joint National Committee on Prevention, Detection, Evaluation, and Treatment of High Blood Pressure
MCA	middle cerebral artery
MRA	magnetic resonance angiography
MRI	magnetic resonance imaging
MRV	magnetic resonance venography
NBCA	N-butyl cyanoacrylate
NIHSS	National Institutes of Health Stroke Scale
NINDS	National Institute of Neurological Disorders and Stroke
PCA	posterior cerebral artery
P-Comm	posterior communicating artery
PCWP	pulmonary capillary wedge pressure
PICA	posterior inferior cerebellar artery
PROGRESS	Perindopril Protection Against Recurrent Stroke Study
PT(INR)	prothrombin time (International Normalized Ratio)
rFVIIa	recombinant activated factor VII
RR	relative risk
SAH	subarachnoid hemorrhage
SCA	superior cerebellar artery
SDH	subdural hematoma
SHEP	Systolic Hypertension in the Elderly Program
SIADH	syndrome of inappropriate antidiuretic hormone secretion
SIVMS	Scottish Intracranial Vascular Malformation Study
STICH	Surgical Trial in Intracerebral Hemorrhage
T1WI	T1-weighted image
T2WI	T2-weighted image
TCD	transcranial Doppler
TIA	transient ischemic attack
t-PA	tissue plasminogen activator
VA	vertebral artery
VGM	vein of Galen malformation
VHL	Von Hippel–Lindau
WI	weighted image

Chapter 1

Intracerebral Hemorrhage

Epidemiology

Intracerebral hemorrhage (ICH) accounts for 10–15% of all strokes. Primary ICH occurs when small intracranial vessels are damaged by chronic hypertension (HTN) or cerebral amyloid angiopathy (CAA), and accounts for 78–88% of all ICH. Secondary causes for ICH are listed in *Table 1.1*.[1]

The incidence of ICH worldwide ranges from 10 to 20 cases per 100 000 population and increases with age. Certain populations, in particular, the Japanese and those of Afro-Caribbean descent, have a heightened incidence of 50–55 per 100 000 that may reflect a higher prevalence of HTN and/or decreased access to healthcare.[1] The incidence of hemorrhage increases exponentially with age and is higher in men than in women.[2]

Clinical presentation

Neurologic deficits from ICH reflect the location of the initial bleeding and associated edema. In addition, seizures, vomiting, headache, and diminished level of consciousness are common presenting symptoms. A depressed level of alertness on initial evaluation occurs infrequently in acute ischemic stroke (AIS) but is seen in approximately 50% of patients with ICH.[3]

Table 1.1 Common secondary causes of intracerebral hemorrhages

Causes	Chapter number	Primary means of diagnosis
Arteriovenous malformation	3	MRI, CA
Intracranial aneurysm	2	MRA, CTA and CA
Cavernous angioma	4	Gradient-echo MRI
Venous angioma	4	MRI with gadolinium, CA
Venous sinus thrombosis	1	MRV, CA
Intracranial neoplasm		MRI with gadolinium
Coagulopathy	1	Clinical history, serologic studies
Vasculitis		Serologic markers, MRI with gadolinium, CA, brain biopsy
Drug use (e.g., cocaine, alcohol)		Clinical history, toxicology screens
Hemorrhagic transformation	1	Non-contrast CT and gradient-echo MRI scans

CA, cerebral angiography.
Adapted with permission from Qureshi *et al.*[1]

Outcomes

Spontaneous, or non-traumatic, ICH has a much poorer outcome than AIS.[1] There is a 62% mortality rate by 1 year, and only about 20% of survivors are living independently by 6 months.[3] About half of the deaths due to ICH over the first 30 days will occur within the first 2 days, largely from cerebral herniation.[3] Later, mortality is more commonly due to medical complications, such as aspiration pneumonia or venous thromboembolism.

The primary predictors for outcomes from ICH are:

- *Lesion size*. Larger hemispheric lesions >30 ml volume have a high mortality rate (**1.1**).

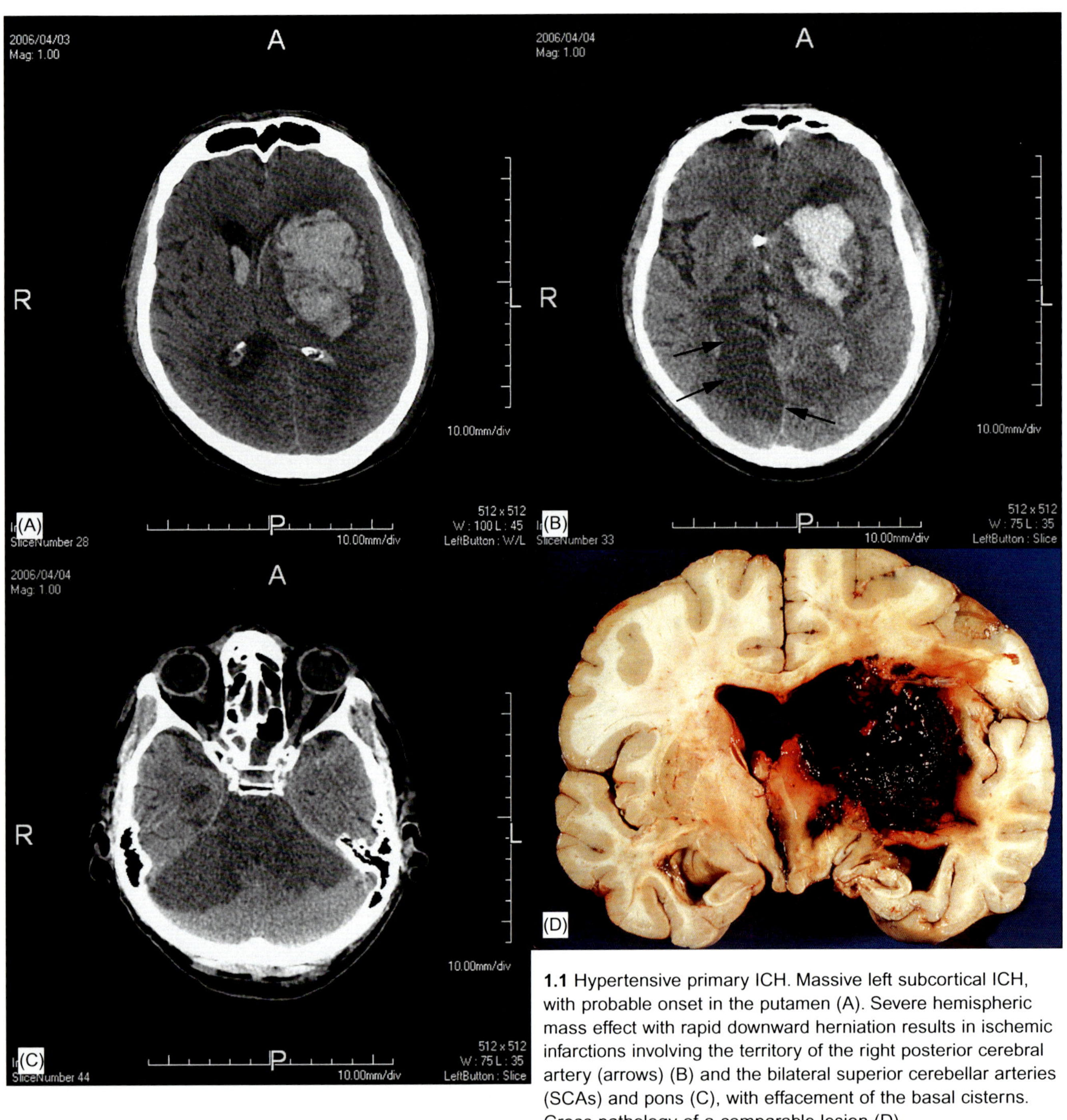

1.1 Hypertensive primary ICH. Massive left subcortical ICH, with probable onset in the putamen (A). Severe hemispheric mass effect with rapid downward herniation results in ischemic infarctions involving the territory of the right posterior cerebral artery (arrows) (B) and the bilateral superior cerebellar arteries (SCAs) and pons (C), with effacement of the basal cisterns. Gross pathology of a comparable lesion (D).

- *Level of consciousness.* Patients with Glasgow Coma Scale (GCS) <9 points and hematoma >60 ml have a 90% mortality rate.[3]
- *Intraventricular component.*[1,4] In one study, intraventricular involvement predicted a mortality rate of 43% at 30 days, versus 9% without ventricular involvement.[5]
- *Lesion location.* Deep hemispheric lesions (e.g., brainstem, thalamus) have a poorer prognosis than subcortical or cerebellar hematomas.[2] Even 5–10 ml of hemorrhage into the brainstem can be devastating (**1.2**).
- *Age.* Advanced age, >80 years, carries a higher risk of mortality.

Risk factors

Hypertension

By far the most important modifiable risk factor for spontaneous ICH is HTN.[3] Primary hypertensive hemorrhage results from the rupture of small penetrating arteries originating in the anterior, middle (i.e., lenticulostriate), and posterior cerebral (i.e., thalamostriate) arteries and the pons (i.e., paramedian perforators) (**1.3**). HTN causes vessel rupture at or near the bifurcation of affected vessels, where degeneration of components of the arterial wall (media and smooth muscle) are identified.[1] The annual risk of recurrent hemorrhage is 2% without antihypertensive treatment.[6]

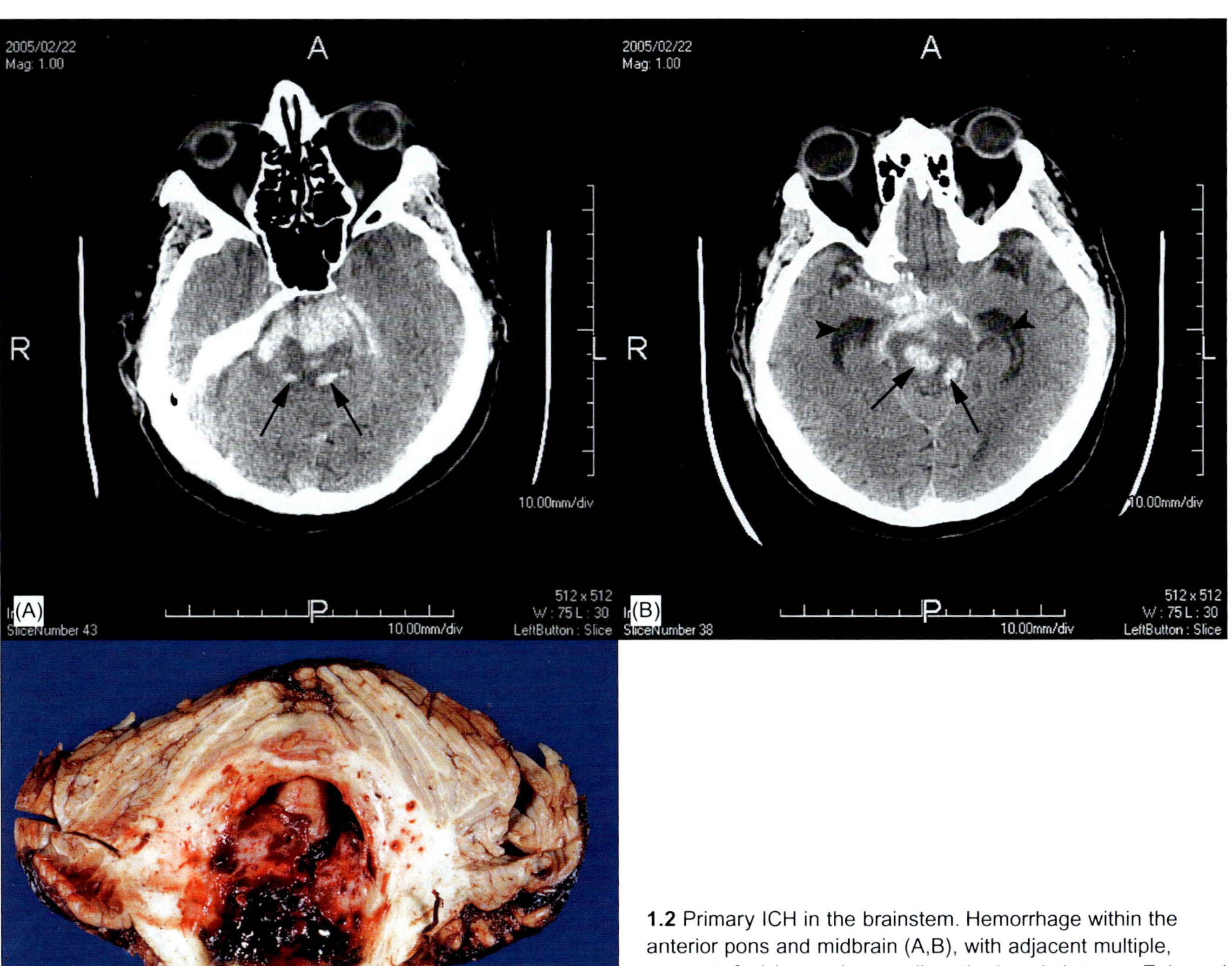

1.2 Primary ICH in the brainstem. Hemorrhage within the anterior pons and midbrain (A,B), with adjacent multiple, punctate foci (arrows), as well as the basal cisterns. Enlarged temporal horns of the lateral ventricles (B, arrowheads) are a sign of obstructive hydrocephalus. Gross pathology of a pontine hemorrhage (C).

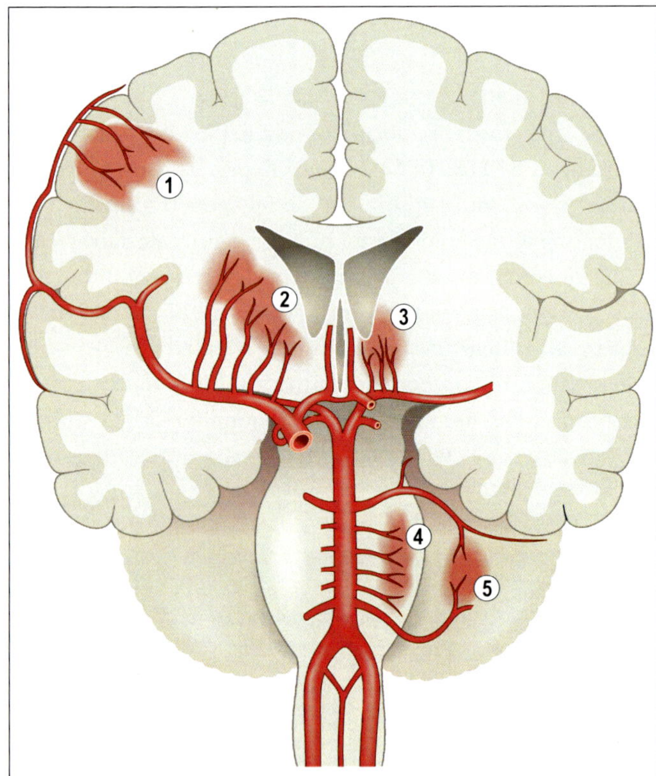

1.3 Common sites for primary ICH. Small, penetrating arterial branches are the source of the vast majority of primary ICH: (1) penetrating cortical branches of the major intracranial arteries; (2) lenticulostriate branches; (3) thalamoperforator branches; (4) paramedian pontine branches; and (5) penetrating branches from the major cerebellar arteries (from Qureshi *et al.*[1] with permission).

Cerebral amyloid angiopathy

Cerebral amyloid angiopathy (CAA) is a leading cause, along with HTN, for spontaneous ICH in patients >60 years old. It is a degenerative condition in which β-amyloid protein deposits within the walls of blood vessels of the cerebral cortex and leptomeninges predispose to leakage of blood into brain parenchyma (**1.4**).[7] The diagnostic criteria are a combination of clinical, neuroimaging, and pathologic findings (*Table 1.2*).[8] The annual risk of recurrent hemorrhage is 10.5%.[9]

Table 1.2 Boston criteria for diagnosis of CAA-related hemorrhage

1. **Definite CAA – Full post-mortem examination demonstrating:**
   - Lobar, cortical, or corticosubcortical hemorrhage
   - Severe CAA with vasculopathy
   - Absence of other diagnostic lesion
2. **Probable CAA with supporting pathology – Clinical data and pathologic tissue (evacuated hematoma or cortical biopsy) demonstrating:**
   - Lobar, cortical, or corticosubcortical hemorrhage
   - Severe CAA with vasculopathy
   - Absence of other diagnostic lesion
3. **Probable CAA – Clinical data and MRI or CT demonstrating:**
   - Multiple hemorrhages restricted to lobar, cortical, or corticosubcortical regions (cerebellar hemorrhage allowed)
   - Age ≥55 years
   - Absence of other cause of hemorrhage*
4. **Possible CAA – Clinical data and MRI or CT demonstrating:**
   - Single lobar, cortical, or corticosubcortical hemorrhage
   - Age ≥55 years
   - Absence of other cause of hemorrhage*

**Other causes of ICH*: supratherapeutic anticoagulation (prothrombin time (International Normalized Ratio) PT(INR)) >3.0); antecedent head trauma or ischemic stroke; central nervous system (CNS) tumor, vascular malformation, or vasculitis; and blood dyscrasia, or coagulopathy.
Adapted with permission from Knudsen *et al.*[8]

Antithrombotic agents

- Oral anticoagulation with warfarin increases the risk of ICH two to five times and is directly related to the intensity of anticoagulation.[10] In contrast to primary ICH, the bleeding associated with warfarin may persist for 12–24 hours.[10] A fatal outcome occurs in two-thirds of patients with an International Normalized Ratio (INR) >3.0 at presentation.[11]
- Antiplatelet agents: aspirin use alone may be a weaker risk factor for continued bleeding due to ICH and poor outcomes;[12] however, combination antiplatelet treatment with aspirin and clopidogrel increases the risk for ICH over either agent alone.[13]

Alcohol

Alcohol impairs coagulation and injures cerebral vessels. Recent heavy alcohol exposure (e.g., during the preceding week) is a risk factor for ICH.[14]

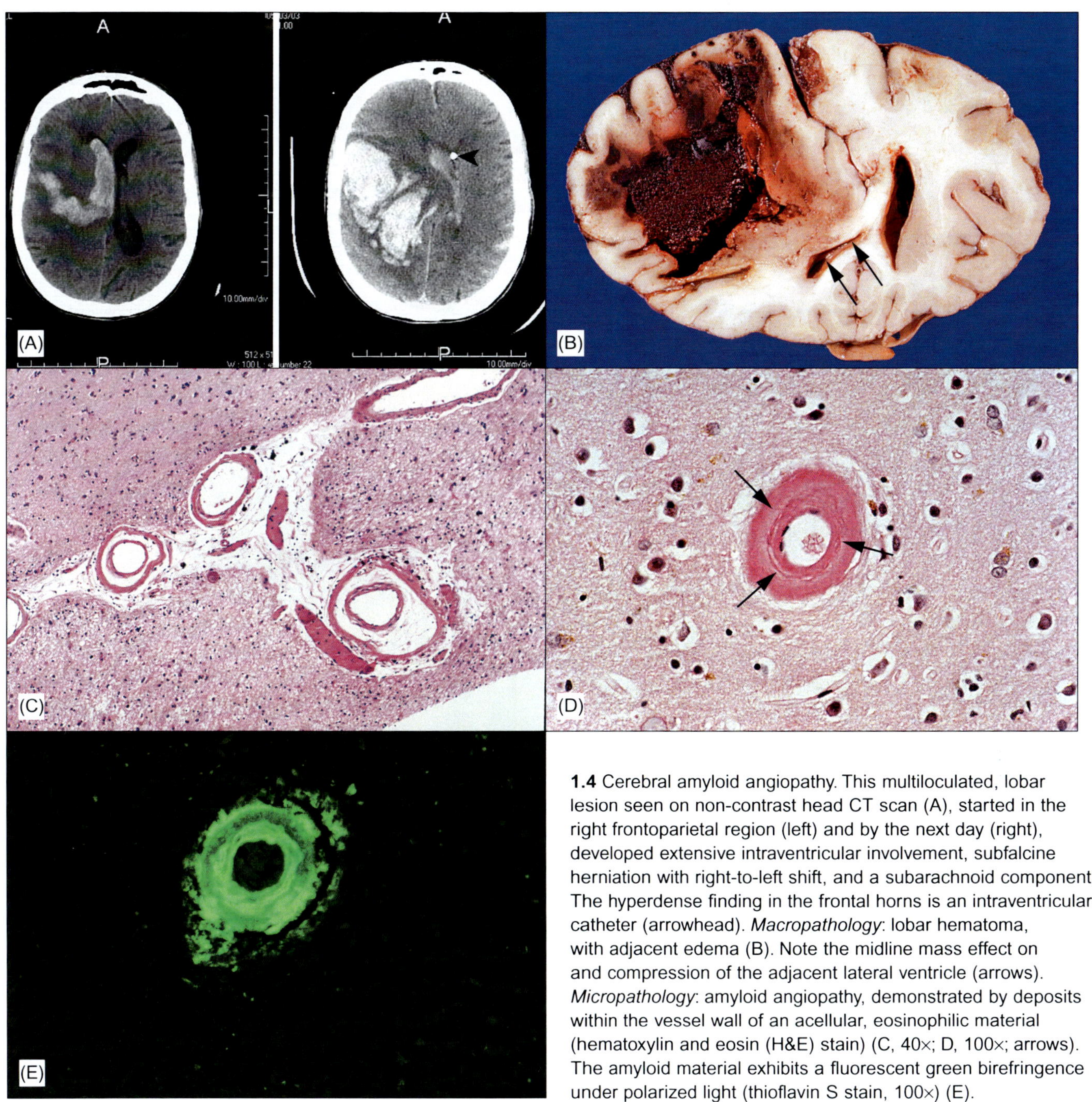

1.4 Cerebral amyloid angiopathy. This multiloculated, lobar lesion seen on non-contrast head CT scan (A), started in the right frontoparietal region (left) and by the next day (right), developed extensive intraventricular involvement, subfalcine herniation with right-to-left shift, and a subarachnoid component. The hyperdense finding in the frontal horns is an intraventricular catheter (arrowhead). *Macropathology*: lobar hematoma, with adjacent edema (B). Note the midline mass effect on and compression of the adjacent lateral ventricle (arrows). *Micropathology*: amyloid angiopathy, demonstrated by deposits within the vessel wall of an acellular, eosinophilic material (hematoxylin and eosin (H&E) stain) (C, 40×; D, 100×; arrows). The amyloid material exhibits a fluorescent green birefringence under polarized light (thioflavin S stain, 100×) (E).

Other risk factors

Illicit drug use and coagulopathic disorders (*Table 1.3*) are associated with an increased risk of ICH. Over-the-counter stimulants, particularly if taken in excessive quantities, may predispose to ICH (**case study 1**). A large case–control study associated phenylpropanolamine use with ICH in young patients.[15]

Pathogenesis

Up to 70% of patients with primary ICH develop some measurable amount of lesion expansion over the initial few hours (**1.5**).[16] Hematoma growth is an independent determinant of both mortality and functional outcome after ICH.[16,17] The mass effect of primary bleeding may cause lesions to migrate and dissect through less dense white matter, with patches of intact brain tissue surrounding a hematoma (**1.6**). Although continued bleeding from the primary lesion source is one mechanism for expansion, another could be the mechanical disruption of local vessels by which multiple adjacent microbleeds develop, accumulate, and contribute to overall lesion volume (**1.2**A,B).

Table 1.3 Coagulation disorders associated with intracerebral hemorrhage

Excessive anticoagulation with warfarin, and other antithrombotic agents
- Aspirin use (RR = 1.35)
- Aspirin plus warfarin (RR = 2.4)
- Warfarin (RR = 2.5)
- Clopidogrel

Coagulation factor deficiencies (VIII, IX) and mutations (XIII)
Thrombocytopenia, especially <10 000/mm^3
Systemic disease
- Hepatic and renal failure
- Leukemia
- Bone marrow failure
- Cancer chemotherapy

Platelet dysfunction
- Idiopathic thrombocytopenic purpura
- HELPP syndrome (hemolysis, elevated liver enzymes, low platelets)
- Essential thrombocythemia

Prothrombotic states
- Disseminated intravascular coagulation
- Thrombotic thrombocytopenic purpura

Genetic polymorphisms
- Factor XIII
- α_1-antichymotrypsin
- Apolipoprotein E (α_2, α_4)

Hereditary disorders of hemostasis
- Von Willebrand's disease
- Afibrinogemia
- Glanzmann's thrombasthenia (GpIIb/IIIa receptor dysfunction)

RR, relative risk.
Adapted with permission from Coull and Skaff.[46]

A hematoma incites local edema and neuronal damage in the adjacent brain parenchyma (**1.7**). This edema typically increases in size over an interval as long as 3 weeks following the initial bleeding, with the greatest growth rate over the first 2 days.[2] Thrombin within the hematoma plays a central role in promoting perihematomal edema.[2] Hemoglobin and its products, heme and iron, are potent mitochondrial toxins, thereby increasing cell death.[18]

Lesion locations

Subcortical intracerebral hemorrhage

The most common site for hypertensive hemorrhage is the putamen, but ICH frequently occurs in all other subcortical locations (**1.8**).

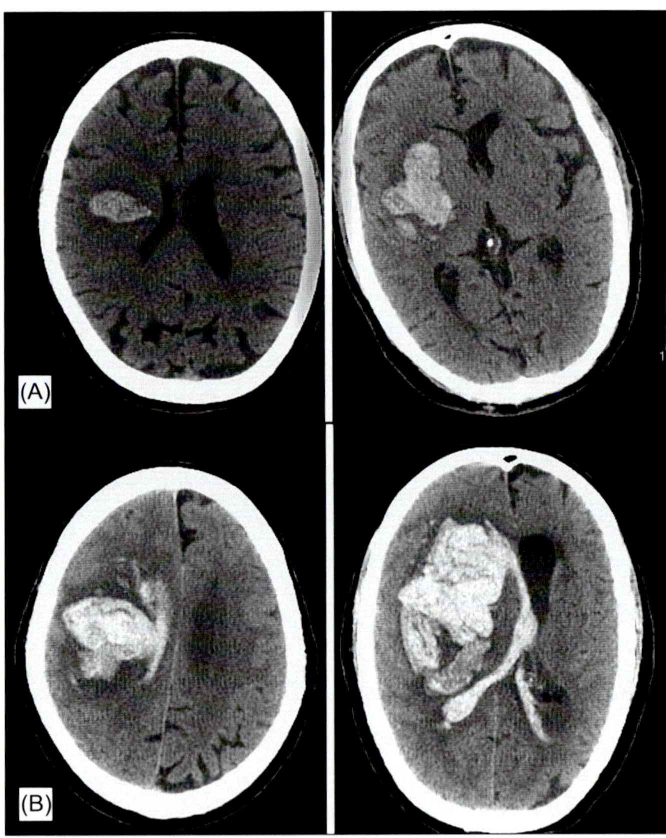

1.5 Early expansion of subcortical hemorrhage. The time elapsed between the two CT studies (A,B) was 80 minutes. First, a patient presenting with headache, dysarthria, and left hemiparesis, due to a right subcortical hemorrhage (A); the second scan was obtained due to rapidly deteriorating mental status and a dilated right pupil from uncal herniation (B). Note significant intraventricular extension, and diffuse edema effacing sulci throughout the right hemisphere.

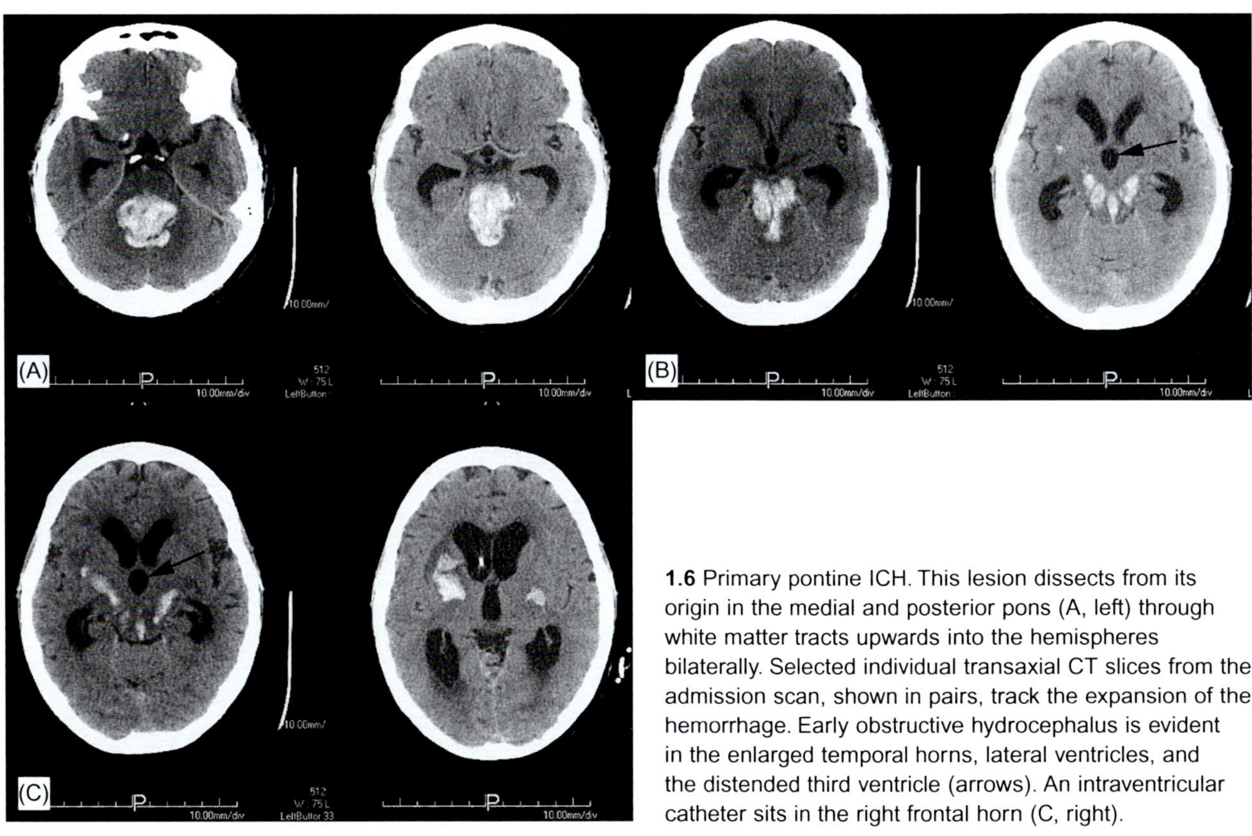

1.6 Primary pontine ICH. This lesion dissects from its origin in the medial and posterior pons (A, left) through white matter tracts upwards into the hemispheres bilaterally. Selected individual transaxial CT slices from the admission scan, shown in pairs, track the expansion of the hemorrhage. Early obstructive hydrocephalus is evident in the enlarged temporal horns, lateral ventricles, and the distended third ventricle (arrows). An intraventricular catheter sits in the right frontal horn (C, right).

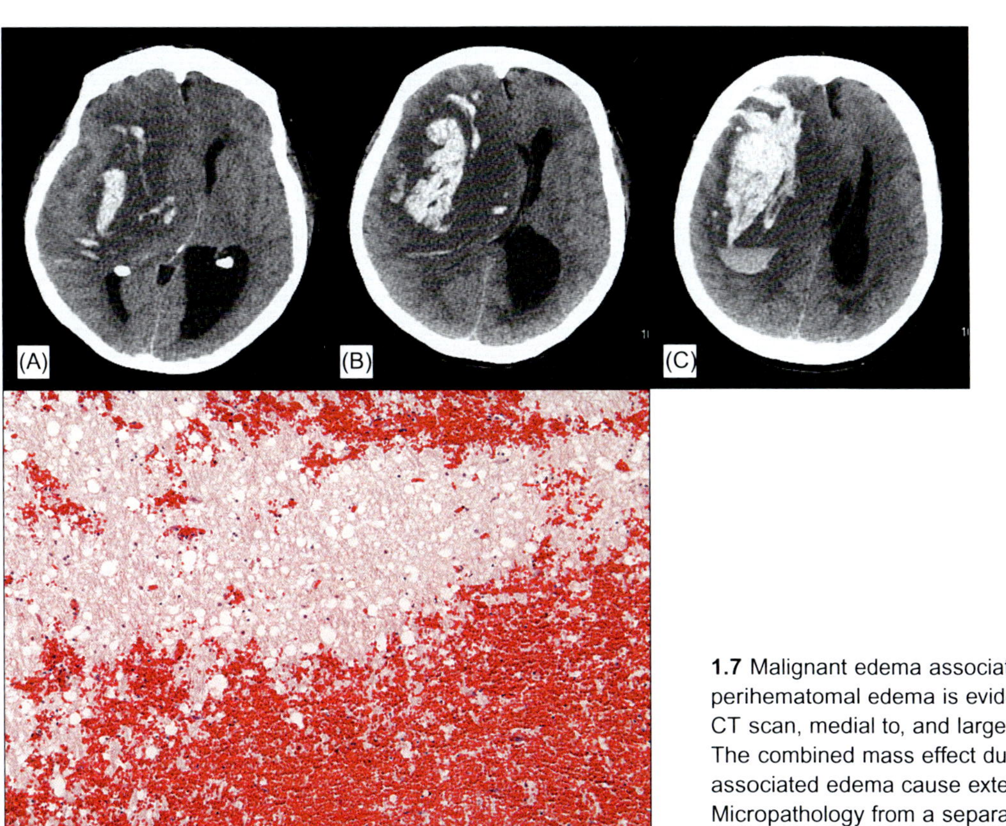

1.7 Malignant edema associated with primary ICH. Massive perihematomal edema is evident as wide hypodense regions on CT scan, medial to, and larger than, the primary hemorrhage. The combined mass effect due to the hemorrhage and its associated edema cause extensive subfalcine herniation (A–C). Micropathology from a separate case (D) shows the appearance of edema surrounded by red blood cells, the latter scattered along the upper margin and lower half of this image (H&E, 40×).

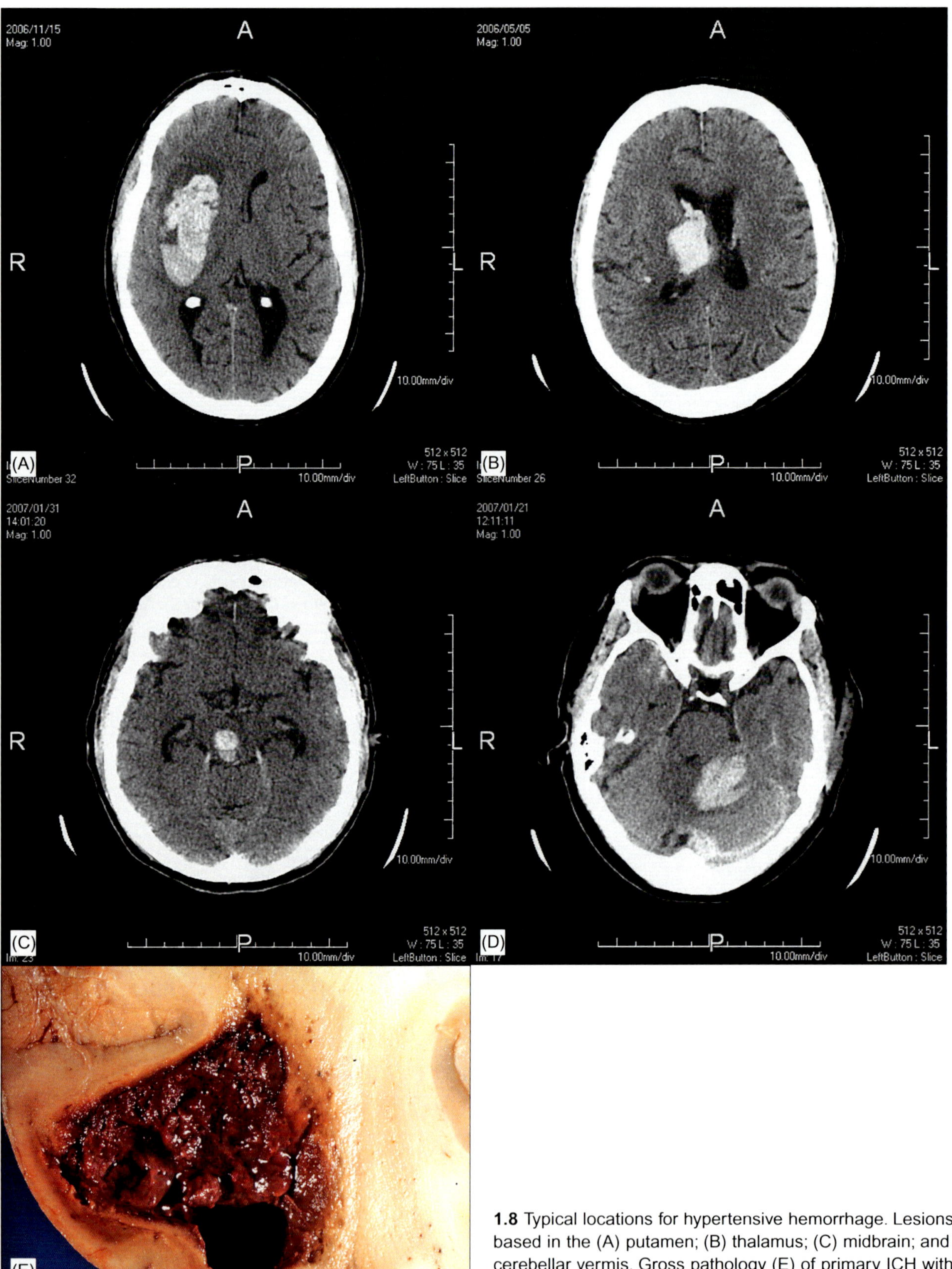

1.8 Typical locations for hypertensive hemorrhage. Lesions based in the (A) putamen; (B) thalamus; (C) midbrain; and (D) cerebellar vermis. Gross pathology (E) of primary ICH within the white matter just below the cortical surface.

Lobar (cortical) intracerebral hemorrhage

Lesions in the peripheral brain parenchyma are typically due to HTN and/or CAA (**1.9**). Larger lesions may also involve subcortical structures, the ventricular system (see **1.4**A, **1.9**B), and even rupture into the subdural and subarachnoid spaces (see **1.4**A, **1.9**E).

Multifocal intracerebral hemorrhage

Hemorrhages may occur in both lobar and subcortical locations, most likely due to HTN (**1.10**). A differential diagnosis of multifocal ICH is provided (*Table 1.4*; see also **2.1**).[20]

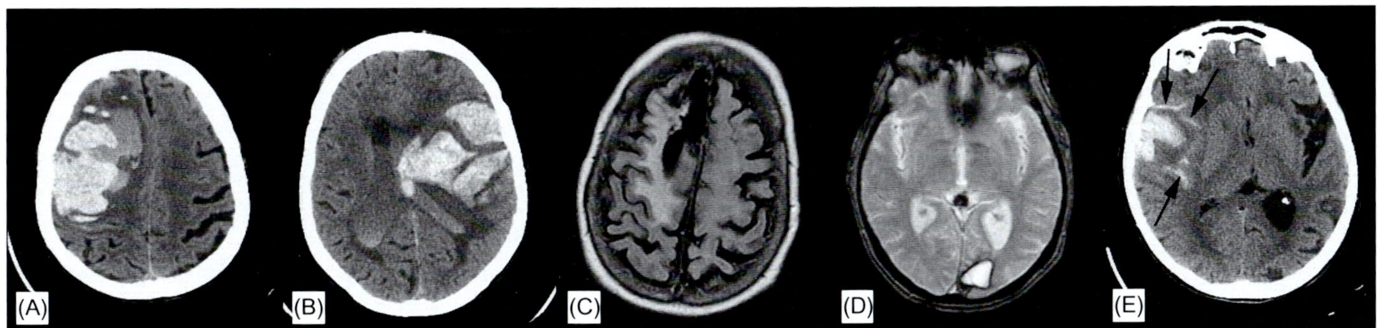

1.9 Lobar ICH. Primary hemorrhages involving the following lobes: (A) right frontal (CT scan); (B) left frontoparietal, with significant involvement of the lateral ventricles (CT); (C) chronic, right medial frontal, with associated hyperintense white matter disease (T2-FLAIR MRI sequence); (D) left occipital (GE-MRI); and (E) right temporal, with subarachnoid involvement (arrows) (CT).

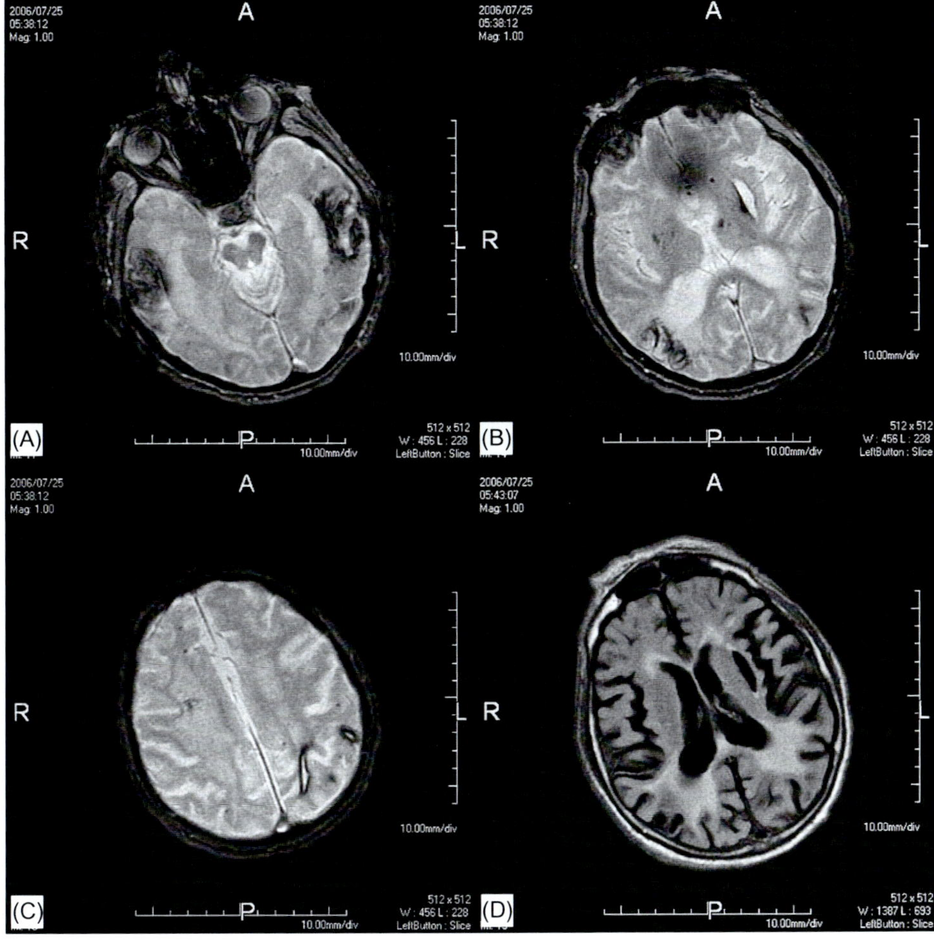

1.10 Multifocal ICH. Bilateral temporal lobe hemorrhages, with multifocal 'slit-like' subcortical and cortical lesions, as well as microhemorrhages registering on GE-MRI sequence as areas of reduced signal (A–C). The T2-FLAIR (D) demonstrates widespread white matter disease, particularly in the bilateral parieto-occipital regions.

Table 1.4 Differential diagnosis, multifocal simultaneous intracerebral hemorrhages

I. Vascular/coagulopathy
   a. Hypertension
      i. Primary
      ii. Iatrogenic, e.g., sympathomimetic drugs
   b. Vasculitis
   c. Cerebral amyloid angiopathy
   d. Coagulopathy
      iii. Antithrombotic and thrombolytic agents
      iv. Blood dyscrasias, e.g., leukemia
      v. Systemic disease, e.g., liver disease
   e. Cerebral venous thrombosis
II. Neoplastic
   a. Metastasis
      i. Bronchogenic carcinoma
      ii. Renal cell carcinoma
      iii. Choreocarcinoma
      iv. Malignant melanoma
   b. Primary
      i. Glioblastoma
      ii. Oligodendroglioma
III. Head trauma

Adapted with permission from Finelli.[19]

Intraventricular hemorrhage

Hemorrhage may dissect from the brain parenchyma into the adjacent ventricular space, carrying a poor prognosis (**1.11**; see also **1.4**A, **1.5**B, **1.6**B, **1.16**A,B).[12] Hemorrhage may also be isolated to the intraventricular space (**1.11**D),[20] and lesions can expand substantially by rupturing into the ventricular system (**1.12**). Ventricular involvement may cause obstructive hydrocephalus and can result in long-term cognitive impairment.[5]

Other common causes of hemorrhage

Microhemorrhage

Microhemorrhage most often results from the rupture of small intracranial blood vessels or vascular malformations, such as cavernous malformations or capillary telangiectasias (see *Table 1.5*). These lesions are usually asymptomatic. The local deposition of hemosiderin, a product of blood degradation, creates a permanent signal reduction best detected by gradient-echo (GE) magnetic resonance imaging (MRI) sequences (**1.13**). Risk factors for microhemorrhage are advanced age, HTN, smoking, and previous ischemic stroke and/or ICH.[21]

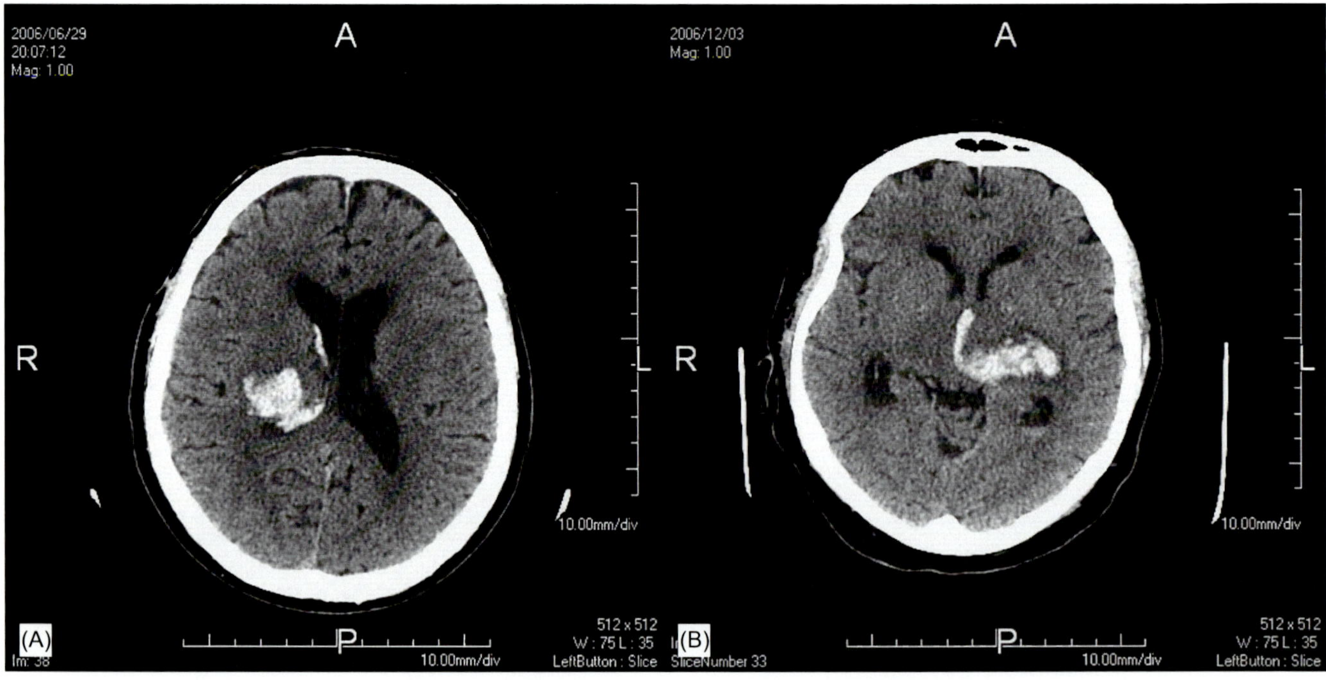

1.11 *Caption overleaf*

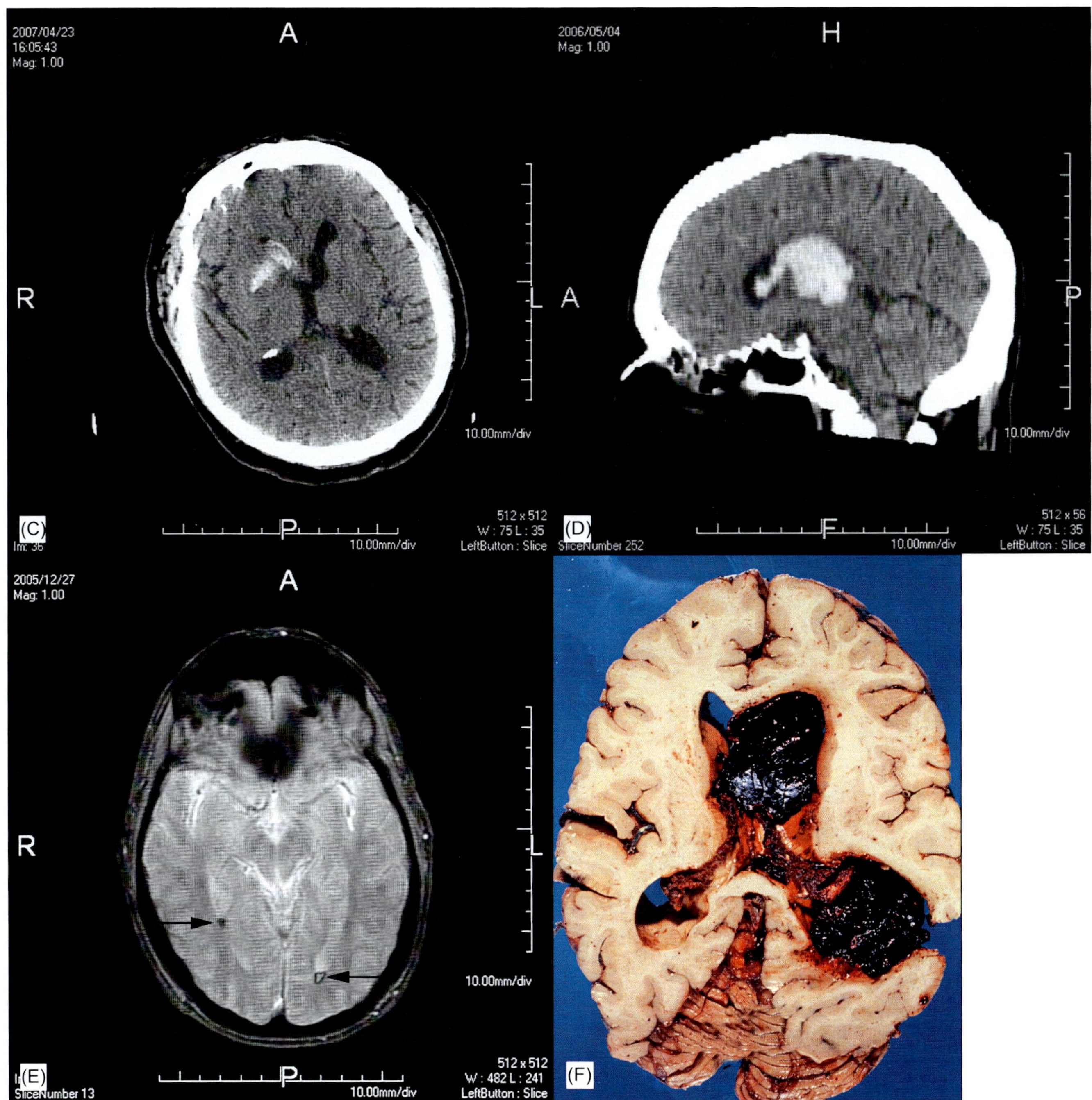

1.11 Intraventricular hemorrhage. Examples of primary hypertensive lesions 'creeping' into the intraventricular space on head CT scans of the periventricular white matter (A), the thalamus (B), and the head of the caudate nucleus (C). Another lesion (from **1.8**B) is shown here on a reconstructed sagittal CT to occupy predominantly the right lateral ventricle (D). An isolated, idiopathic intraventricular hemorrhage without a parenchymal component, on a GE-MRI sequence (E); note layering of blood in the posterior horns of the lateral ventricles (arrows). Gross pathology of extensive intraventricular hemorrhage, with ventricular dilatation consistent with obstructive hydrocephalus (F).

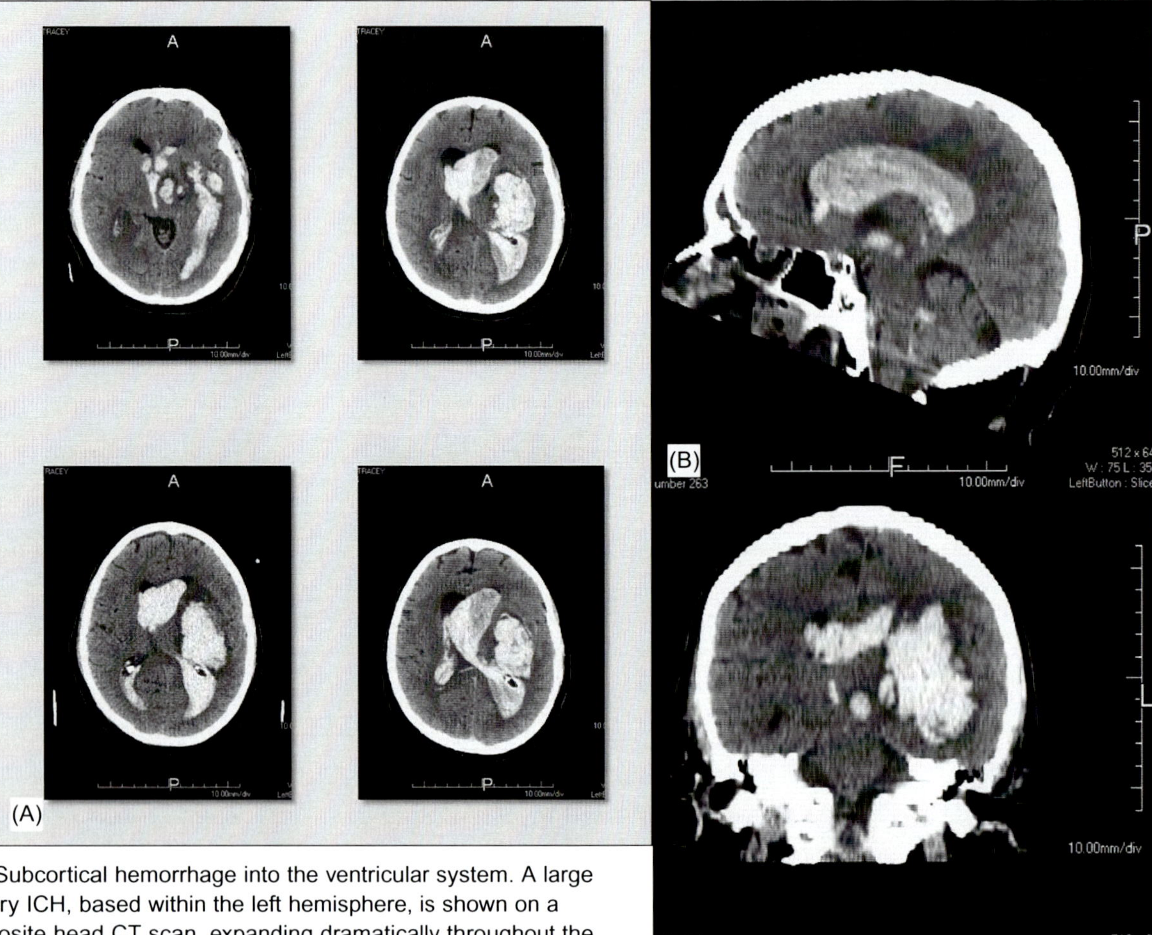

1.12 Subcortical hemorrhage into the ventricular system. A large primary ICH, based within the left hemisphere, is shown on a composite head CT scan, expanding dramatically throughout the ventricular system (A). Other images are reconstructed sagittal (B) and coronal (C) sections of the CT.

Table 1.5 Common causes of cerebral microhemorrhage

- Hypertension
- Cerebral amyloid angiography
- CADASIL (cerebral autosomal dominant arteriopathy with subcortical infarcts and leukoencephalopathy)
- Vascular malformations:
  - Cavernous malformation
  - Capillary telangiectasia
- Head trauma, with diffuse axonal injury
- Calcium or iron deposits, typically in the basal ganglia, may mimic microhemorrhage

Adapted with permission from Viswanathan and Chabriat.[21]

The clinical relevance of microhemorrhage includes:

- Association with cognitive impairment.
- Increased risk for developing acute hemorrhage during thrombolytic treatment administered for AIS.[22]
- Increased long-term risk for ICH in patients exposed chronically to antithrombotic agents.[21]

Hemorrhagic infarction

Hemorrhagic infarction (HI) (**1.14**) is defined as bleeding into an AIS, which:

- does not contribute to mass effect;
- does not impact upon short-term clinical outcomes;
- is linked to a higher baseline stroke severity and early computed tomography (CT) changes;

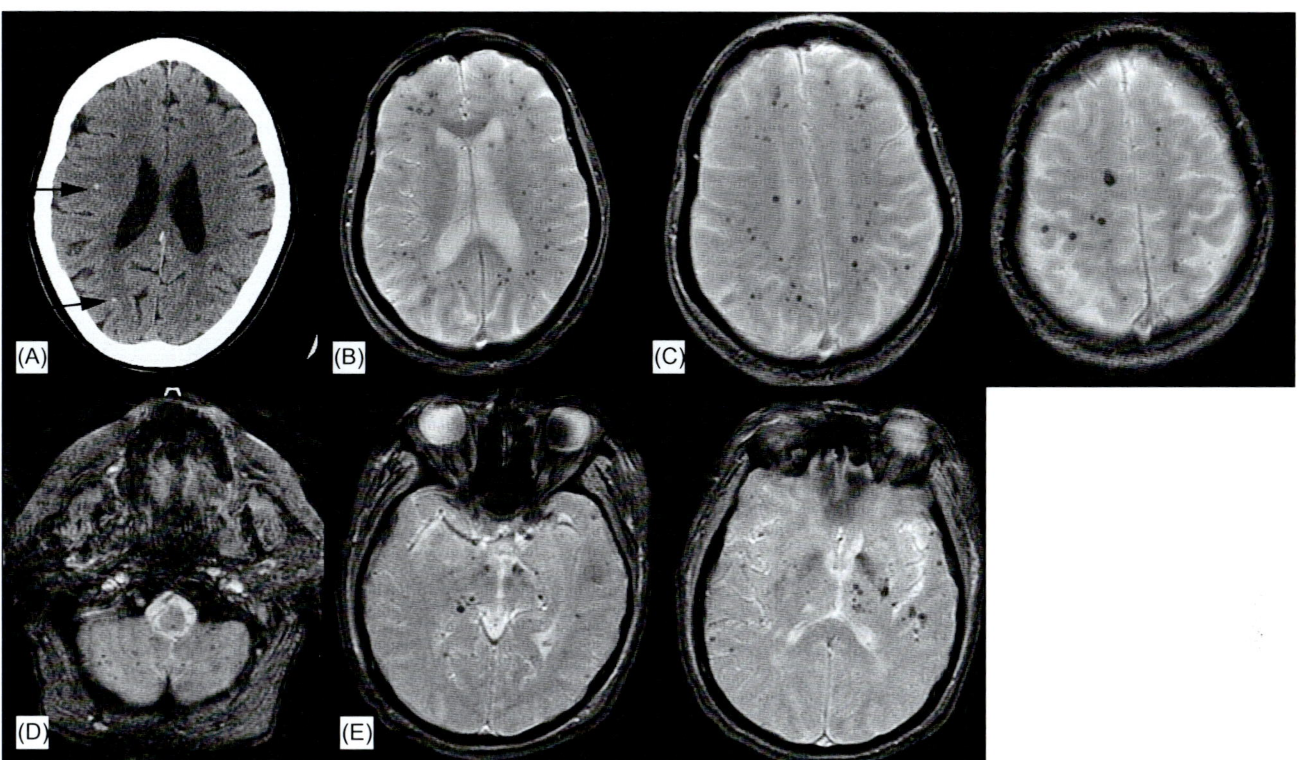

1.13 Microhemorrhages. The non-contrast head CT scan hints at punctuate hemorrhages, with two hyperdense lesions in the right hemisphere (arrows) (A), while subsequent GE-MRI sequence documents dozens of microhemorrhages, located predominantly in the white matter of the cerebral hemispheres (B,C). In a second patient (D,E), lesions are predominantly situated within the posterior fossa, as well as the basal ganglia and temporal lobes, on GE-MRI.

- is more common in large strokes where there is widespread loss of the blood–brain barrier, resulting in extravasation of blood into the initial lesion;
- is statistically independent of exposure to tissue plasminogen activator (t-PA).[23]

Also referred to as hemorrhagic transformation, HI is considered a natural consequence of AIS, attributable to a local ischemic vasculopathy, with intact hemostatic control. The ECASS (European Cooperative Acute Stroke Study) clinical trials[24,25] further segregated HI into two groups:

- *HI-1:* small petechiae (**1.14**A).
- *HI-2:* more confluent petechiae (**1.14**B–D).

The GE-MRI sequence is particularly useful in visualizing such lesions (**1.14**D). The pathology of HI is shown (**1.14**E,F).

Hemorrhage after thrombolysis for acute ischemic stroke

Following exposure to intravenous (IV) t-PA, there are two types of clinically significant hemorrhages, parenchymal and extra-ischemic hematomas.[23] Parenchymal hematoma (PH) denotes a larger extravasation of blood than HI, initiated by an ischemic lesion. The ECASS clinical trials segregated these hemorrhages into two groups:

- *PH-1:* the blood clot does not exceed 30% of infarcted volume and has only a mild space-occupying effect (**1.15**).
- *PH-2:* a dense clot exceeds 30% of infarct volume, with significant mass effect (**1.16**).

PHs are:

- Linked to thrombolytic drug exposure and dose, edema or early mass effect on initial head CT scan, stroke

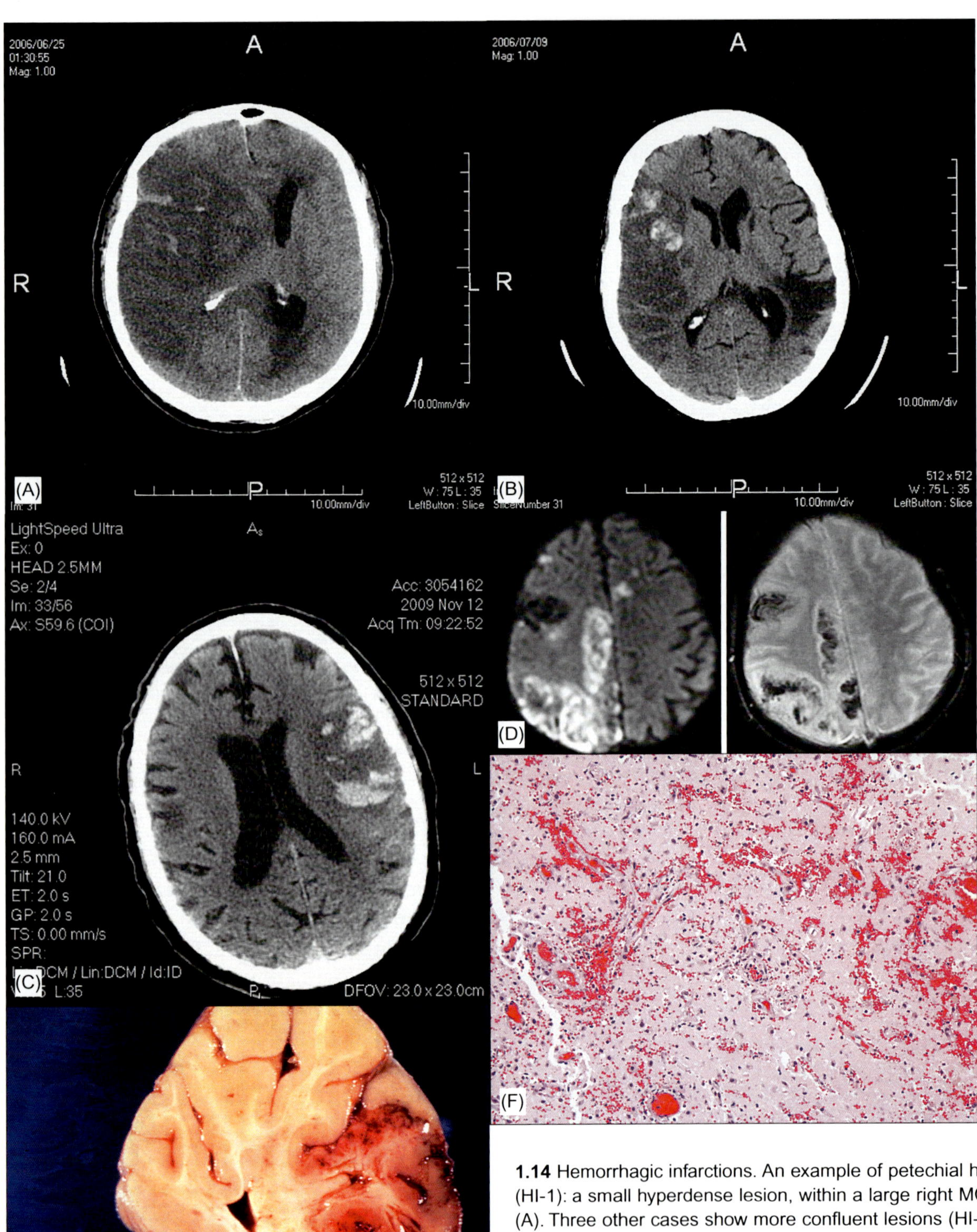

1.14 Hemorrhagic infarctions. An example of petechial hemorrhage (HI-1): a small hyperdense lesion, within a large right MCA-territory AIS (A). Three other cases show more confluent lesions (HI-2): a hyperdense region on CT scan (B) within a subacute, hypodense right hemispheric ischemic stroke, with a smaller contralateral area of encephalomalacia; (C) patchy hemorrhage into a left MCA-territory AIS; and (D) multifocal lesions on diffusion-weighted (DW) (left) and GE (right) MRI sequences, in a patient on warfarin with atrial fibrillation. Gross pathology of HI (E), particularly evident along the cortical ribbon. Micropathology (F) shows red blood cells interspersed within infarcted, pale brain tissue (H&E, 40×).

severity, and age.[23,26] IV thrombolytic treatment for stroke increases the risk of PH by a factor of 12, as compared with IV t-PA given for acute myocardial infarction.[23]

- Associated with significant adverse clinical outcomes, particularly for PH-2 lesions.[24]
- Associated with the use of unfractionated heparin, particularly during intra-arterial thrombolysis (**case study 2**).[27]
- Potentially related to time-to-recanalization (i.e., prolongation of arterial recanalization may increase the likelihood of PH).[23]

Significant clinical deterioration associated with PH is known as 'symptomatic hemorrhage,' an important outcome measure in acute stroke treatment. One common definition for symptomatic hemorrhage is a clinical deterioration of >4 points on the National Institutes of Health Stroke Scale (NIHSS) associated with hemorrhage seen on CT scan within 36 hours of stroke onset.[27] Various predictors for symptomatic hemorrhage include hyperglycemia, concurrent heparin use, the timing of successful recanalization, a history of diabetes and cardiac disease, leukoariosis, early signs of infarct on CT scans, and elevated pretreatment mean blood pressure.[28] Neurosurgical evacuation typically is not a helpful treatment for symptomatic hemorrhage, because the lesion is frequently large and multifocal.

Extra-ischemic hematomas are: located remotely from the initial ischemic stroke lesion; may be isolated or multifocal, with or without mass effect (**1.17**);[23] and associated with concurrent coagulopathy and previously occult vasculopathies, such as CAA, microhemorrhages, or hypertensive vasculopathy.

In the NINDS (National Institute of Neurological Disorders and Stroke) trial of IV t-PA for AIS, the incidence of extra-ischemic cerebral hematomas was 1.3%.[29]

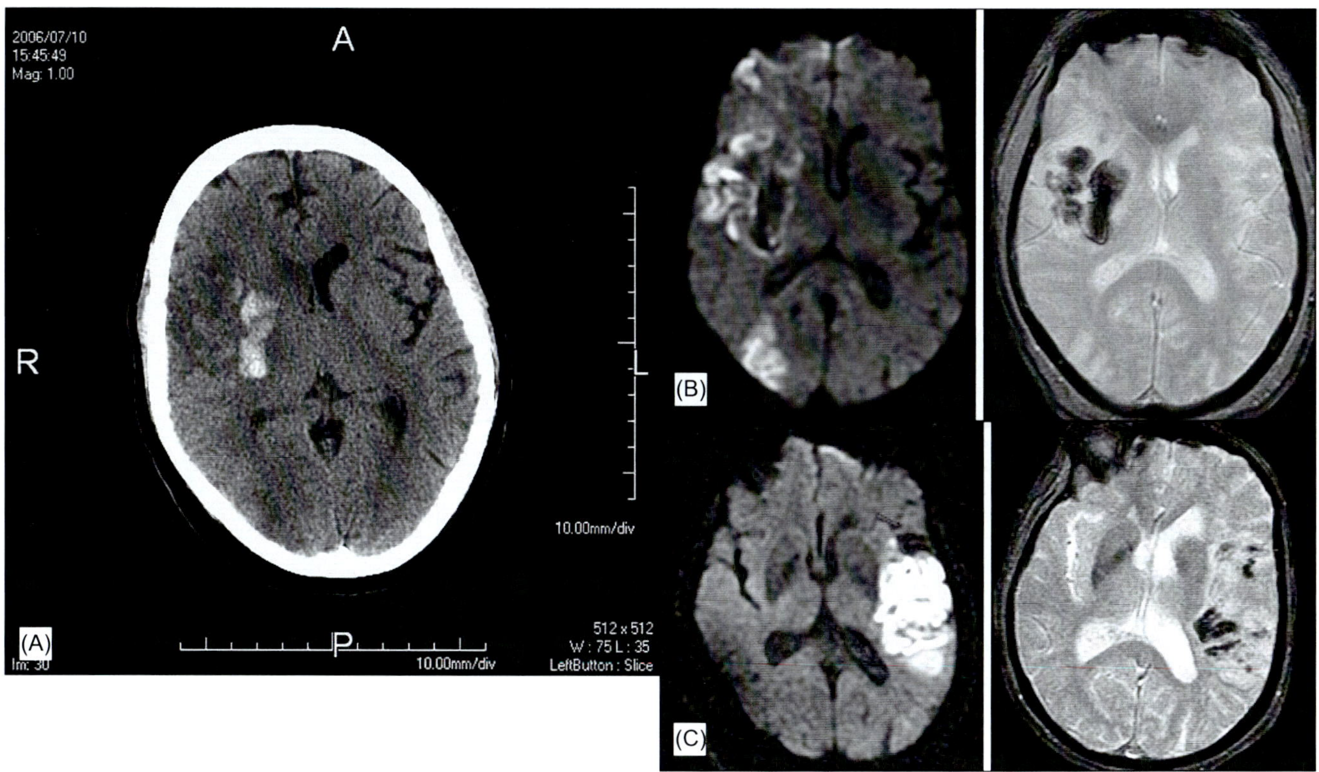

1.15 Parenchymal hemorrhages (PH-1). Patchy hemorrhage, without significant mass effect, into a right MCA-distribution ischemic stroke, treated with IV t-PA; this lesion is shown on CT scan (A), as well as DW (B, left), and GE (B, right) MRI. A second patient (C) who received IV and intra-arterial t-PA for a left M2 occlusion is shown: DW (left) and GE (right) MRI.

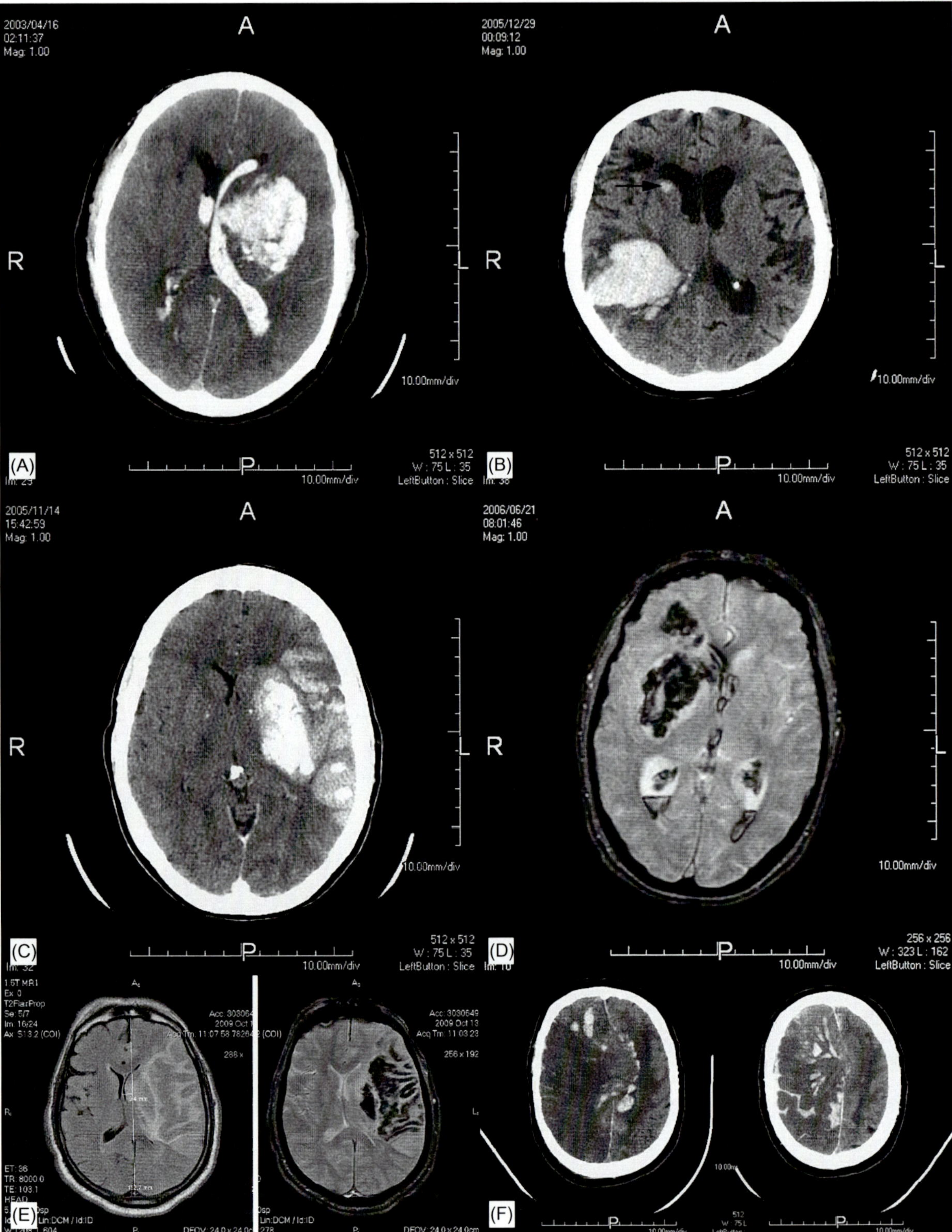

1.16 Parenchymal hemorrhages (PH-2). Six different patients who deteriorated from hemorrhage into ischemic strokes, following treatments with: (A) mechanical embolectomy, with late recanalization; (B) IV t-PA: note a small hemorrhagic component within the head of the caudate nucleus (arrow); (C) intra-arterial t-PA: note hyperdense contrast dye staining the putaminal and cortical regions of the hemorrhage; (D) IV t-PA (GE-MRI); (E) IV and IA t-PA, with substantial hemorrhage into a left hemispheric stroke (FLAIR sequence, left; GE, right), probably contributing to the midline mass effect of this lesion and (F) IV t-PA: multifocal hemorrhages within a right hemispheric stroke with malignant edema, subarachnoid involvement, and severe subfalcine herniation. All of these lesions were associated with a >4-point deterioration on the NIHSS and are therefore classified as symptomatic hemorrhages.

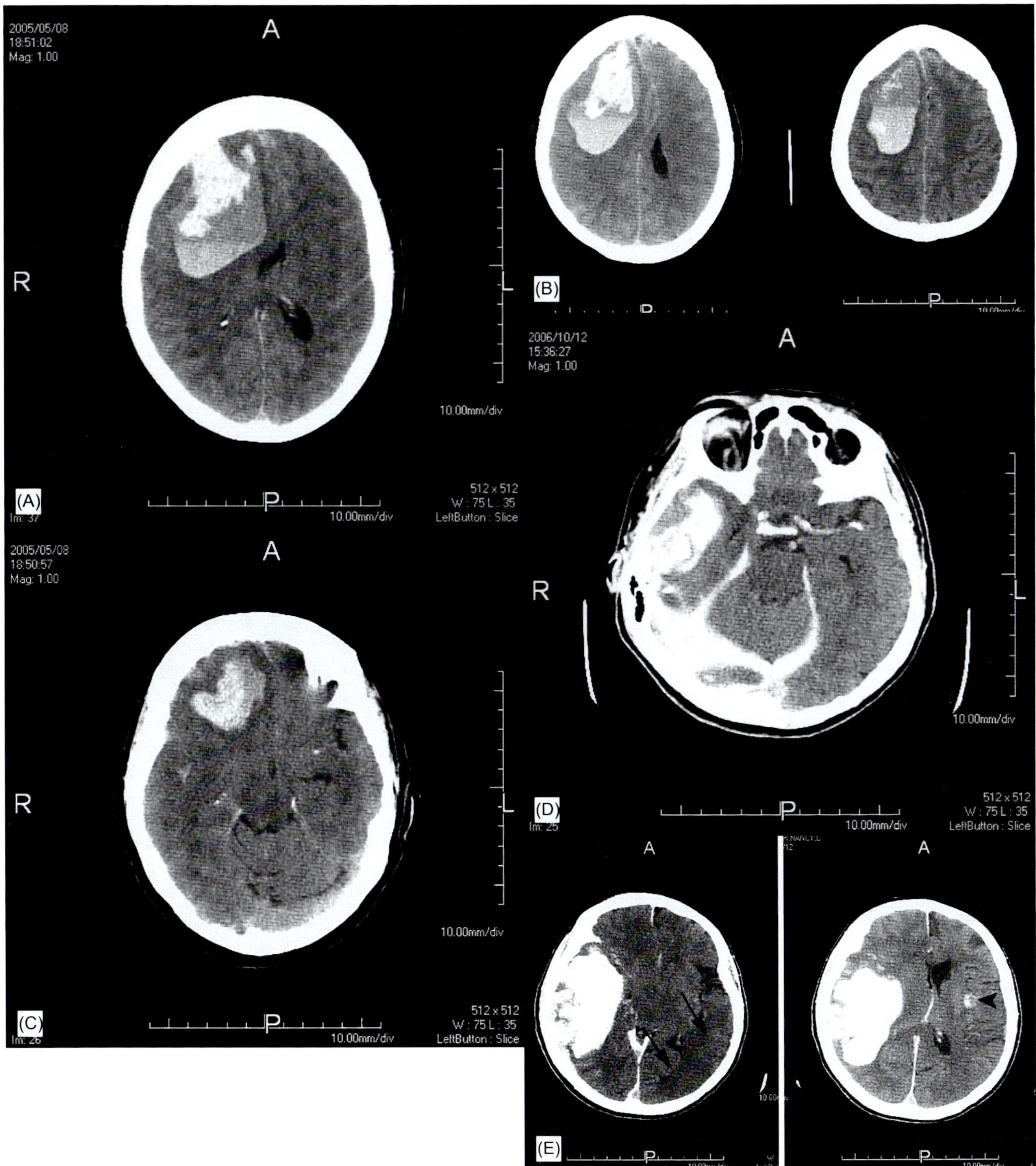

1.17 Extra-ischemic hematomas.

Patient 1 (A–C): this patient was taking clopidogrel and aspirin following coronary angioplasty and stenting for an acute myocardial infarction. Four days later, the patient acutely developed a left hemispheric stroke syndrome, and was treated with IV t-PA. The large right frontal hemorrhage (volume estimated at 55 ml) shows a fluid–fluid level within the lesion (A,B). A second, separate focus of hemorrhage was identified in the basal forebrain (C). Diffuse hemispheric edema is present bilaterally.

Patient 2 (D,E). This patient presented with an NIHSS score of 14 points due to a left M1 occlusion. Endovascular mechanical embolectomy partially recanalized the lesion, but the patient rapidly deteriorated, due to massive contralateral hemorrhage based in the right temporal lobe. The high density of the hemorrhage is intensified by iodinated contrast dye used during the intra-arterial procedure. The CT scans document subarachnoid involvement along the cerebellar tentorium (D) and ischemic stroke in the inferior division of the left MCA (arrows) (E, left), as well as a small hemorrhage consistent with HI-1 (arrowhead) (E, right).

Cerebral venous thrombosis

Venous occlusive intracranial disease is associated with oral contraceptive use,[30] the immediate post-partum period, and a wide range of hypercoagulable medical conditions. Significant cerebral venous thrombosis involves one or more of the major venous sinuses and typically results in parenchymal hemorrhage. By definition, the territories of the ischemic and hemorrhagic lesions are in a venous, rather than arterial, distribution. Involvement of the deep venous system (**case study 3**) carries a much worse prognosis than if only the superficial sinuses (**1.18, 1.19**) and/or cortical veins (**1.20**) are involved.[31,32] Magnetic resonance venography (MRV) is commonly used to identify major venous sinus occlusions.

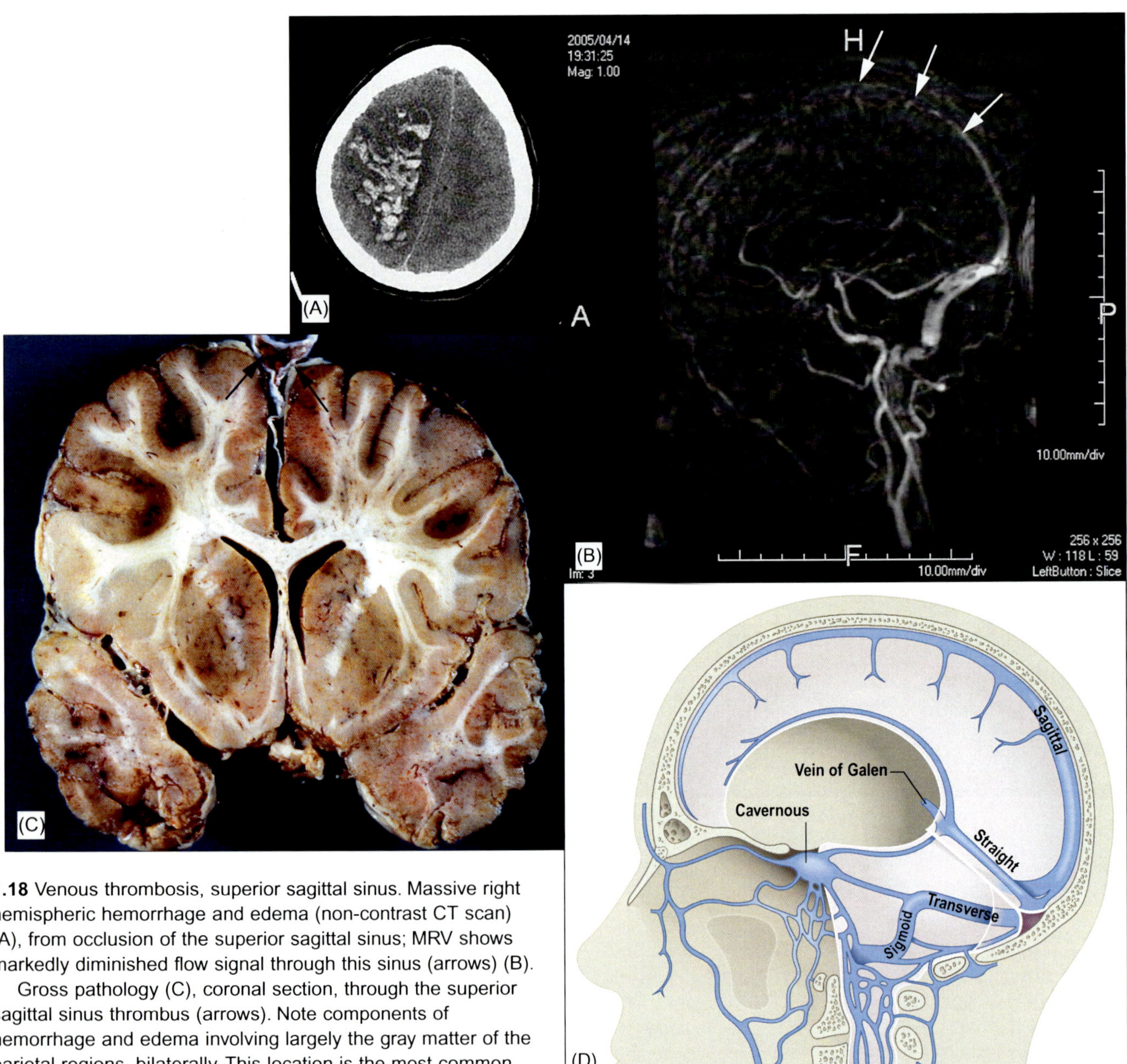

1.18 Venous thrombosis, superior sagittal sinus. Massive right hemispheric hemorrhage and edema (non-contrast CT scan) (A), from occlusion of the superior sagittal sinus; MRV shows markedly diminished flow signal through this sinus (arrows) (B).

Gross pathology (C), coronal section, through the superior sagittal sinus thrombus (arrows). Note components of hemorrhage and edema involving largely the gray matter of the parietal regions, bilaterally. This location is the most common site for thrombosis among the major intracranial venous sinuses (D) (adapted from Gost-Bierska *et al.*,[32] with permission).

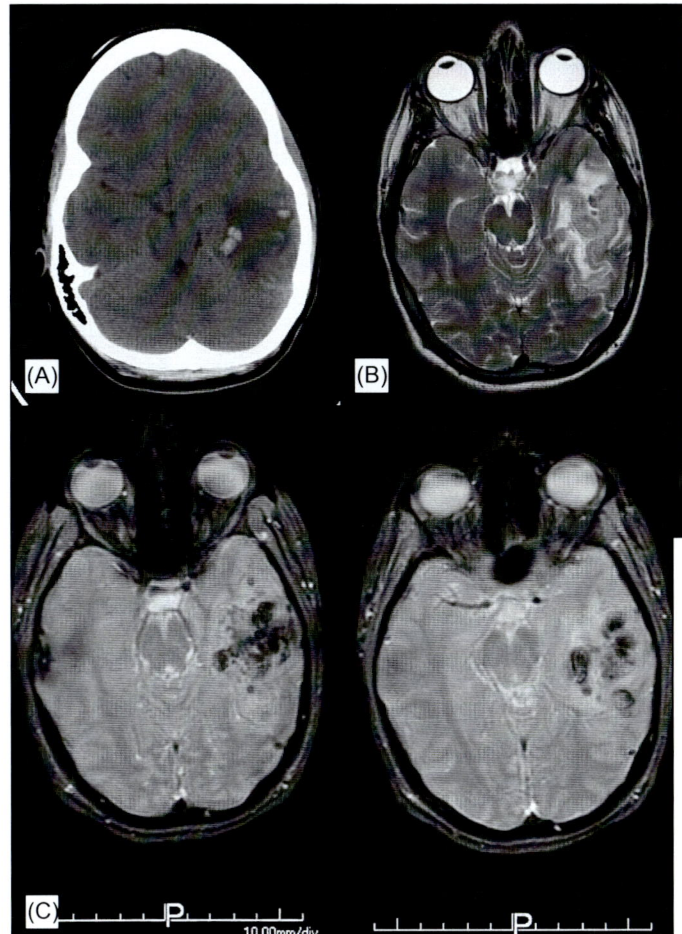

1.19 Venous thrombosis, left transverse sinus. This CT scan (A) demonstrates hemorrhage into a hypodense lesion in a non-arterial distribution, in a young patient presenting with aphasia and headache. The left temporal lesion is better delineated on MRI sequences; (B) vasogenic edema on T2-weighted imaging (T2WI), and (C) multifocal hemorrhage on GE-MR. This temporal lobe lesion was due to occlusion of the adjacent transverse sinus, evident as absent flow on MRV; compare to intact flow through the right transverse sinus (arrows) (D).

Diagnosis

Computed tomography

Head CT scans are the standard for detecting acute ICH. Lesion volume is estimated using a validated method, providing critical prognostic information during the initial clinical evaluation.[33] An equation for the volume of a three-dimensional ellipsoid ($4/3 \times \pi \times (r)^3$) is converted to approximate the lesion volume (**1.21**), as follows:

$(x \times y \times z)/2$
x = length of lesion (cm)
y = width of lesion (cm)
z = height (number of transverse CT scan cuts in cm).

The presence of early hydrocephalus (**1.22**) and intraventricular blood (**1.11**) are also easily appreciated with CT scans. Over time, the hyperdense lesion of a primary ICH fades, and the underlying local brain injury appears hypodense (**1.23**).

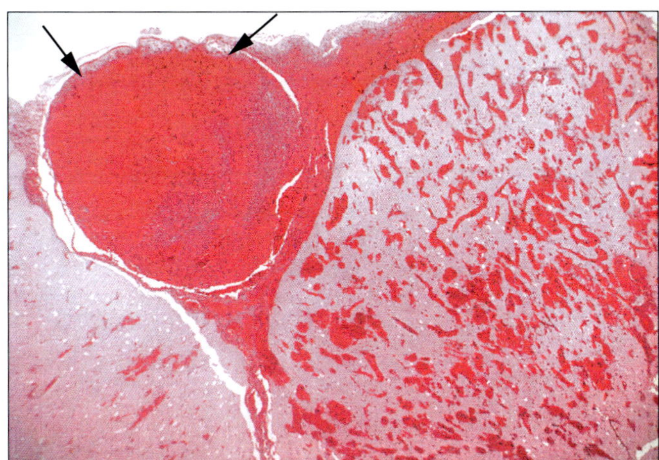

1.20 Isolated cortical vein thrombosis. Micropathology isolates in cross-section a fresh thrombus occluding a single cortical vein (arrows) (H&E, 40×). Acute hemorrhage is evident as red blood cells interspersed within the brain tissue, immediately below and to the right of the occluded vein.

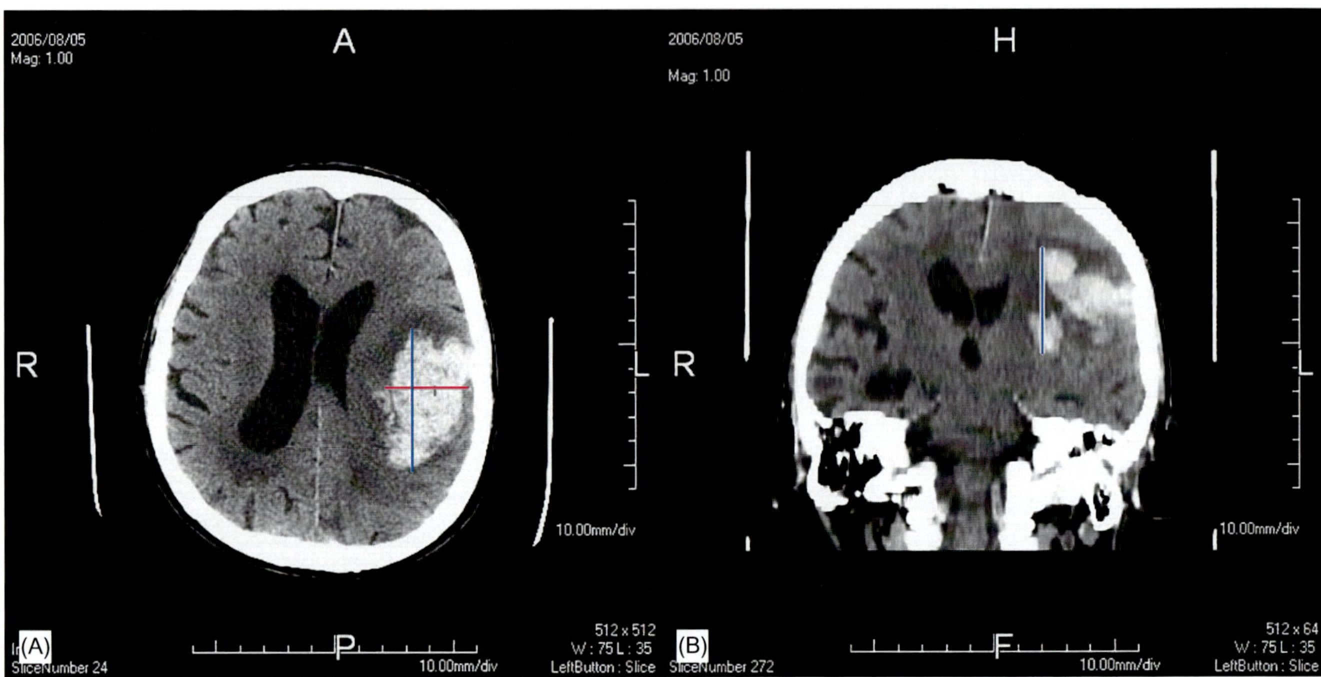

1.21 Measurement of hemorrhage volume. On CT scan, this primary ICH has a width (red line) by length (blue line) measurements of ≥3 cm ×6 cm (A). A reconstructed coronal view of the lesion provides the height of the lesion (blue line), at ≥4 cm (B). A centimeter-scale ruler is situated along the right margins (perihematomal edema, the hypodense rim surrounding the hematoma, is not included in measuring the volume). Lesion height is approximated by counting the number of adjacent transaxial centimeter-wide cuts in which the hyperdensity of the hemorrhage extends. In this case, the volume is approximated as {(3×6×4), divided by 2} ≈36 ml, consistent with a large hemorrhage.

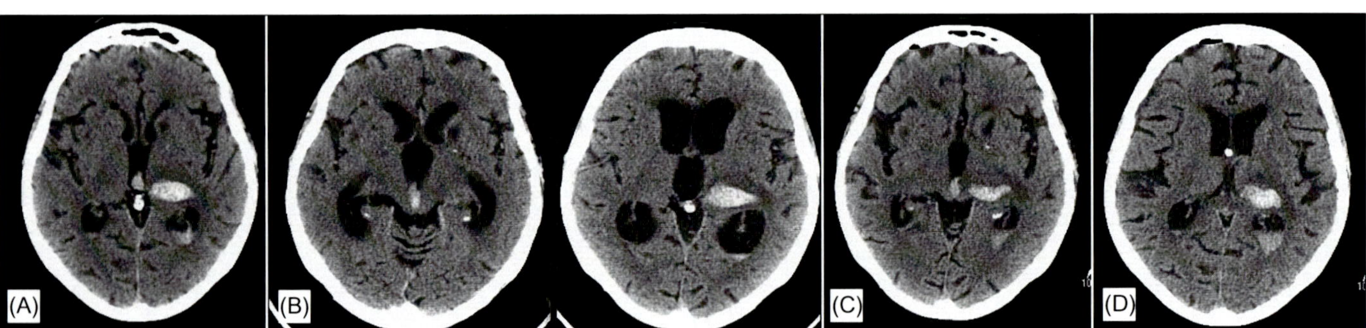

1.22 Acute obstructive hydrocephalus. Admission CT scan shows a small hemorrhage based in the left thalamus (A). Only 8 hours later (B), the third and lateral ventricles are dilated, with 'squaring off' of the frontal horns (right), consistent with acute hydrocephalus due to occlusion of the aqueduct of Sylvius (left). Following external ventricular drain placement on the next day (C,D), the third ventricle and the frontal and temporal horns normalized. The tip of the drain is hyperdense, situated between the frontal horns (D).

Magnetic resonance imaging

Brain MRI scans offer some advantages over CT imaging, particularly: in monitoring the time course following an acute ICH; in detecting underlying causes for ICH (*Table 1.1*), such as cavernous malformations or primary or metastatic neoplasms; and in differentiating regions of ischemic infarction versus local hemorrhage, such as in cases of HI. The GE-MRI sequence accurately detects quiescent, old subclinical microhemorrhages that are frequently identified in patients with chronic HTN or CAA (**1.13**). In selected patients (e.g., with cavernous malformation, see Chapter 4), an MRI scan may obviate the need for conventional angiography.

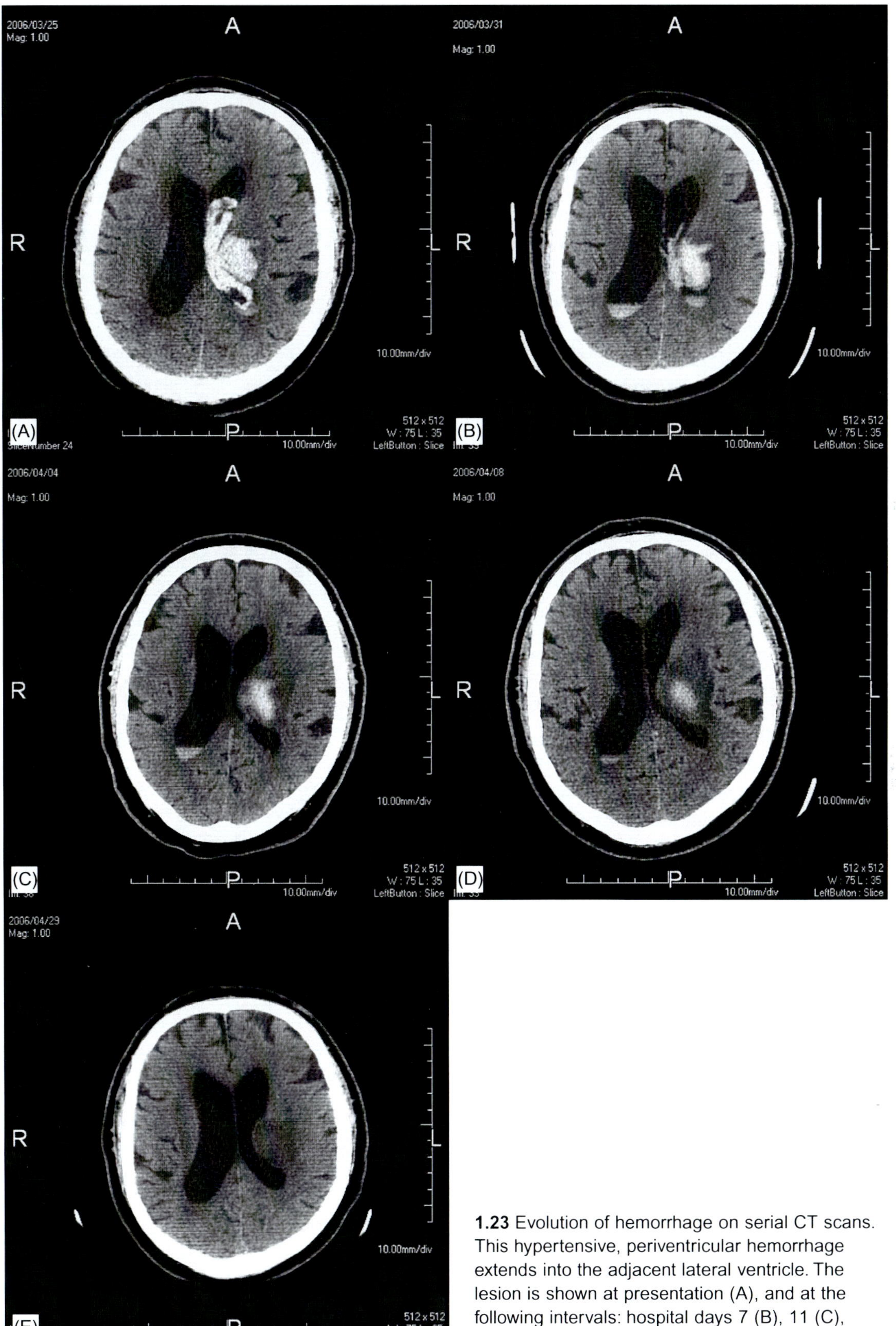

1.23 Evolution of hemorrhage on serial CT scans. This hypertensive, periventricular hemorrhage extends into the adjacent lateral ventricle. The lesion is shown at presentation (A), and at the following intervals: hospital days 7 (B), 11 (C), 15 (D), and 36 (E).

Perihematomal edema registers on both CT as hypodense regions (**1.7**), and MRI scans as increased signal intensity on T2-weighted or FLAIR (fluid attenuated inversion recovery) sequences (**1.19**B).

Conventional cerebral angiography

Angiography offers the potential for detecting underlying neurovascular lesions not identified by other imaging modalities. A large prospective study evaluating the positive yield for angiography in the evaluation of ICH suggested that this invasive study should be ordered in younger patients (≤45 years of age) and those with lobar and/or intraventricular hemorrhages, where identification of an underlying large vessel lesion, particularly an intracranial aneurysm or arteriovenous malformation, is more likely (**case study 4**).[34] Conversely, angiography is not recommended for older patients with HTN whose lesion sites are typical for hypertensive ICH.[3]

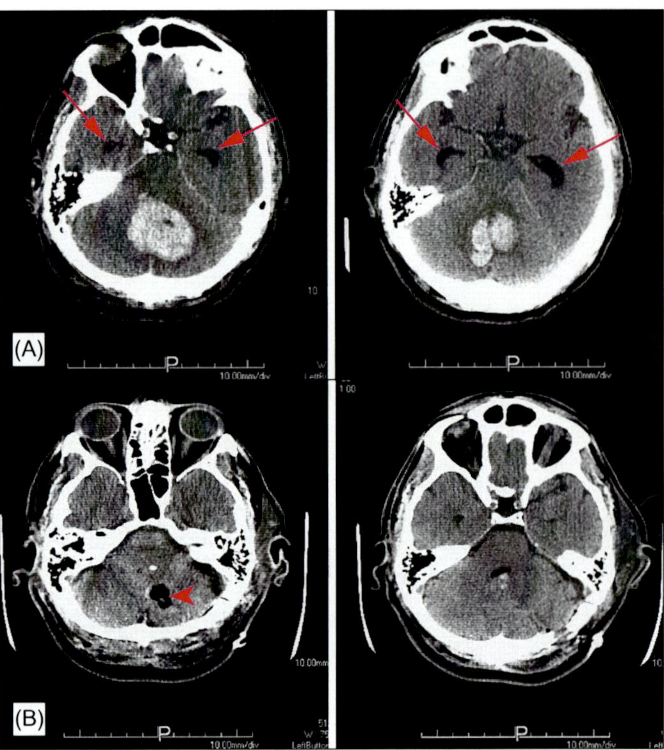

1.24 Cerebellar hemorrhage, treated with neurosurgery. Head CT scan shows a large, primary ICH based in the cerebellar vermis, causing effacement of the basal cisterns around the pons and early obstructive hydrocephalus, with markedly enlarged temporal horns (arrows) (A). The patient underwent emergent craniotomy over the next few hours, and subsequent CT scan the following day (B) shows recovery of basal cisterns, reduction in ventricular size, and a pocket of air in the left cerebellar hemisphere (arrowhead), with some edema in the left middle cerebellar peduncle. Note the craniotomy defect from the left suboccipital approach.

Management

Primary treatment

There are no evidence-based primary treatments that improve early outcomes for acute ICH.[3] Clinical trials have shown that early treatment with recombinant activated factor VII (rFVIIa) prevents early ICH expansion,[17,35] but clinical outcomes were not improved over placebo in a pivotal Phase 3 trial.[36] A promising area for rFVIIa may be in the treatment of warfarin-associated ICH.[10,37]

Neurosurgical interventions

The single mandated indication for neurosurgical decompression is cerebellar hemorrhage (**1.24**).[1] Early craniotomy, prior to brainstem compression, is critical. The best surgical candidates are patients with an initial GCS <14 and hematoma volume >40 ml, while those with higher GCS and smaller lesions are likely to have a good outcome with conservative, non-surgical management.[38]

Neurosurgical evacuation of clot in primary hemispheric ICH has had mixed results in randomized and non-randomized clinical trials. The leading study, I-STICH (International Surgical Trial in Intracerebral Haemorrhage), identified neutral outcomes for early evacuation.[2,39] Nonetheless, a role for neurosurgical decompression to reduce clot size may exist in highly selected patients, particularly younger patients (e.g., <60 years old) who have peripheral, lobar ICH (**case study 5**). Less invasive surgical interventions, such as catheter-based clot aspiration or thrombolysis, are being studied.[40]

Intraventricular ICH may contribute to elevated intracranial pressure (ICP) by causing obstructive hydrocephalus. The amount of ventricular blood to cause hydrocephalus need not be great (**1.22**). In this setting, external drainage of cerebrospinal fluid via ventricular catheter may be indicated to reduce ICP.

Medical management

The appropriate management of HTN, a common accompaniment of acute ICH, is a controversial topic[1,3] and is being addressed in pilot studies.[3] Guidelines from the American Stroke Association discuss specific blood pressure targets and commonly considered agents: beta-blockers (labetalol, esmolol), calcium channel blockers (nicardipine), angiotensin converting enzyme (ACE) inhibitors (enalapril), and hydralazine. Other agents such as nitroprusside are effective as second-line options but carry the risk of significant vasodilation.[3]

Mass effect causing significant elevation of ICP, with the risk for cerebral herniation syndromes, may be managed emergently with osmotic agents, such as mannitol and/or hypertonic saline, and hyperventilation.[1,3] However, these approaches have never been formally studied in clinical trials.

Seizures occur in 10% of patients with primary ICH, usually at onset or within the initial 24 hours, and reflect cortical involvement of the lesion.[39,41] Anticonvulsant agents are empirically recommended for patients with significant hematomas in peripheral territories in the cerebral hemispheres. The appropriate duration of anticonvulsant use has not been established. For patients who are seizure-free, guidelines suggest discontinuation of the anti-epileptic drug after the first month post-hemorrhage.[3]

Neurointensivist management of ICH in an intensive care unit (ICU) setting may improve patient outcomes.[42]

Secondary stroke prevention

Various clinical trials, including SHEP (Systolic Hypertension in the Elderly Program)[43] and PROGRESS (Perindopril Protection Against Recurrent Stroke Study),[44] have documented the critical role of antihypertensive agents in both primary and secondary stroke prevention of ICH. The JNC-7 report (Seventh Report of the Joint National Committee on Prevention, Detection, Evaluation, and Treatment of High Blood Pressure) provides an extensive overview of the role of HTN in stroke risk, specific drug classes, lifestyle modifications, and target blood pressures. In general, lower blood pressures are associated with a proportional reduction of recurrent stroke and stroke mortality.[45]

Case studies

Case study 1. Autopsy, subcortical hemorrhage

A 36-year-old patient with a known history of HTN and reportedly excessive use of a weight-loss agent and stimulant, xenedrine, presented with an evolving large, left subcortical ICH. Despite aggressive neurocritical care, with ICP monitoring, cerebrospinal fluid (CSF) drainage and hypertonic saline, the patient died from cerebral herniation 7 days into the hospitalization.

A CT scan (**CS 1.1**) on hospital day 5 showed the mass effect on the midbrain (**CS 1.1**A) and, with associated edema, upon the lateral ventricle (**CS 1.1**B). The small hemorrhage

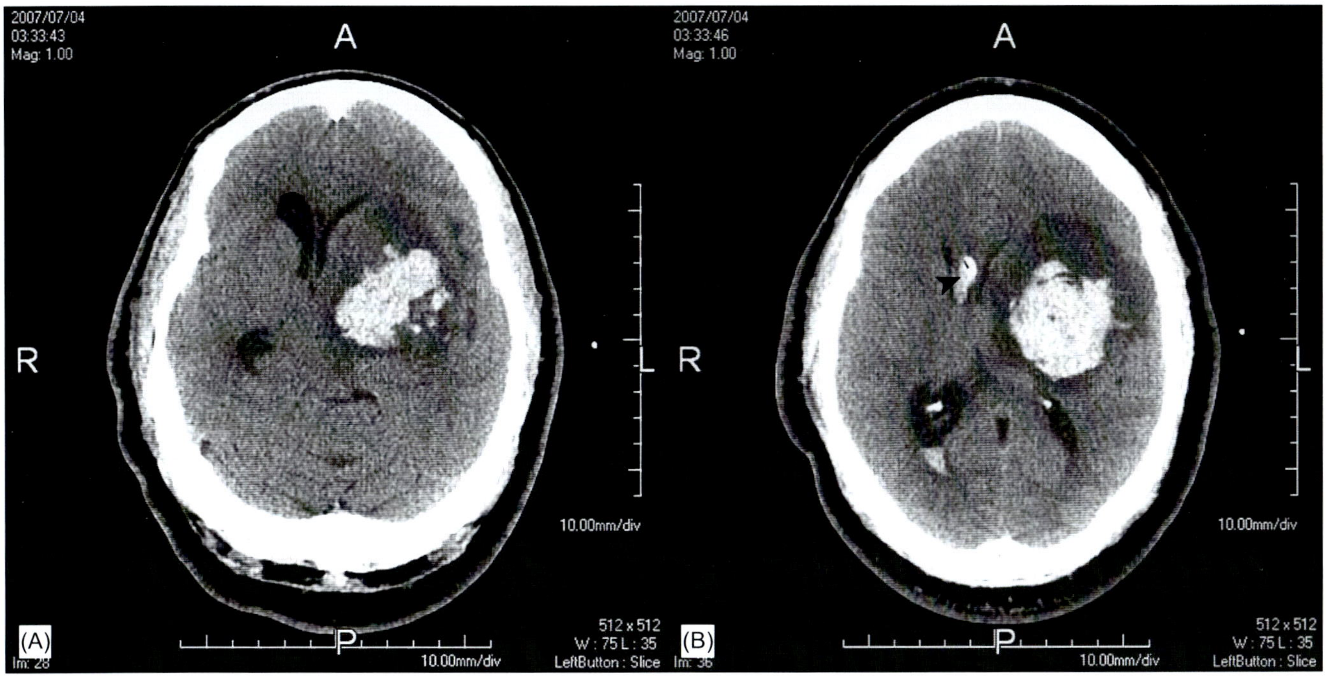

CS 1.1

between the frontal horns (arrowhead) (**CS 1.1**B) was caused by the catheter tip of an external ventricular drain.

At autopsy, the patient's heart showed severe obstructive ventricular hypertrophy (**CS 1.2**). The brain slices (**CS 1.3**) show: disintegration of the entire subcortical tissue at the site of hemorrhage, with associated perihematomal edema, left uncal herniation (arrowhead), and obliteration of midline basal ganglia and diencephalic structures (**CS 1.3**A); severe left-to-right midline mass effect on a more posterior slice (**CS 1.3**B); and Duret hemorrhages within the deformed midbrain (arrowheads) (**CS 1.3**C). The external ventricular drain within the right frontal horn caused a local hemorrhage in the right corpus callosum (arrowhead) (**CS 1.3**B) (pathology courtesy of Dean Uphoff, MD).

Comments

Undertreated HTN as well as 'innocuous,' unregulated over-the-counter stimulants and homeopathic agents may contribute to very harmful complications at any age, demonstrated here by a severe cardiomyopathy and massive ICH. A relatively younger brain might not readily accommodate the mass effect of acute ICH as well as an older, atrophic one. Emergent, decompressive neurosurgical evacuation for deep, hemispheric hematomas has not proven to improve clinical outcomes.[39]

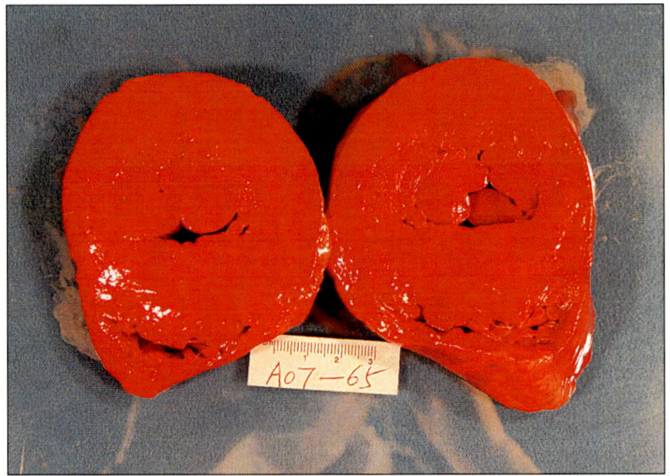

CS 1.2

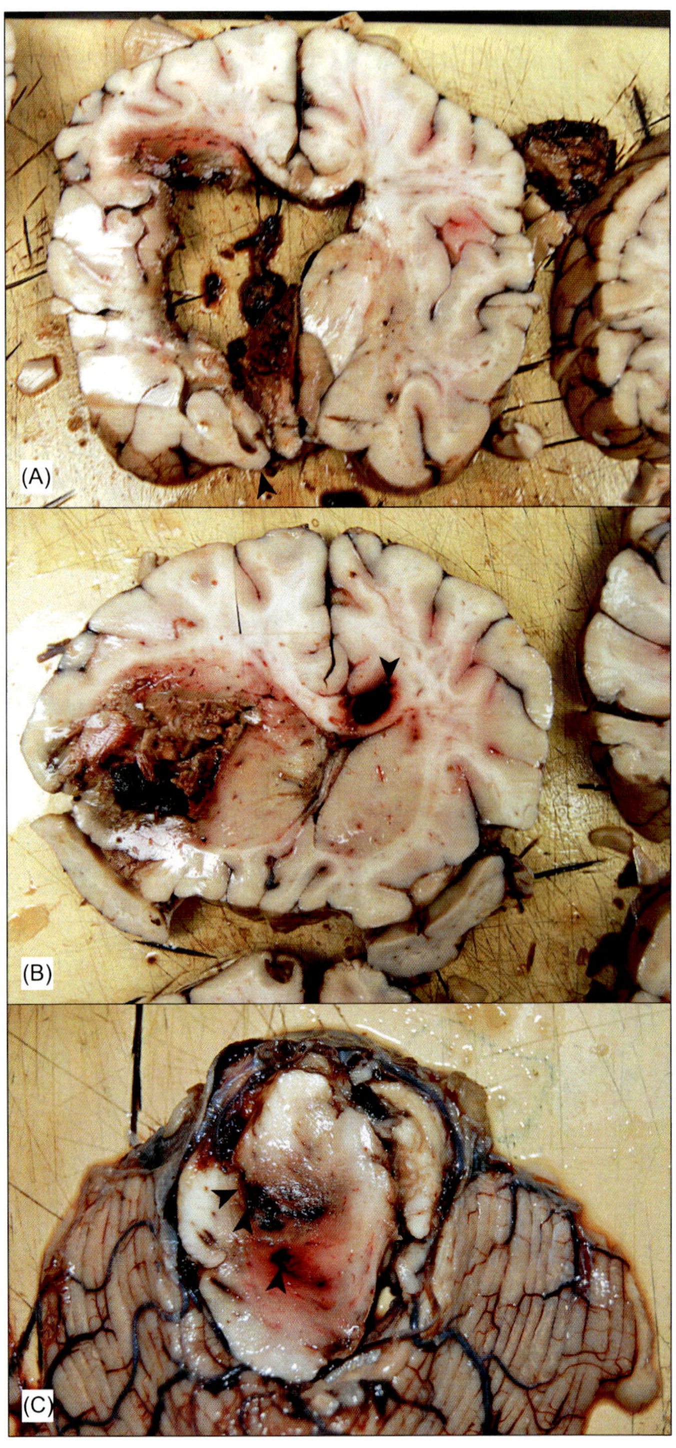

CS 1.3

Case study 2. Parenchymal hemorrhage associated with anticoagulation

A 59-year-old patient developed symptomatic hemorrhage while being anticoagulated with IV unfractionated heparin for an AIS within the territory of the left middle cerebral artery at an outside hospital. IV heparin had been started, because an MRI study from another institution (not shown) reportedly documented a cervical dissection of the left internal carotid artery. On the admission head CT scan following transfer (**CS 2.1**), the hematoma demonstrates major mass effect upon the midbrain (A), of the pineal gland, with a midline shift of approximately 3 mm (**CS 2.1**B), and the lateral ventricle (**CS 2.1**C).

Owing to a worsening sensorium and early imaging, both of concern for impending herniation, an emergent decompressive craniotomy was undertaken in order to remove the clot and reduce mass effect. The post-craniotomy head CT scans taken the next day (**CS 2.2A–C**, left images) are juxtaposed with those done 1 week later (**CS 2.2A–C**, right images), at the same three levels as in **CS2.1**. Pockets of postoperative air within the lesion site at 1 day largely resolve within the first week. Improvement of the midline mass effect and recovery of the basal cisterns are noted. The initial left middle cerebral artery stroke, most evident at the level of the ventricles (C), now appears as a well-delineated hypodensity in the frontoparietal region.

At 1 year follow-up, the patient is ambulatory and largely independent, despite dense right arm paresis as well as severe expressive (greater than receptive) aphasia.

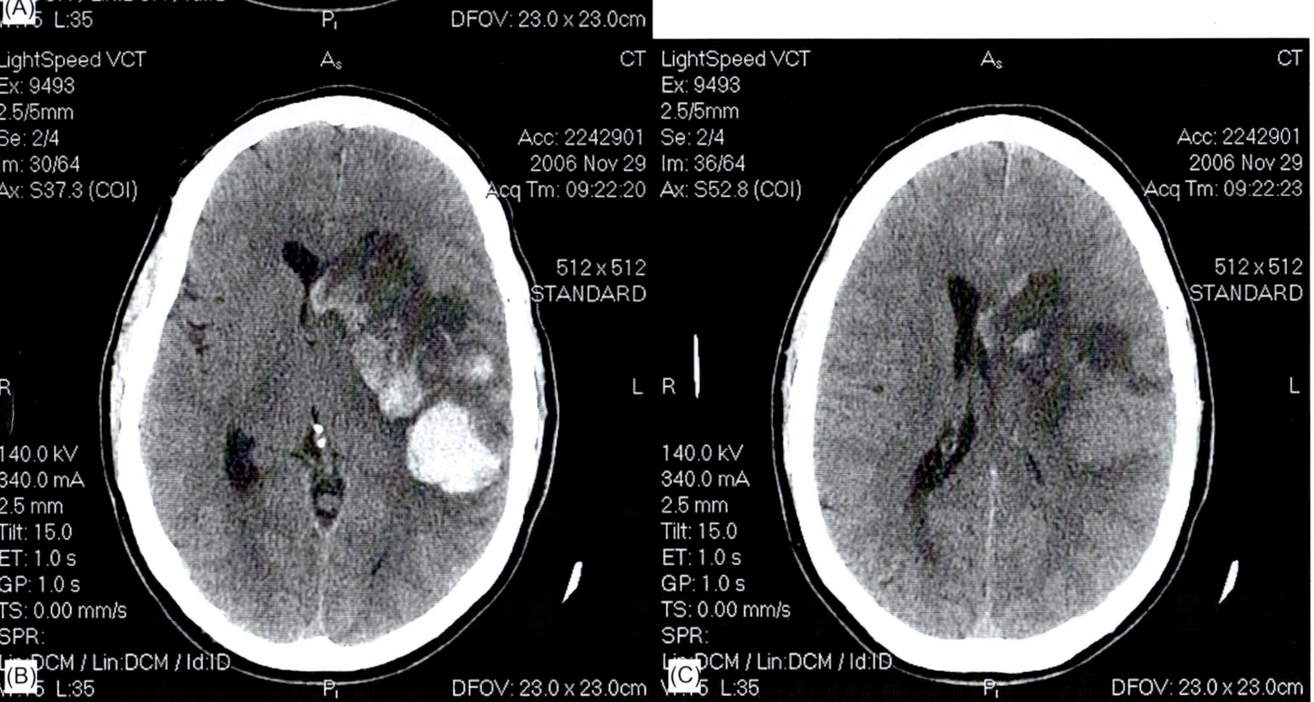

CS 2.1

Comments

The emergent concern was that worsening sensorium was a sign of increasing mass effect upon the upper brainstem and of early uncal herniation. The neurosurgical decompression was probably life saving, but would not improve the disability from this large dominant-hemisphere stroke. The decision to pursue surgery related largely to the patient's young age and excellent pre-stroke health.

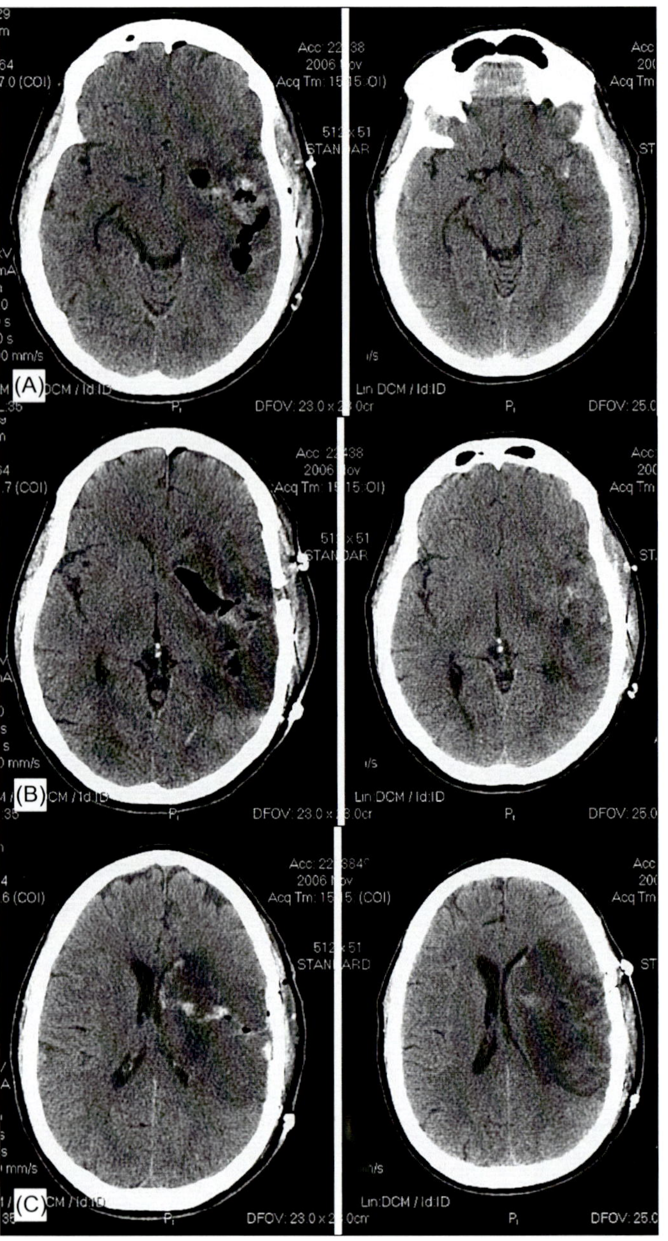

CS 2.2

Case study 3. Deep venous sinus thrombosis

A healthy 45-year-old woman with no significant past medical history, except for use of oral contraceptives, presented with lethargy and obtundation. Uncertainty of the diagnosis at another hospital led to an emergent transfer to a regional Stroke Center. A deep venous sinus thrombosis was suspected based upon the diffuse subcortical venous congestion seen on MRI (**CS 3.1**): on the FLAIR sequence (**CS 3.1**A), there is heightened signal intensity in the left, greater than right, basal ganglia and thalami; and on T1-weighted image (T1WI) with gadolinium contrast (**CS 3.1**B), the periventricular veins are dilated.

The patient rapidly deteriorated despite treatment with IV heparin. Cerebral angiography was undertaken with the plan to directly reopen the deep venous system. A lateral view of the venous circulation (**CS 3.2**) showed normal drainage and wide patency of the superficial venous system and dural sinus; however, it also showed stagnation, with no opacification, of essentially the entire deep venous system, including the internal cerebral veins, the vein of Galen, and the straight sinus (compare with **1.18**D).

Attempts were made over 3 hours to try to re-establish flow in the deep venous system (**CS 3.3**). Local thrombolytic infusion with 12 mg of t-PA, delivered directly into the proximal straight sinus, with an approach from the right transverse sinus, partially established an irregular channel with limited antegrade flow across this sinus (**CS 3.3**A; the sinus is shown on subtracted (left) and unsubtracted (right) views). Markers of the microcatheter are noted in the middle and distal straight sinus (arrowheads). An additional attempt was made with a 4-mm balloon angioplasty (**CS 3.3**B, shown inflated on subtracted views, left) and, to demonstrate relation to the skull base (unsubtracted views, right; arrowheads point to end-markers of the balloon), that was also unsuccessful.

This lesion resulted in a central herniation syndrome. The patient progressed to brain death within 2 days.

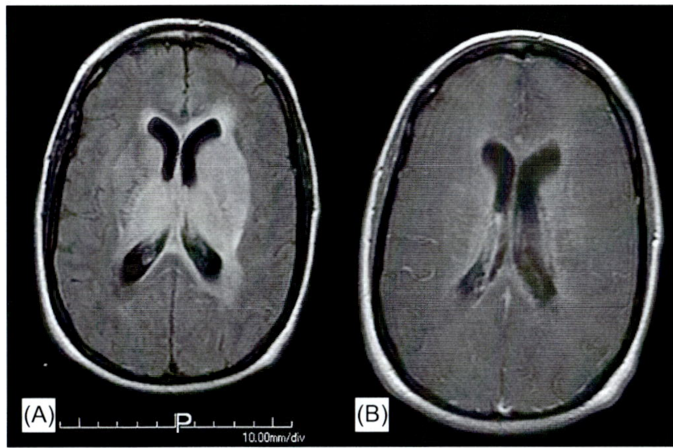

CS 3.1

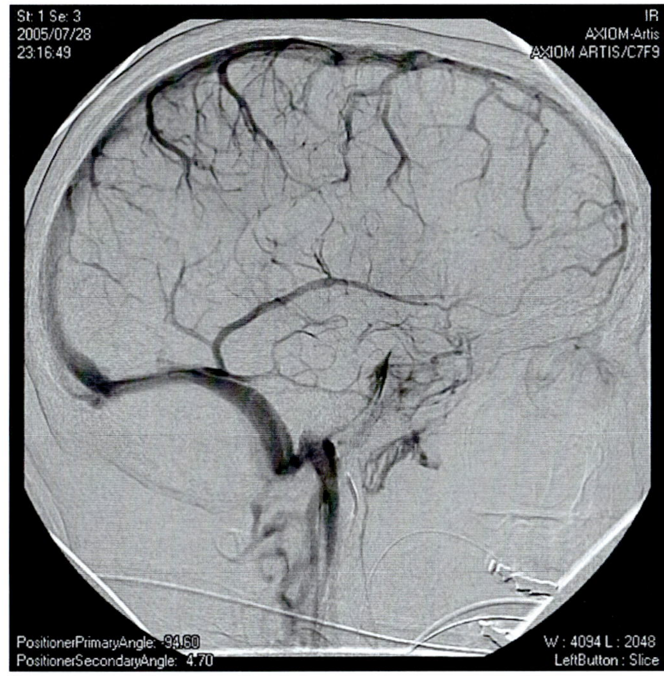

CS 3.2

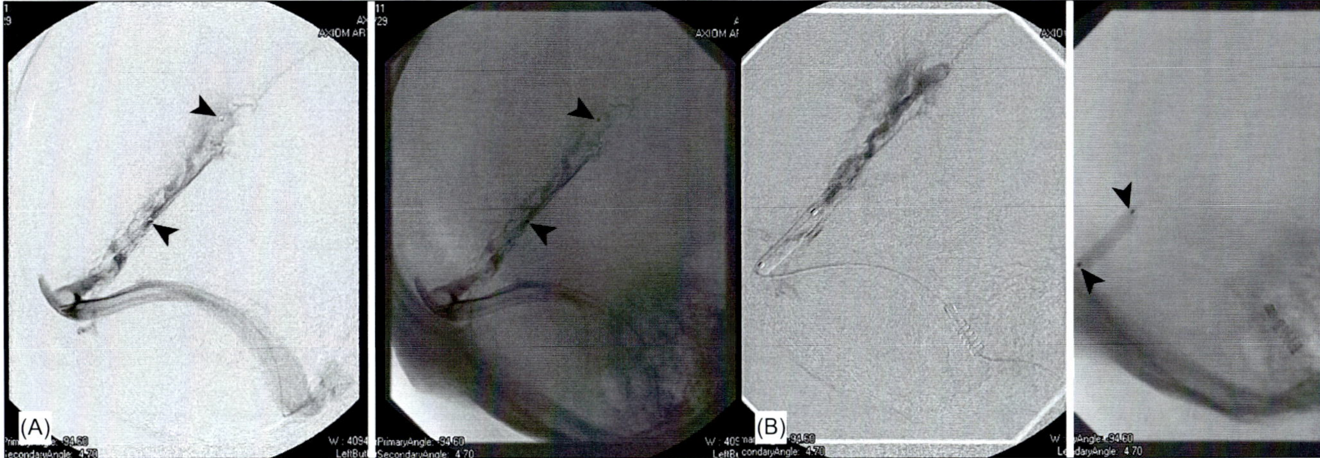

CS 3.3

Case study 4. Atypical lobar hemorrhage

A 40-year-old right-handed patient without a previous history of HTN presented with a lobar hemorrhage in the right frontoparietal region (T2-weighted MRI sequence, **CS 4.1**A). The conventional angiogram shows a parasagittal micro-arteriovenous malformation on lateral projection, as a point of early venous filling (**CS 4.1**B, arrow).

The subsequent composite image (**CS 4.1**C) shows a magnified view of a later phase of this lateral injection lesion (left), and the microcatheter injection (right) shows the point of fistulization (arrow) and again, early venous filling. The microcatheter tip is demonstrated by the white marker (arrowhead). Post-treatment images (D): following glue embolization, the abnormal venous filling is no longer visualized (left), and the glue cast of the arteriovenous malformation is evident on an unsubtracted skull X-ray film (right).

The patient made an outstanding short-term recovery, with only minimal residual paresis of the non-dominant left hand.

Comments

This presentation exemplifies an atypical ICH. The lobar location in a young patient without HTN warrants an angiographic study to search for underlying neurovascular pathology.[34] An underlying vascular malformation of this small size and peripheral location would likely have been missed with non-invasive modalities, specifically CT angiography or MR angiography. Conventional angiography also provides a guide map for endovascular treatment, the only required intervention here (rather than an open craniotomy) to prevent any risk for recurrent hemorrhage.

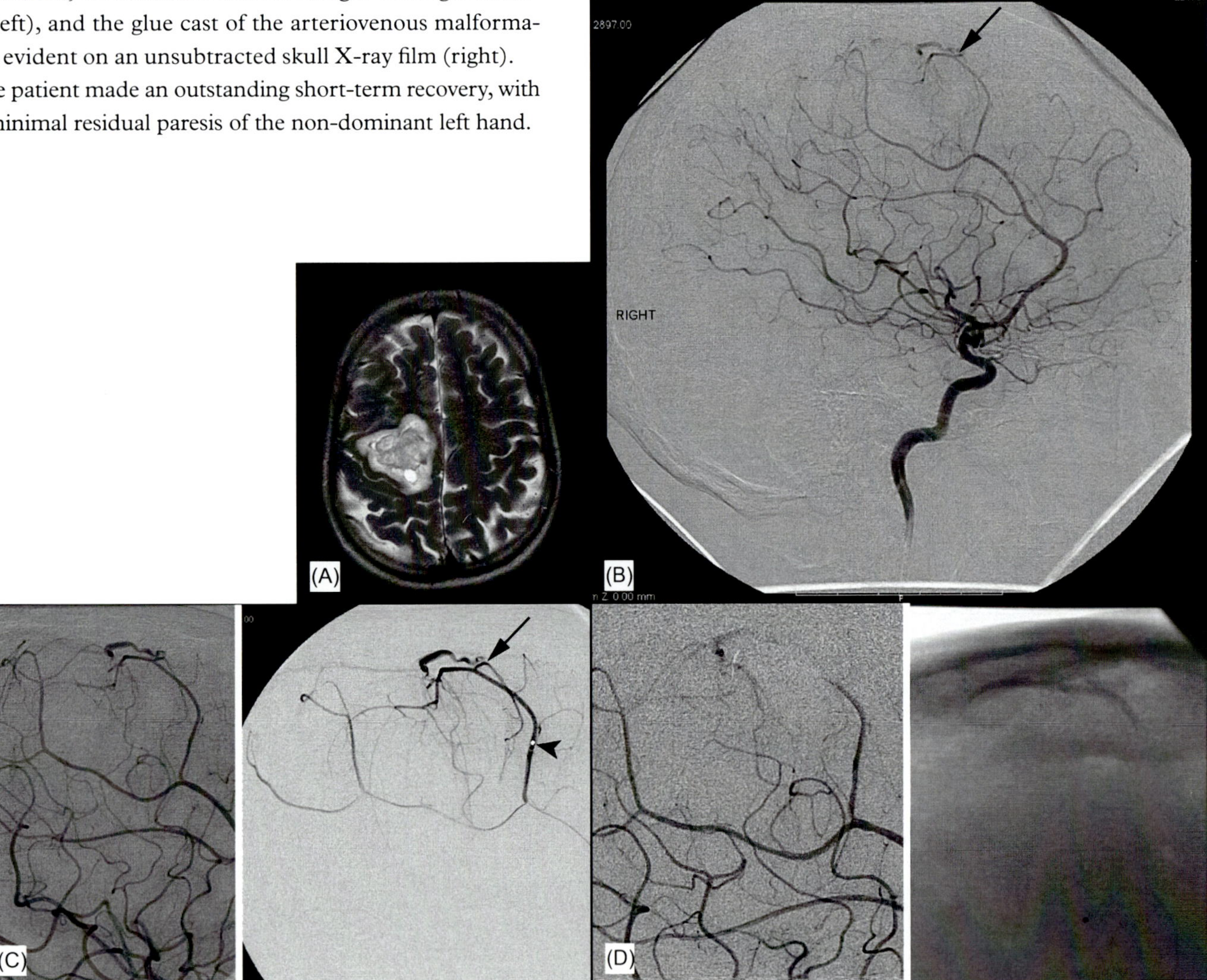

CS 4.1

Case study 5. Lobar hemorrhage treated with neurosurgery

A 75-year-old man presented with a large, loculated left hemispheric hemorrhage involving the occipital, temporal, and parietal lobes (**CS 5.1**), causing severe midline mass effect (**CS 5.1**A), in particular with torque of the midbrain and trapping of the contralateral lateral ventricle (arrow). This patient underwent an emergent decompressive craniotomy, with a follow-up CT scan (**CS 5.1**B) shown at these same levels, the midbrain (left) and the calcified pineal gland (arrowhead) (right), with resolution of much of the midline mass effect.

Micropathology (**CS 5.2**) from the resected brain tissue shows evidence for CAA: swollen capillary walls, laden with amyloid (arrowheads), in both the brain parenchyma (H&E, 100×) (**CS 5.2**A) and the meninges (**CS 5.2**B, H&E, 40×). The β-amyloid within several arterial walls of the meninges stains brown (**CS 5.2**C, immunoperoxidase stain for β-amyloid, 40×) (pathology courtesy of Dean Uphoff, MD).

Comments

The leading causes for lobar hemorrhage in elderly patients are HTN and CAA. This patient had neither previous history of, nor neuroimaging features consistent with, HTN, making CAA the leading diagnosis. Neurosurgery was undertaken as a life-saving therapeutic endeavor, not a diagnostic one.

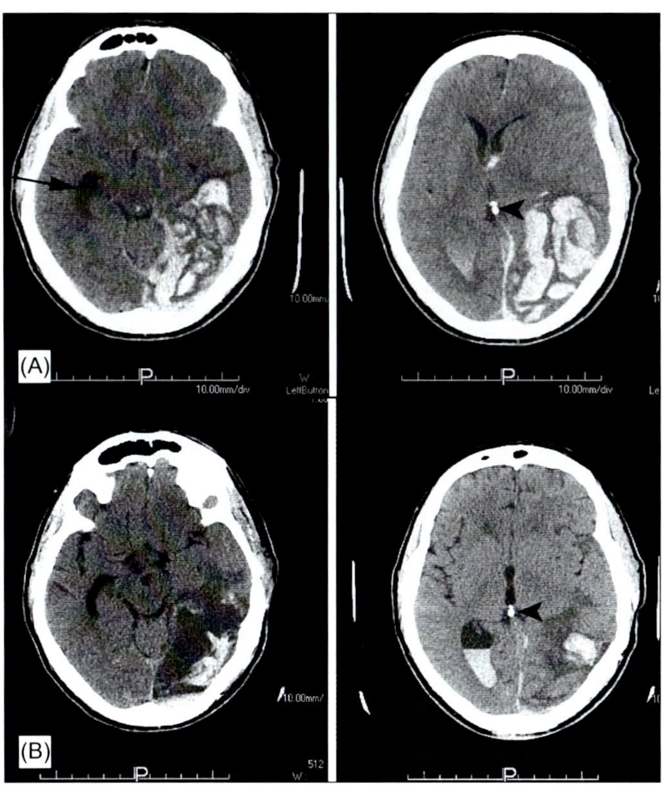

CS 5.1

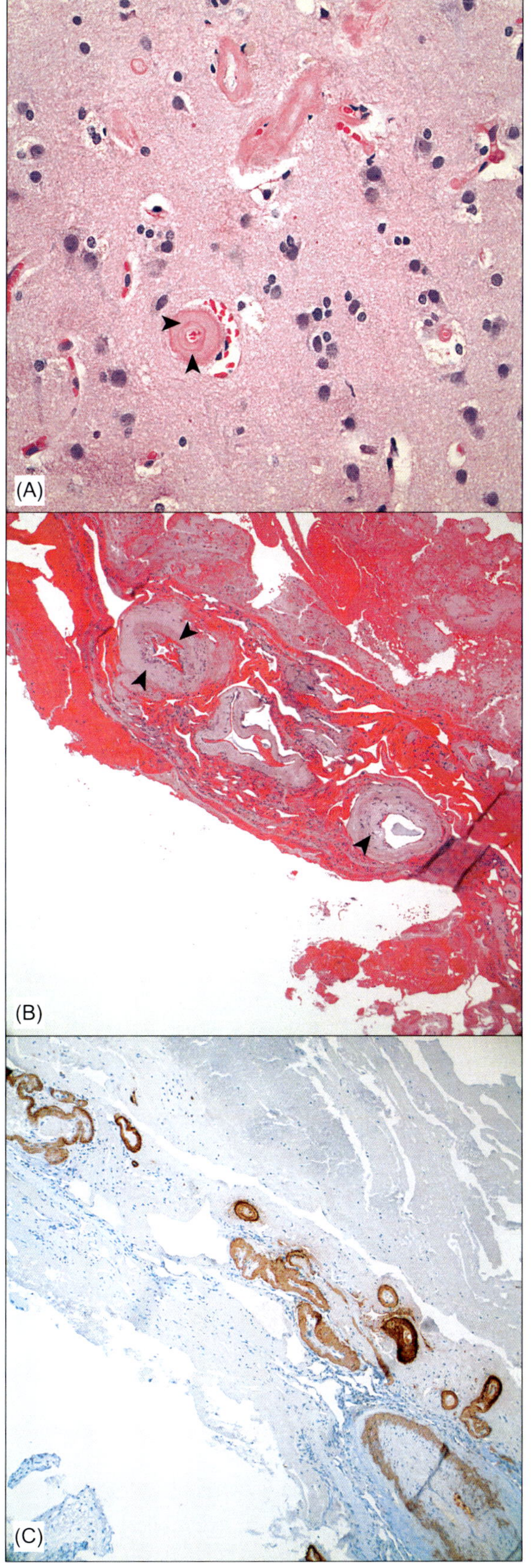

CS 5.2

References

1. Qureshi A, Tuhrim S, Broderick J, Batjer H, Hondo H, Hanley D. Spontaneous intracerebral hemorrhage. *N Engl J Med* 2001; **344**: 1450–60.
2. Juvela S, Kase C. Advances in intracerebral hemorrhage management. *Stroke* 2006; **37**: 301–4.
3. Broderick J, Connolly S, Feldmann E, *et al.* Guidelines for the management of spontaneous intracerebral hemorrhage in adults: 2007 update: a guideline from the American Heart Association/American Stroke Association Stroke Council. *Stroke* 2007; **38**: 2001–23.
4. Broderick J, Adams H, Jr, Barsan W, *et al.* Guidelines for the management of spontaneous intracerebral hemorrhage: a statement for healthcare professionals from a special writing group of the Stroke Council, American Heart Association. *Stroke* 1999; **30**: 905–15.
5. Tuhrim S, Horowtiz D, Sacher M, Godbold J. Validation and comparison of models predicting survival following intracerebral hemorrhage. *Crit Care Med* 1995; **23**: 950–4.
6. Arakawa S, Saku Y, Ibayashi S, Nagao T, Fujishima M. Blood pressure control and recurrence of hypertensive brain hemorrhage. *Stroke* 1998; **29**: 1806–9.
7. Greenberg SM. Cerebral amyloid angiopathy: prospects for clinical diagnosis and treatment. *Neurology* 1998; **51**: 690–94.
8. Knudsen K, Rosand J, Karluk D, Greenberg S. Clinical diagnosis of cerebral amyloid angiopathy: validation of the Boston criteria. *Neurology* 2001; **56**: 537–9.
9. O'Donnell H, Rosand J, Knudsen K, *et al.* Apolipoprotein E genotype and the risk of recurrent lobar intracerebral hemorrhage. *N Engl J Med* 2000; **342**: 240–5.
10. Aguilar M, Hart R, Kase C, *et al.* Treatment of warfarin-associated intracerebral hemorrhage: literature review and expert opinion. *Mayo Clin Proc* 2007; **82**: 82–92.
11. Eckman M, Rosand J, Knudsen K, Singer D, Greenberg S. Can patients be anticoagulated after intracerebral hemorrhage? A decision analysis. *Stroke* 2003; **34**: 1710–16.
12. Tuhrim S. Aspirin-use before ICH: a potentially treatable iatrogenic coagulopathy? [Editorial]. *Stroke* 2006; **37**: 4–5.
13. Diener H-C, Bogousslavsky J, Brass L, *et al.* Aspirin and clopidogrel compared with clopidogrel alone after recent ischaemic stroke or transient ischaemic attack in high-risk patients (MATCH): randomised, double-blind, placebo-controlled trial. *Lancet* 2004; **364**: 331–7.
14. Ariesen MJ, Claus SP, Rinkel GJE, Algra A. Risk factors for intracerebral hemorrhage in the general population: a systematic review. *Stroke* 2003; **34**: 2060–5.
15. Kernan W, Viscoli C, Brass L, *et al.* Phenylpropanolamine and the risk of hemorrhagic stroke. *N Engl J Med* 2000; **343**: 1826–32.
16. Davis SM, Broderick J, Hennerici M, *et al.* Hematoma growth is a determinant of mortality and poor outcome after intracerebral hemorrhage. *Neurology* 2006; **66**: 1175–81.
17. Mayer S. Ultra-early hemostatic therapy for intracerebral hemorrhage. *Stroke* 2003; **34**: 224–9.
18. Selim M. Deferoxamine mesylate: a new hope for intracerebral hemorrhage: from bench to clinical trials. *Stroke* 2009; **40**(Suppl 1): S90–S91.
19. Finelli P. A diagnostic approach to multiple simultaneous intracerebral hemorrhages. *Neurocrit Care* 2006; **4**: 267–71.
20. Gates P. Intraventricular hemorrhages. In: Bogousslavsky J, Caplan L, eds. *Stroke Syndromes*, 2nd edn. Cambridge: Cambridge University Press; 2001: 612–17.
21. Viswanathan A, Chabriat H. Cerebral microhemorrhage. *Stroke* 2006; **37**: 550–5.
22. Wardlaw J, Lewis S, Keir S, Dennis M, Shenkin S. Cerebral microbleeds are associated with lacunar stroke defined clinically and radiologically, independently of white matter lesions. *Stroke* 2006; **37**: 2633–6.
23. Trouillas P, von Kummer R. Classification and pathogenesis of cerebral hemorrhages after thrombolysis in ischemic stroke. *Stroke* 2006; **37**: 556–61.
24. Fiorelli M, Bastianello S, von Kummer R, *et al.* Hemorrhagic transformation within 36 hours of a cerebral infarct: relationships with early clinical deterioration and 3-month outcome in the European Cooperative Acute Stroke Study I (ECASS I) cohort. *Stroke* 1999; **30**: 2280–4.
25. Larrue V, von Kummer R, Muller A, Bluhmki E. Risk factors for severe hemorrhagic transformation in ischemic stroke patients treated with recombinant tissue plasminogen activator: a secondary analysis of the European–Australasian Acute Stroke Study (ECASS II). *Stroke* 2001; **32**: 438–41.
26. Khatri P, Wechsler L, Broderick J. Intracranial hemorrhage associated with revascularization therapies. *Stroke* 2007; **38**: 431–40.

27. Kase CS, Furlan AJ, Wechsler LR, *et al.* Cerebral hemorrhage after intra-arterial thrombolysis for ischemic stroke: the PROACT II trial. *Neurology* 2001; **57**: 1603–10.
28. Neumann-Haefelin T, Hoelig S, Berkefeld J, *et al.* Leukoaraiosis is a risk factor for symptomatic intracerebral hemorrhage after thrombolysis for acute stroke. *Stroke* 2006; **37**: 2463–6.
29. The National Institute of Neurological Disorders and Stroke rt-PA Stroke Study Group. Intracerebral hemorrhage following intravenous t-PA therapy for ischemic stroke. *Stroke* 1997; **28**: 2109–18.
30. Martinelli I, Sacchi E, Landi G, Tailoi E, Duca F, Nammucci P. High risk of cerebral-vein thrombosis in carriers of a prothrombin-gene mutation and in users of oral contraceptives. *N Engl J Med* 1998; **338**: 1793–7.
31. Ferro JM, Canhao P, Stam J, Bousser M-G, Barinagarrementeria F, for the ISCVT Investigators. Prognosis of cerebral vein and dural sinus thrombosis: results of the International Study on Cerebral Vein and Dural Sinus Thrombosis (ISCVT). *Stroke* 2004; **35**: 664–70.
32. Gosk-Bierska I, Wysokinski W, Brown R, Jr., *et al.* Cerebral venous sinus thrombosis: incidence of venous thrombosis recurrence and survival. *Neurology* 2006; **67**: 814–19.
33. Broderick J, Brott T, Duldner J, Tomsick T, Huster G. Volume of intracerebral hemorrhage: a powerful and easy-to-use predictor of 30-day mortality. *Stroke* 1993; **24**: 987–93.
34. Zhu X, Chan M, Poon W. Spontaneous intracranial hemorrhage: which patients need diagnostic cerebral angiography? A prospective study of 206 cases and review of the literature. *Stroke* 1997; **28**: 1406–9.
35. Mayer S, Brun N, Begtrup K, *et al.* Recombinant activated factor VII for acute intracerebral hemorrhage. *N Engl J Med* 2005; **352**: 777–85.
36. Mayer SA, Brun NC, Begtrup K, et al. Efficacy and safety of recombinant activated factor VII for acute intracerebral hemorrhage. *N Engl J Med* 2008; **358**: 2127–37.
37. Steiner T, Rosand J, Diringer M. Intracerebral hemorrhage associated with oral anticoagulant therapy: current practices and unresolved questions. *Stroke* 2006; **37**: 256–62.
38. Kobayashi S, Sato A, Kageyama Y, Nakamura H, Watanabe Y, Yamaura A. Treatment of hypertensive cerebellar hemorrhage – surgical or conservative management? *Neurosurgery* 1994; **32**: 246–50.
39. Mendelow A, Gregson B, Fernandes H, *et al.* Early surgery versus initial conservative treatment in patients with spontaneous supratentorial intracerebral haematomas in the International Surgical Trial in Intracerebral Haemorrhage (STICH): a randomised trial. *Lancet* 2005; **365**: 387–97.
40. Montes J, Wong J, Fayad P, Awad I. Stereotactic computed tomographic-guided aspiration and thrombolysis of intracerebral hematoma: protocol and preliminary experience. *Stroke* 2000; **31**: 834–40.
41. Bladin C, Alexandrov A, Bellavance A, *et al.* Seizures after stroke: a prospective multicenter study. *Arch Neurol* 2000; **57**: 1617–22.
42. Diringer M, Edwards D. Admission to a neurologic/neurosurgical intensive care unit is associated with reduced mortality rate after intracerebral hemorrhage. *Crit Care Med* 2001; **29**: 635–40.
43. SHEP Cooperative Research Group. Prevention of stroke by antihypertensive drug treatment in older persons with isolated systolic hypertension: final results of the Systolic Hypertension in the Elderly Program (SHEP). *JAMA* 1991; **263**: 3255–64.
44. PROGRESS Group. Randomised trial of a perindopril-based blood-pressure-lowering regimen among 6105 individuals with previous stroke or transient ischaemic attack. *Lancet* 2001; **358**: 1033–41.
45. Chobanian A, Bakris G, Black H, *et al.* Seventh report of the Joint National Committee on Prevention, Detection, Evaluation, and Treatment of High Blood Pressure (JNC 7 – Complete Version). *Hypertension* 2003; **42**: 1206–52.
46. Coull B, Skaff P. Disorders of coagulation. In: Bougousslavsky J, Caplan L, eds. *Uncommon Causes of Stroke*. New York: Cambridge University Press; 2001: 86–95.

Further reading

Broderick J, Connolly S, Feldmann E, *et al.* Guidelines for the management of spontaneous intracerebral hemorrhage in adults: 2007 update: a guideline from the American Heart Association/American Stroke Association Stroke Council. *Stroke* 2007; **38**: 2001–23.

Mayer S. Ultra-early hemostatic therapy for intracerebral hemorrhage. *Stroke* 2003; **34**: 224–9.

PROGRESS Group. Randomised trial of a perindopril-based blood-pressure-lowering regimen among 6105 individuals with previous stroke or transient ischaemic attack. *Lancet* 2001; **358**: 1033–41.

Qureshi A, Tuhrim S, Broderick J, Batjer H, Hondo H, Hanley D. Spontaneous intracerebral hemorrhage. *N Engl J Med* 2001; **344**: 1450–60.

Trouillas P, von Kummer R. Classification and pathogenesis of cerebral hemorrhages after thrombolysis in ischemic stroke. *Stroke* 2006; **37**: 556–61.

Viswanathan A, Chabriat H. Cerebral microhemorrhage. *Stroke* 2006; **37**: 550–5.

Resources for patients

Intracerebral hemorrhage

American Stroke Association (www.strokeassociation.org)
National Stroke Association (www.stroke.org)
www.strokecenter.org/pat/ich.htm

Cerebral amyloid angiopathy

http://angiopathy.org/

Chapter 2

Intracranial Aneurysms and Subarachnoid Hemorrhage

Epidemiology

Subarachnoid hemorrhage (SAH) is the extravasation of blood into the cerebrospinal fluid spaces of the central nervous system. The most common causes are head trauma (**2.1**) and the rupture of intracranial aneurysms (IA) (**2.2**).[1] Non-traumatic SAH results from a ruptured IA in 80% of cases, while 20% are due predominantly to non-aneurysmal perimesencephalic SAH.[2-4]

Aneurysmal SAH accounts for only 1–7% of all new strokes, with an aggregate worldwide incidence of 10.5 cases per 100 000 person-years.[2,5] However, because of poor outcomes, high mortality rate, and young age of onset, SAH results in a loss of productive life-years comparable with that for ischemic stroke.[6] SAH accounts for 27% of all stroke-related years of potential life lost before 65 years of age.[6] Increasing age is associated with non-traumatic SAH, with a mean age of presentation of 55 years. The risk for SAH in women is 1.6 times that of men and for black people 2.1 times that of white people.[7]

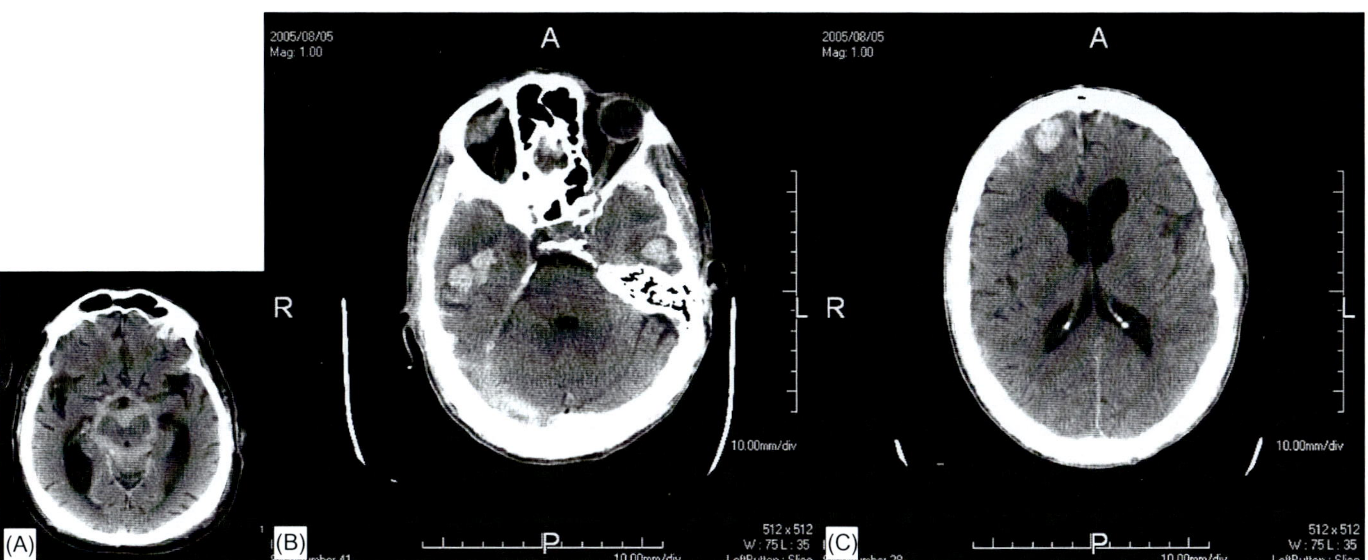

2.1 Traumatic SAH. Subarachnoid blood from closed head injury may be associated with diffuse SAH in the basal cisterns (A); this lesion occurred when an elderly patient fell down a flight of steps. In a second case, traumatic brain injury from a motor vehicle accident (B,C), there is diffuse parenchymal hemorrhage in the temporal and frontal lobes, more apparent than the minor subarachnoid component along the right cerebellar tentorium and around the lobar lesions.

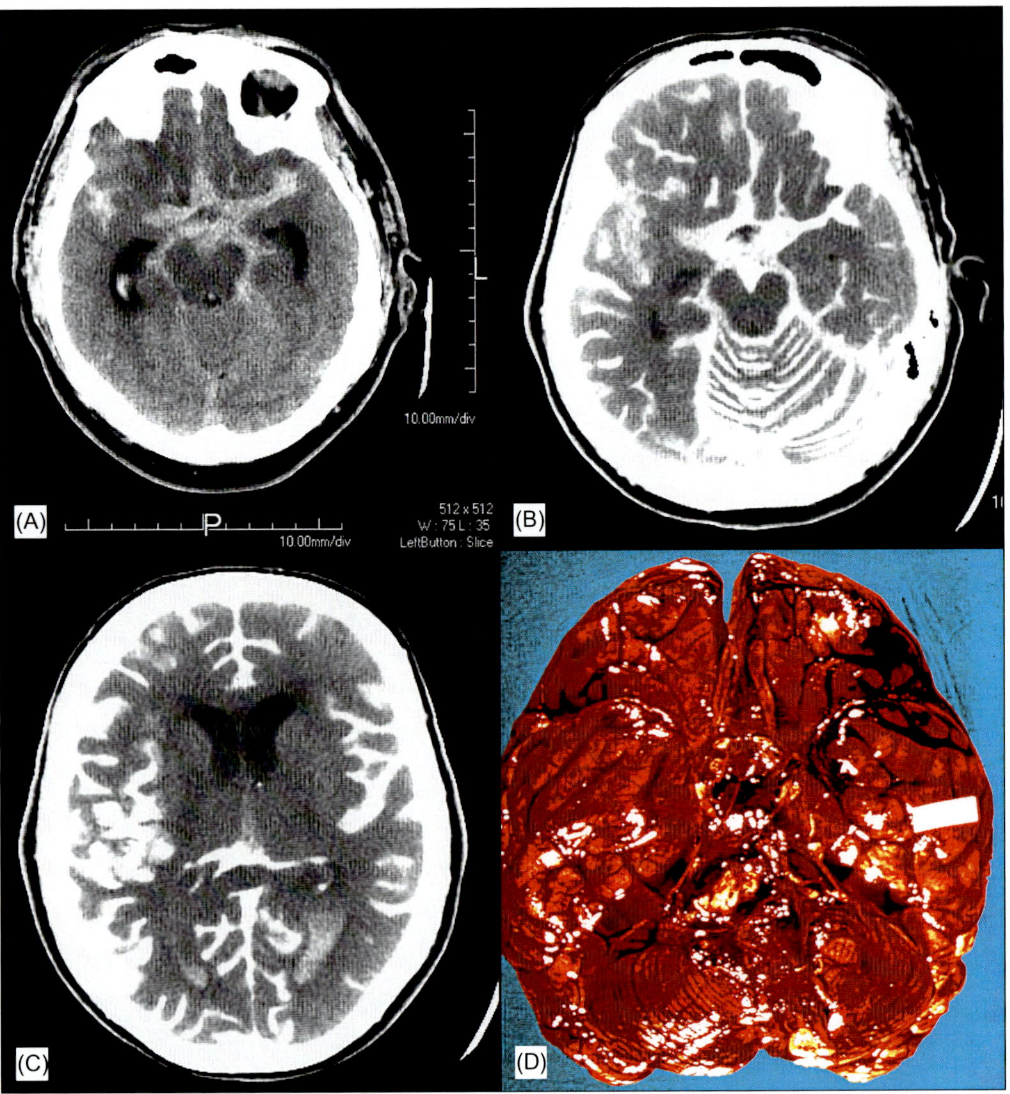

2.2 Typical aneurysmal SAH. A non-contrast CT scan demonstrates widespread, extensive SAH from a ruptured aneurysm of the A-Comm (A), with the circle of Willis here resembling a crab and enlarged temporal horns of the lateral ventricles. A second patient's CT scan with contrast (B,C) shows extensive blood within the majority of hemispheric sulci, as well as some layering in the posterior horns of the lateral ventricles. Gross pathology from a patient who died from SAH (D), with the entire surface of the brain covered with blood.

Risk factors

Modifiable risk factors for aneurysmal SAH are:

- cigarette smoking;
- hypertension;
- cocaine use;
- heavy, recent alcohol use.[2,8]

Smoking confers a 3–10-fold higher risk of aneurysmal SAH than among non-smokers, and is dose dependent.[8] Smoking may contribute to IA formation by decreasing the effectiveness of α_1-antitrypsin, an inhibitor of proteolytic enzymes such as elastase. Excessive proteolysis may then result in degradation of arterial wall connective tissue, promoting aneurysm formation.

Inherited connective tissues disorders such as Ehlers–Danlos syndrome (type IV), pseudoxanthoma elasticum, and fibromuscular dysplasia are associated with the development of IA and SAH.[1] In familial intracranial aneurysm syndromes, individual patients and at least two first-degree relatives harbor an IA. However, the inheritance pattern is often unclear.[8] Patients with a history of a familial IA syndrome have a higher risk for aneurysm formation and are at risk of rupture at both a smaller aneurysm size and an earlier age than patients with sporadic IAs.[8–10]

Pathogenesis

Aneurysms arise much more commonly from intracranial arteries than from extracranial arteries of similar size. This discrepancy is due to the thinner walls of intracranial arteries, which have an attenuated tunica media and lack an external elastic lamina.[8] Microscopic examinations show that the typical saccular, or 'berry' IA, has a very thin or no tunica media and a severely fragmented or absent internal elastic lamina (**2.3**). An aneurysm's wall consists of only intima and adventitia, with variable amounts of interposed fibrohyaline tissue. High pulsatile pressure is maximal at the branching points of the proximal arteries around the circle of Willis (**2.3**).[11] These arterial bifurcations are the chief sites of atherosclerotic aneurysm formation, and the point of rupture is usually at the dome of the lesion.

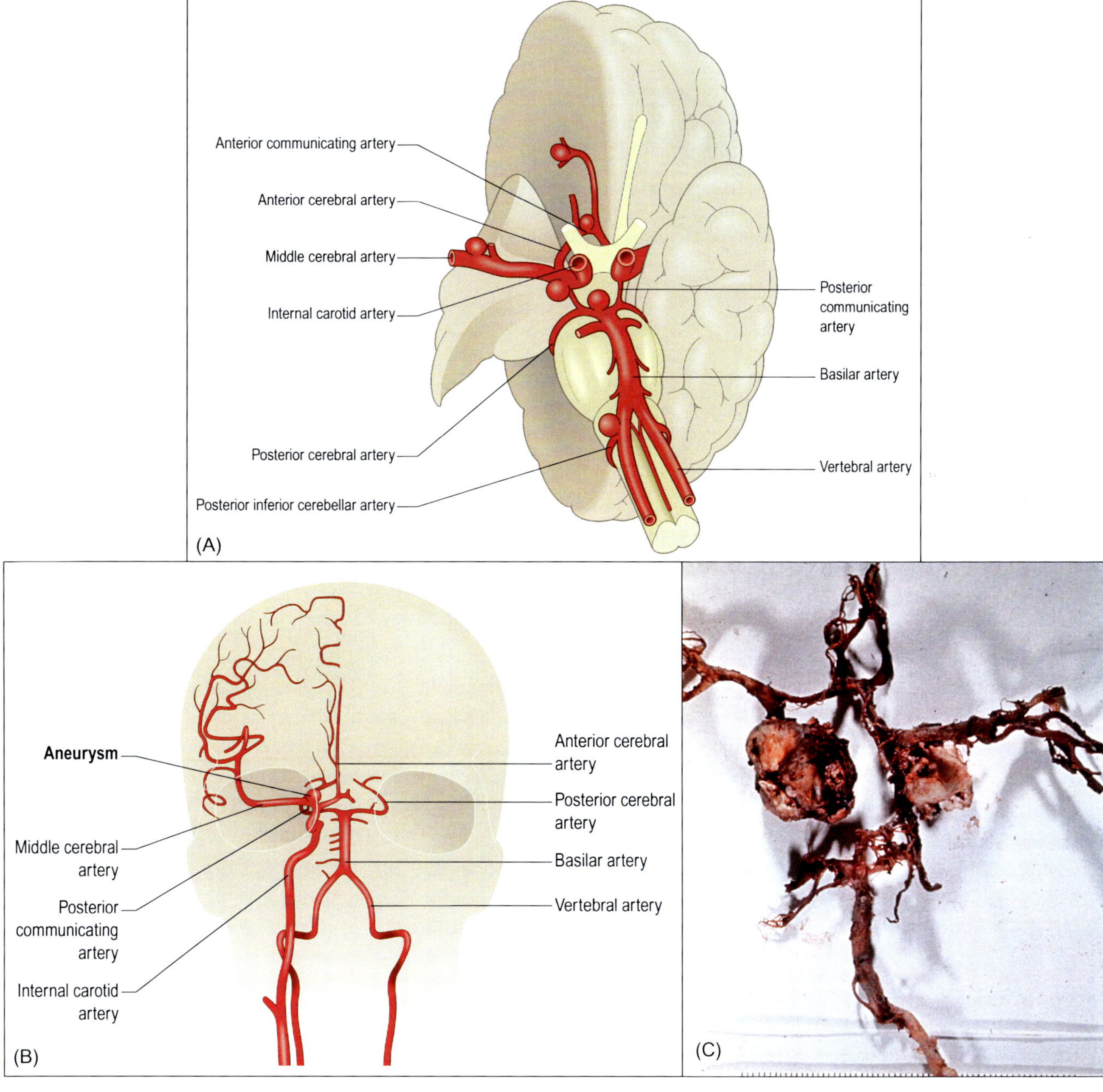

2.3 Common sites and pathology of intracranial aneurysms. The branch points around the circle of Willis are the most common locations for IAs (A) (adapted from Schievink[8]). The circle of Willis, where aneurysms commonly develop, lies directly behind the orbits (B, adapted from Ellegala and Day[11]). This anatomic dissection of the circle of Willis demonstrates at least two giant aneurysms, situated around the distal internal carotid artery (ICA) and posterior communicating artery (P-Comm) junctions (C).

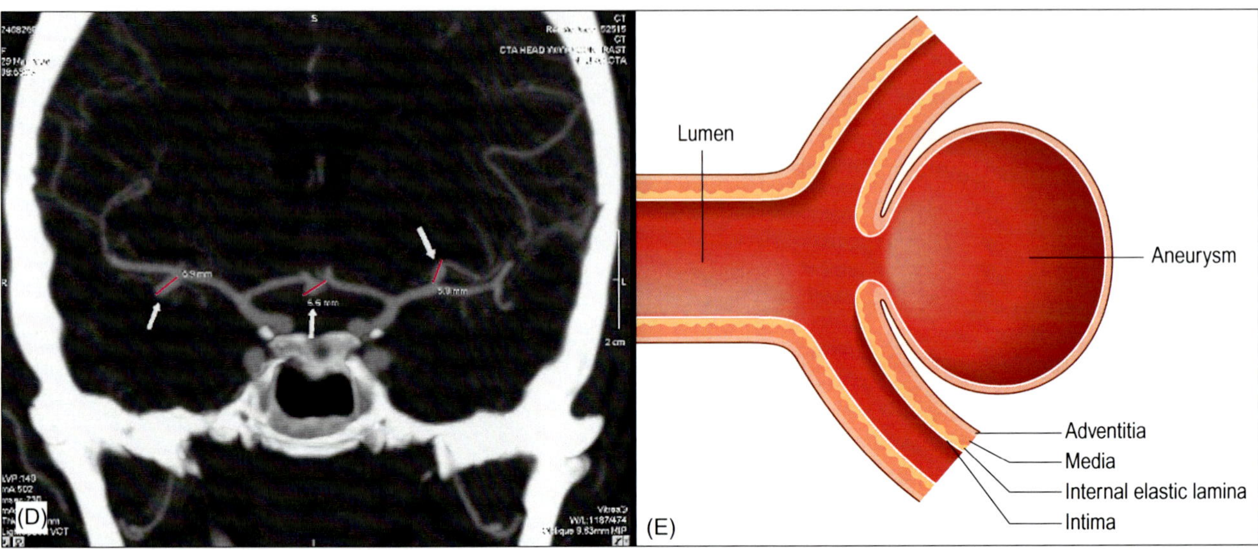

2.3 (*continued*) Common sites and pathology of intracranial aneurysms. A CTA, coronal slice (D), shows three unruptured aneurysms around the first- and second-order intracranial branches, at the MCA (M1–M2) bifurcations bilaterally and, centrally, an inferior-pointing A-Comm lesion, with estimates of their diameters. The diagram (E) demonstrates the loss of the internal elastic lamina and media in an aneurysm. The other wall layers are designated for intima and adventitia (adapted from Osborn[53]).

Clinical presentation

Common presenting symptoms of SAH are severe headache ('the worst headache of one's life') with nausea, vomiting, and a diminished level of consciousness, with or without focal neurologic deficits. Neurologic deficits may result from direct pressure from the aneurysm, increased intracranial pressure, and/or intracerebral hematoma in cases where the rupture directs blood into the brain parenchyma as well as the subarachnoid space.

- Non-specific findings on examination:
  - nuchal rigidity;
  - diminished level of consciousness.
- Findings related to rapidly increased intracranial pressure:
  - papilledema;
  - sixth-nerve palsy;
  - retinal, subhyaloid, and vitreous hemorrhages indicate a more abrupt increase in intracranial pressure and increased mortality (**2.4**).[2]
- Neurologic signs indicating the location of an aneurysm:
  - third-nerve palsy from the direct mass effect of a posterior communicating artery aneurysm upon this cranial nerve;
  - sixth-nerve palsy;
  - nystagmus or ataxia from posterior fossa lesions;
  - aphasia, hemiparesis, or visual neglect from proximal middle cerebral artery (MCA) aneurysms;
  - bilateral leg weakness or abulia from aneurysms of the anterior communicating artery (A-Comm).[12]

Neurologic deficits on presentation form the basis for the two leading clinical grading scales for SAH, the Hunt–Hess and the World Federations of Neurological Surgeons (*Table 2.1*).[13,14]

Misdiagnosis of SAH is common.[12,15] A first severe or worst headache should prompt a non-contrast head computed tomography scan (CT) scan, to rule out SAH (**2.5**). However, patients who are misdiagnosed tend to be less ill, and may have an early headache that resolves. These so-called sentinel headaches are believed to result from early bleeding and stretching of the aneurysm's wall but may be indistinguishable from other benign headaches. Several excellent reviews discuss the differential diagnosis for SAH.[2,8,12] Common reasons for misdiagnosis relate to failures to appreciate the clinical spectrum of this disease, the limitation of CT scans in diagnosis, and failure to perform a lumbar puncture or correctly interpret cerebrospinal fluid findings.[2,12] The sensitivity of modern non-contrast CT scans for identifying SAH is >90%;[12] however, patients with atypical headache for whom SAH is in the differential diagnosis and who have a normal CT scan should subsequently undergo a lumbar puncture to increase the accuracy of diagnosis.

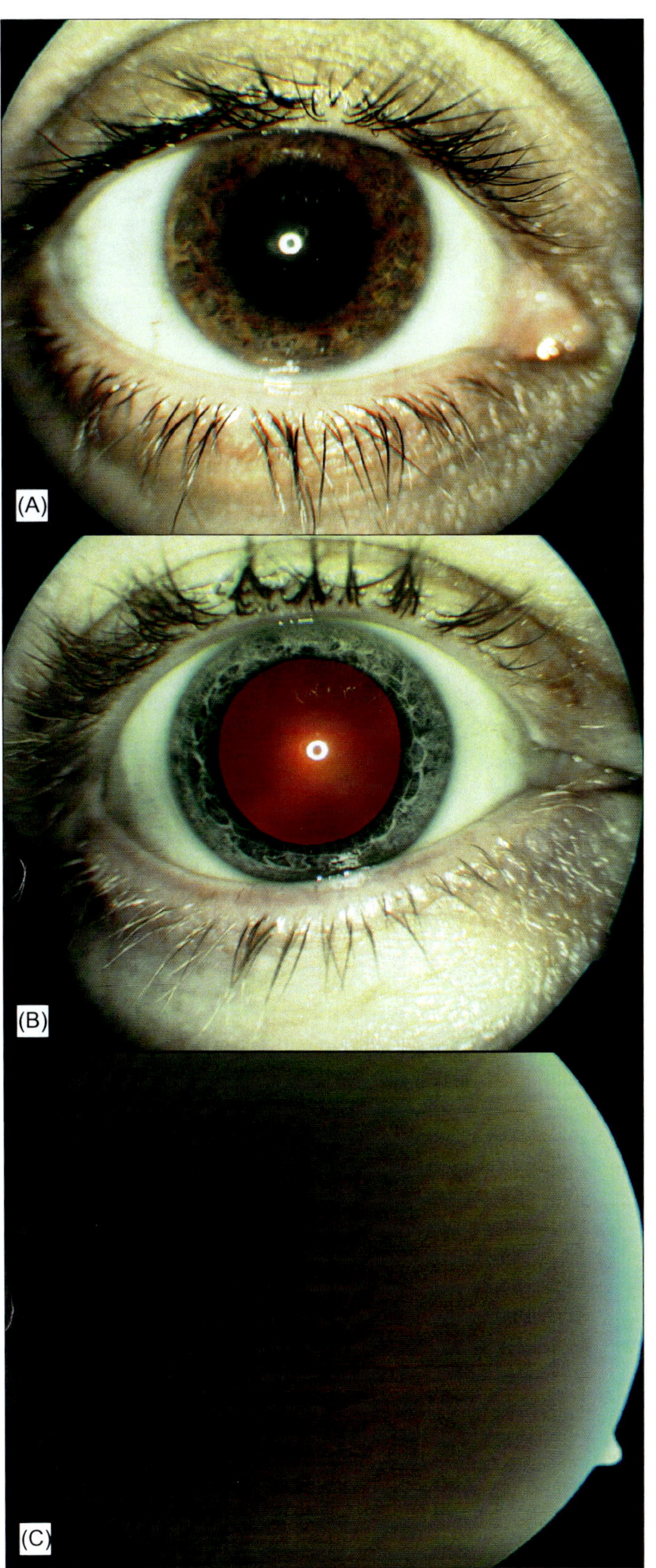

Diagnosis

Before modern CT and magnetic resonance (MR) neurovascular imaging, conventional cerebral angiography was required to identify IAs. Non-invasive CT and MR angiography (MRA) now obviate the need for conventional angiography in most patients.

Magnetic resonance imaging and angiography

This modality misses some smaller aneurysms, usually identifying lesions <5 mm in diameter in prospective studies, but may detect lesions as small as 2 mm. This modality provides excellent anatomical detail for the localization of IAs relative to brain parenchyma, complications (e.g., ischemic stroke, perilesional edema) related to treatments, and occasionally flow dynamics within an IA (**2.6, 2.7**). It is also the best method for demonstrating the presence of a thrombus within an aneurysmal sac (see **3.5**B).[8] However, MRA is not very useful in planning open neurosurgical procedures. Most studies recommend MRA as the screening tool of choice for patients with an inherited risk for aneurysm formation, such as those with a familial IA syndrome[9,10] or polycystic kidney disease.[16–18]

2.4 Terson syndrome. The typical red reflex from the retina is absent on a retroilluminated photograph of the pupil (A) due to extensive vitreal hemorrhage that developed because a ruptured IA caused acutely elevated intracranial and intraocular pressures. (Neuroimaging of this patient is shown in **2.13**.) Compare with a normal red reflex due to the retina in the dilated eye of a different patient (B). An intraocular photograph of the first patient is extremely hazy due to extensive blood diffused throughout the vitreous (C).

Table 2.1 Grading severity of subarachnoid hemorrhage

(A) Hunt and Hess Grading System[14]

Grade	Description*
1	Asymptomatic, or mild headache and slight nuchal rigidity
2	Cranial nerve palsy, moderate–severe headache, nuchal rigidity
3	Mild focal deficit, lethargy, or confusion
4	Stupor, moderate–severe hemiparesis, early decerebrate rigidity
5	Deep coma, decerebrate rigidity, moribund appearance

*Add one grade for serious systemic disease (hypertension, diabetes mellitus (DM), severe atherosclerosis, chronic obstructive pulmonary disease) or severe vasospasm on angiography.

(B) Grading Scale of the World Federation of Neurological Surgeons[13]

Grade	GCS*	Clinical appearance	Grade	SAH	Intraventricular hemorrhage
1	15	No motor deficit	0	Absent	Absent
2	13–14	No motor deficit	1	Minimal	Absent in both lateral ventricles
3	13–14	Motor deficit	2	Minimal	Present in both lateral ventricles
4	7–12	±Motor deficit	3	Thick†	Absent in both lateral ventricles
5	3–6	±Motor deficit	4	Thick†	Present in both lateral ventricles

*Glasgow Coma Scale = Sum of points for eye opening (4 points), best motor response (6 points), and best verbal response (5 points).
†This designation denotes a hemorrhage filling one or more of 10 cisterns or fissures: the frontal interhemispheric fissure, the quadrigeminal cistern, both suprasellar cisterns, both ambient cisterns, both basal Sylvian fissures, and both lateral Sylvian fissures.

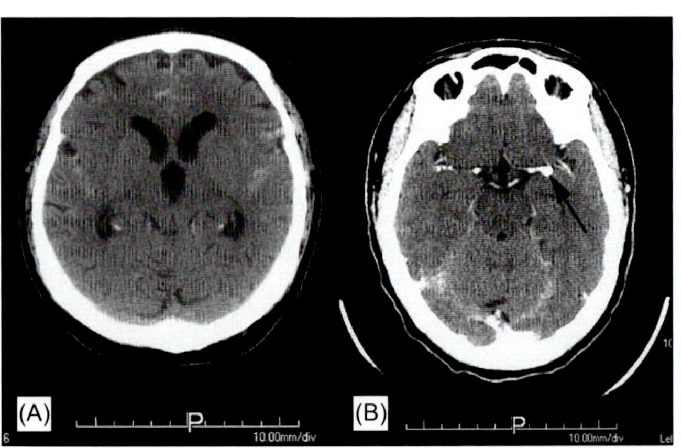

2.5 Subtle CT scans of SAH. (A) Shows subarachnoid blood in both Sylvian fissures as well as in the interhemispheric fissure. Another sign of SAH here is the rounded third ventricle and temporal horns of the lateral ventricles, consistent with early obstructive hydrocephalus. (B) A contrast-enhanced CT scan demonstrates subarachnoid blood along the cerebellar tentorium, and a left MCA-bifurcation IA (arrow) as a possible source.

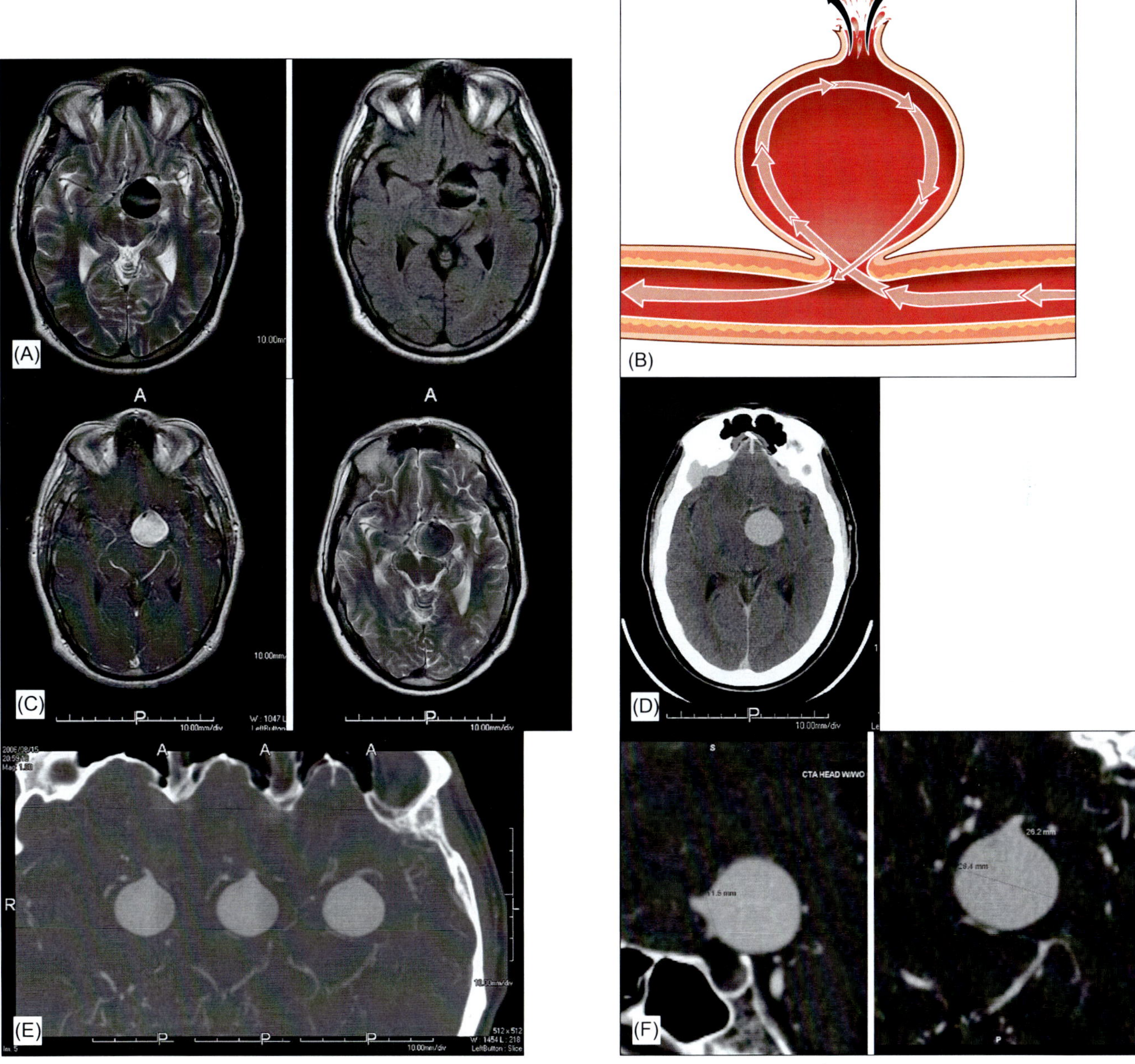

2.6 Giant intracranial aneurysm on MR and CTA. T2-weighted (A, left) and FLAIR (A, right) sequences of an unruptured giant distal left ICA aneurysm suggest a vortex, a swirling of blood flow within the center of this lesion. Particularly within larger aneurysms, the arterial supply enters the lesion on the far (distal) wall of the lesion and exits in a vortex-type pattern via the near (proximal) wall (B, adapted from Osborn[53]). Occasionally, this pattern of flow is appreciated on MR imaging. A gadolinium-enhanced T1-weighted image (left) and unenhanced T2-weighted image (right) demonstrate the lesion's mass effect upon the adjacent left cerebral peduncle (C).

The CT study shows the level of anatomic detail in a non-contrast study (D), and some advantages of a CTA study. Three adjacent transverse cuts of the source images of the CTA (E) demonstrate how the lesion straddles the A1 (medial) and M1 (lateral) segments. The final CTA images (F) measure the width of the aneurysm neck, at 11.5 mm (left) and the overall diameter of the lesion, at 28.4 mm (right). Giant aneurysms are defined by a diameter >25 mm. Because of the extremely wide neck and location of this IA, it was later treated by sacrifice (embolic occlusion) of the parent feeding artery, the left ICA.

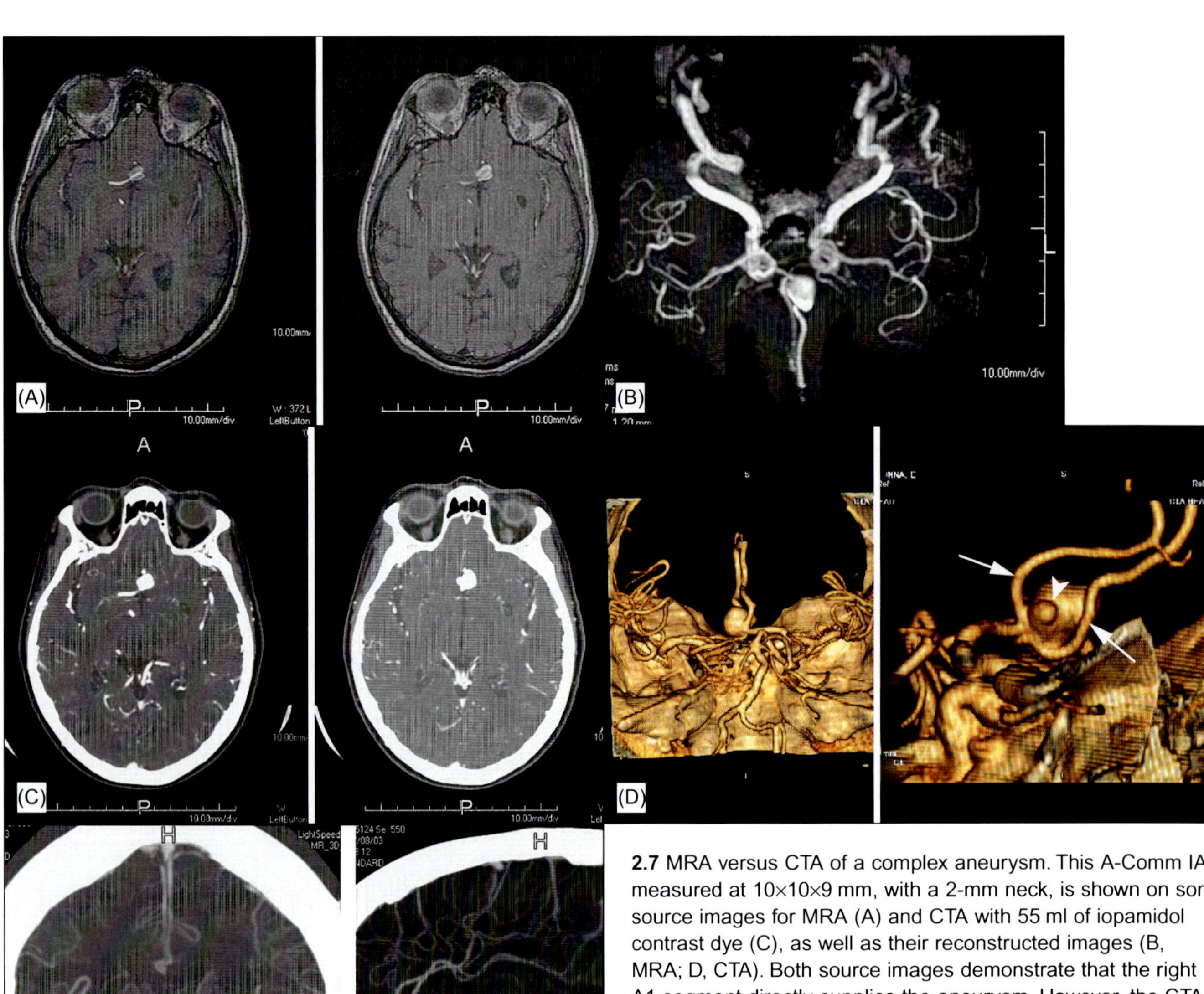

2.7 MRA versus CTA of a complex aneurysm. This A-Comm IA measured at 10×10×9 mm, with a 2-mm neck, is shown on some source images for MRA (A) and CTA with 55 ml of iopamidol contrast dye (C), as well as their reconstructed images (B, MRA; D, CTA). Both source images demonstrate that the right A1 segment directly supplies the aneurysm. However, the CTA provides better morphologic detail of this complex lesion, as well as better resolution regarding the parent and distal lesions surrounding the IA. The bilateral A2 segments both emanate from the sides of this aneurysm (D, right; arrows). The CTA study (E) also enables with coronal (left) and sagittal (right) images, a clear view relating this aneurysm to the skull base. A focal outpouching of the IA, emanating from the right lateral wall, is best visualized on CTA (arrowhead) (D, right). Although the CTA appears to supply better data to plan aneurysm ablation therapies in this comparison with MRA, many imaging-related variables will affect such a comparison of CT and MR modalities, including slice width, imaging technology (e.g., magnet strength), and contrast administration.

Computed tomography and computed tomography angiography

Modern rapid multislice CT scanners (often available in the emergency department) have greatly advanced lesion detection.[19] Helical CT angiography (CTA) quickly enables a three-dimensional anatomical reconstruction of aneurysm morphology (**2.6–2.8**), identifies aneurysm components (including calcification), defines the lesion location in relation to the skull base, and is safer for medically unstable patients than MR imaging (MRI). The presence of aneurysm wall calcification and/or an aneurysm's adjacency to bone, detected more accurately by CT than conventional angiography, may indicate a lesion of higher neurosurgical risk (**2.9**). Finally, CTA is the only option for patients who are excluded from MRA because of metal implantation, including early generation ferromagnetic aneurysm clips as these are an absolute contraindication to MRA.[8] Some of these clips are also problematic in CT and MRI studies because they cause significant streaky metallic artifact that may obscure adjacent structures (**2.10**).

A hyperdense clot adjacent to a common location for an IA in the basal cisterns is typically diagnostic for a ruptured lesion (**2.11**); however, occasionally, rupture may occur with minimal or no subarachnoid component. In that case, a lobar hemorrhage and/or intraventricular bleeding may be suggestive of an underlying aneurysm (**2.12, 2.13**).[20]

Conventional angiography

This catheter-based modality provides high-resolution images of aneurysm morphology, and usually the best information for procedural planning in anticipation of aneurysm treatment.[21] When performed intra-operatively, it confirms complete IA obliteration and patency of adjacent (parent or distal) vasculature (**2.14**). Angiography is also the standard approach to monitoring the status of endovascular coils deposited within an IA, as they cause artifact on other imaging modalities. However, angiography is invasive, and, as iodinated dye does not penetrate the thrombus within an aneurysm, there is the potential to underestimate the overall size of the lesion. Risks related to this procedure include ischemic infarction from catheter-associated embolization, hematoma or pseudoaneurysm formation at the femoral puncture site, and renal failure due to dye exposure.[8] The periprocedural risk of permanent neurologic injury is approximately 0.5% in large prospective series;[22] however, it is likely to be higher in elderly patients with atherosclerotic disease and in patients with generalized connective tissue disorders, such as Ehlers–Danlos syndrome.[1]

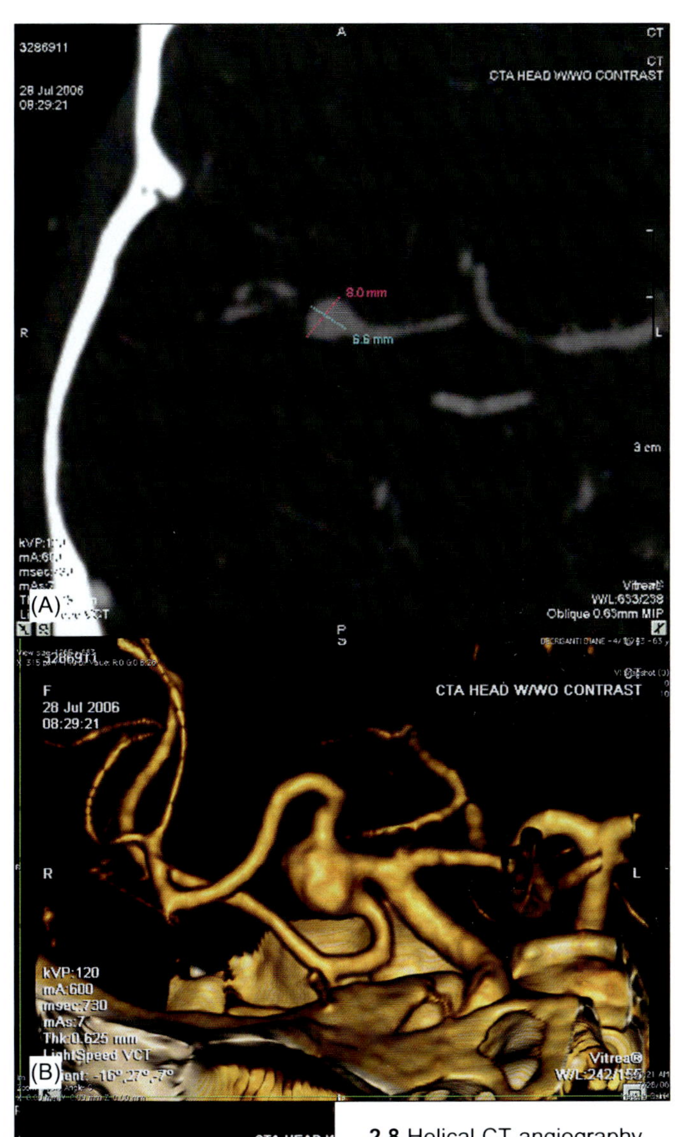

2.8 Helical CT angiography. A complex MCA bifurcation aneurysm is shown on the CTA source images (A) to measure 8.0×6.6 mm. The reformatted image shows the location of this lesion relative to the skull base (B). The aneurysm can then be isolated and rotated, in order to plan treatment (C). In this case, treatment is complicated by the immediate involvement of three arteries, the parent M1 segment (arrow) and the two M2 branches emanating outward (arrowheads).

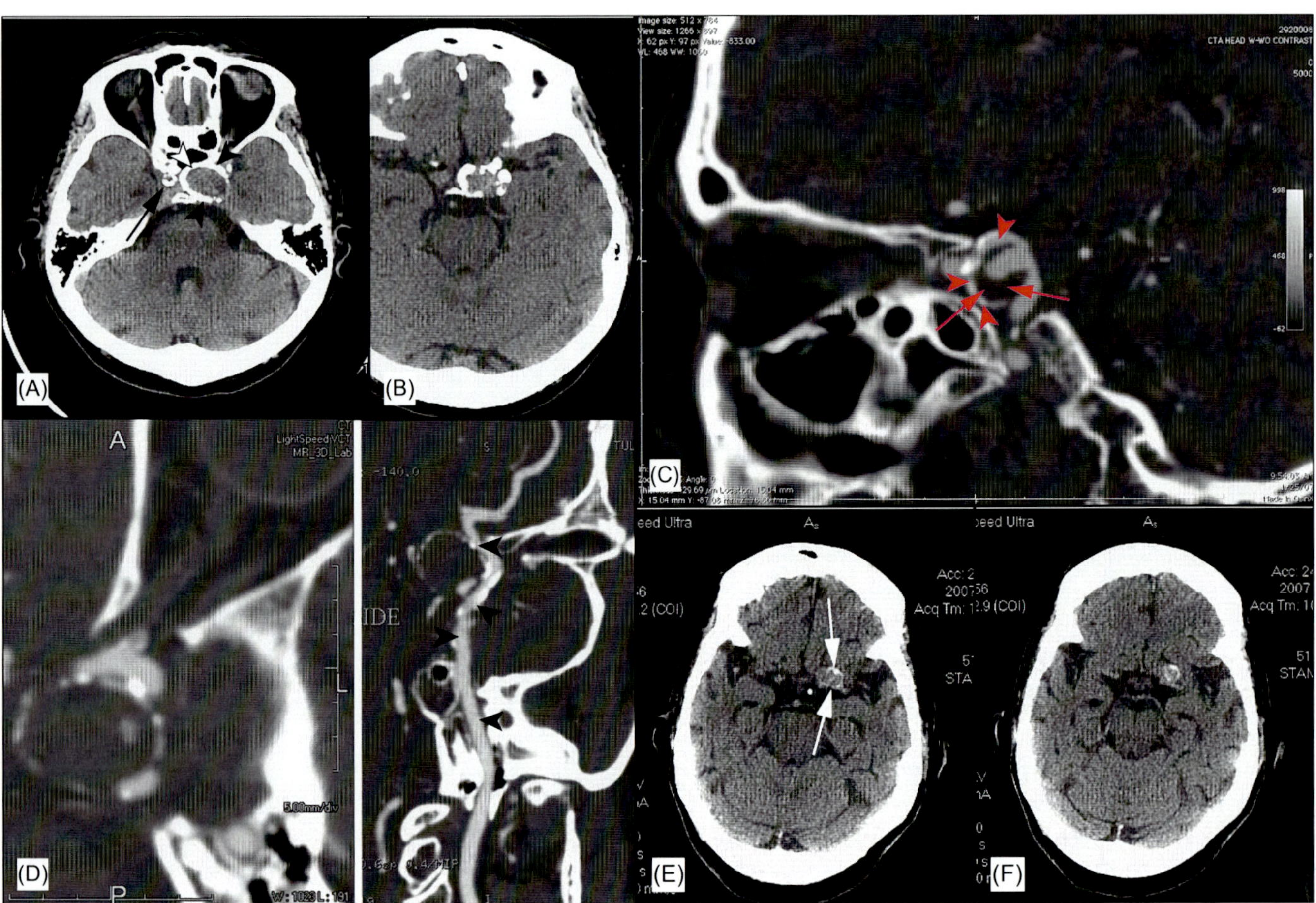

2.9 Calcified aneurysms. The non-contrast CT scan (A,B) shows a giant aneurysm encased in an extensively calcified wall (arrowhead). The wall of the contralateral distal ICA is also calcified (arrow). On a sagittal view of the CTA (C), relatively little contrast penetrates into the upper middle part of the lumen of the aneurysm, due to extensive thrombosis, evident as a gray layer (arrows) between the calcified wall (arrowheads) and the contrast dye. The IA is also shown relative to the orbital apex (the eye is located in the upper right corner; D, left); and, on a sagittal view, relative to its parent ICA (arrowheads) (D, right). A second lesion from a different patient, shown on a non-contrast CT scan (E,F) suggests a calcified IA at the level of the Circle of Willis (arrows).

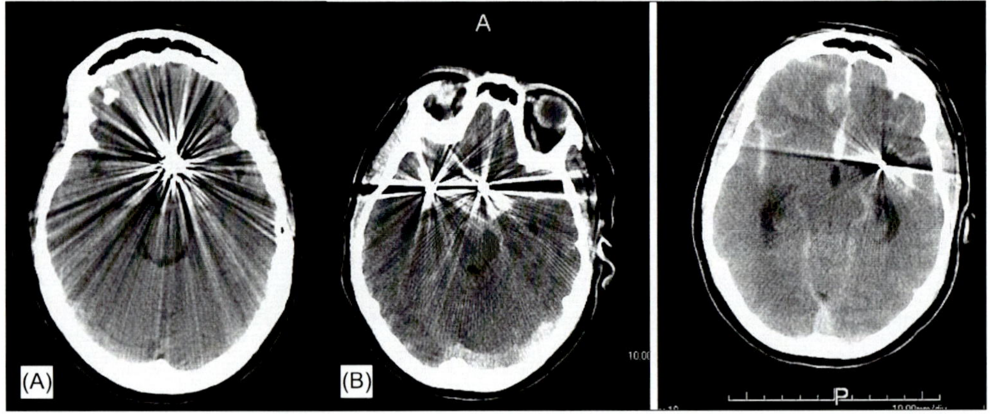

2.10 Artifact from aneurysm coiling. The aneurysm treated with endovascular coiling is a left ICA lesion in the para-ophthalmic region (A). The second patient (B), whose CTA is shown in **2.3**(E), had coiling of all three IAs. Widespread SAH is appreciated (B, right). Catheter-delivered aneurysm coils, often platinum based, create the same metallic artifact on CT scans as surgical clips.

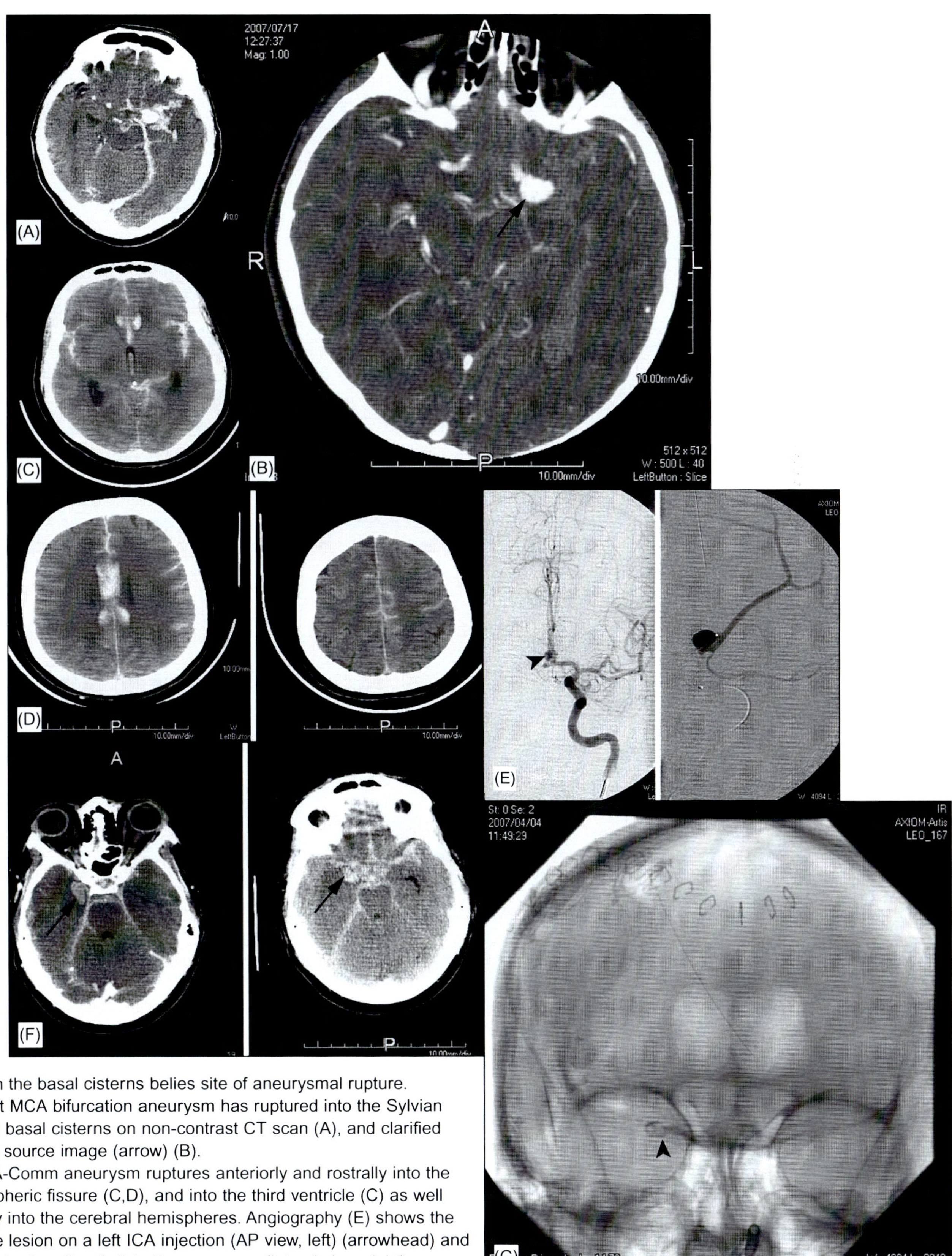

2.11 Clot in the basal cisterns belies site of aneurysmal rupture.

(1) A left MCA bifurcation aneurysm has ruptured into the Sylvian fissure and basal cisterns on non-contrast CT scan (A), and clarified with a CTA source image (arrow) (B).

(2) An A-Comm aneurysm ruptures anteriorly and rostrally into the interhemispheric fissure (C,D), and into the third ventricle (C) as well as diffusely into the cerebral hemispheres. Angiography (E) shows the responsible lesion on a left ICA injection (AP view, left) (arrowhead) and in a microinjection directly into the aneurysm (lateral view, right).

(3) A right P-Comm aneurysm is visualized to the right of the circle of Willis on an admission CT scan (arrows) (F). This lesion was clipped (G); the surgical clip on fluoroscopy is seen behind the medial right orbit (arrowhead).

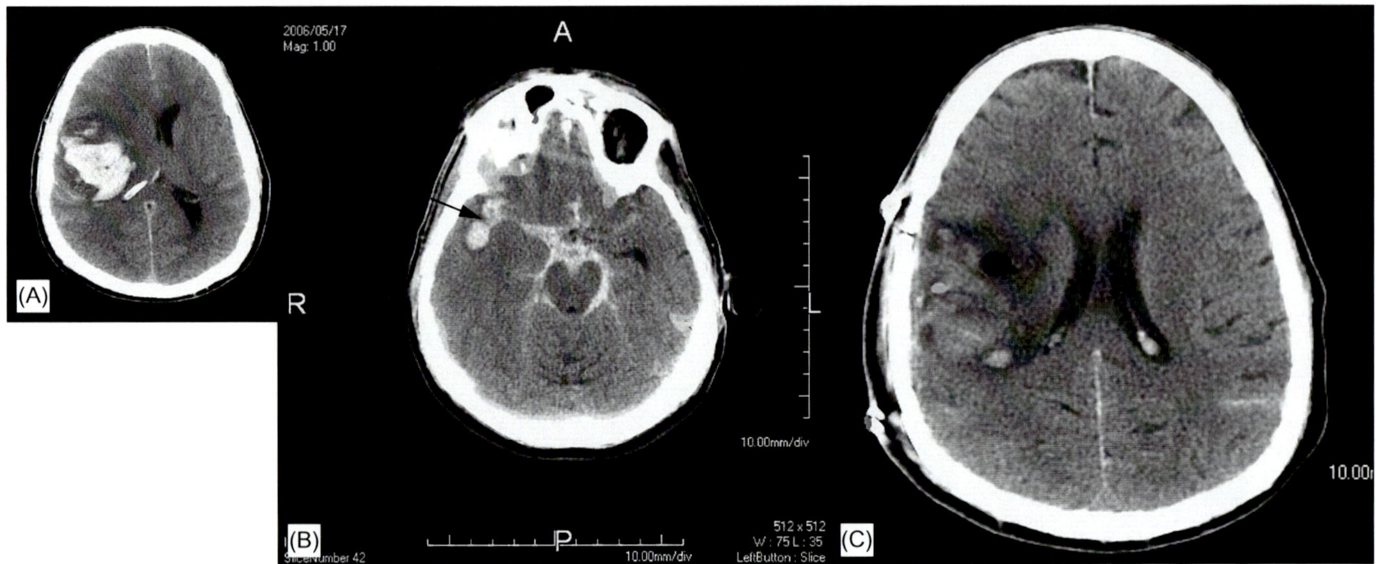

2.12 Hemispheric hemorrhage from MCA aneurysm from an arteriovenous malformation. A large right hemispheric ICH (A) resulted from rupture of a right MCA aneurysm (arrow) (B), with significant SAH within the basal cisterns. During a decompressive craniotomy, shown in the postoperative non-contrast CT scan (C), the M2 branch aneurysm had been clipped and coagulated. Compare the midline mass effect and the lateral ventricles post-ICH (A) versus post-craniotomy (C). The clot and lesion within the white matter and adjacent cortex were removed, and the pathology revealed an underlying arteriovenous malformation. The IA was located in a feeding artery to the arteriovenous malformation.

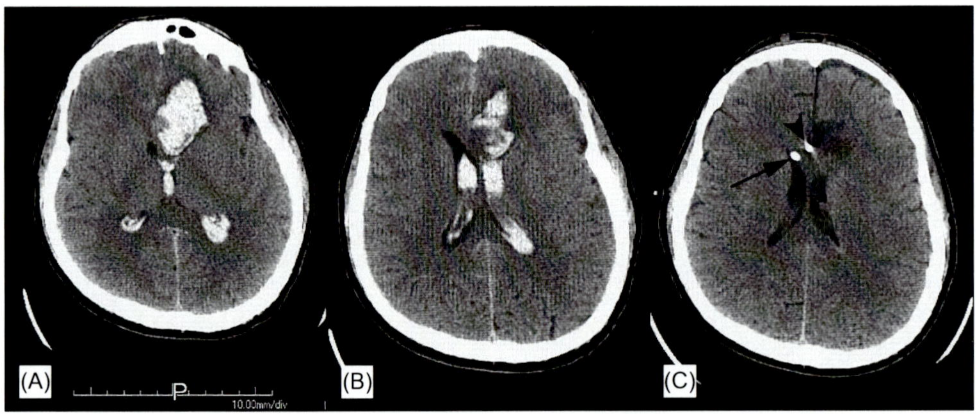

2.13 Parenchymal hemorrhage from ruptured aneurysm. This A-Comm aneurysm (A,B) ruptured upward into the right anterior corpus callosum and frontal lobe, with significant involvement of adjacent lateral ventricle (B) but with minimal subarachnoid bleeding into the interhemispheric fissure, and none into the basal cisterns. At 7 days posthemorrhage (C), much of the blood dissipated, and the hyperdense markers indicates an aneurysm clip (arrowhead) and the tip of an external ventricular drain entering from the right frontal lobe (arrow), as well as a hypodensity indicating a left medial frontal (subcortical, anterior cerebral artery (ACA) perforator) infarct.

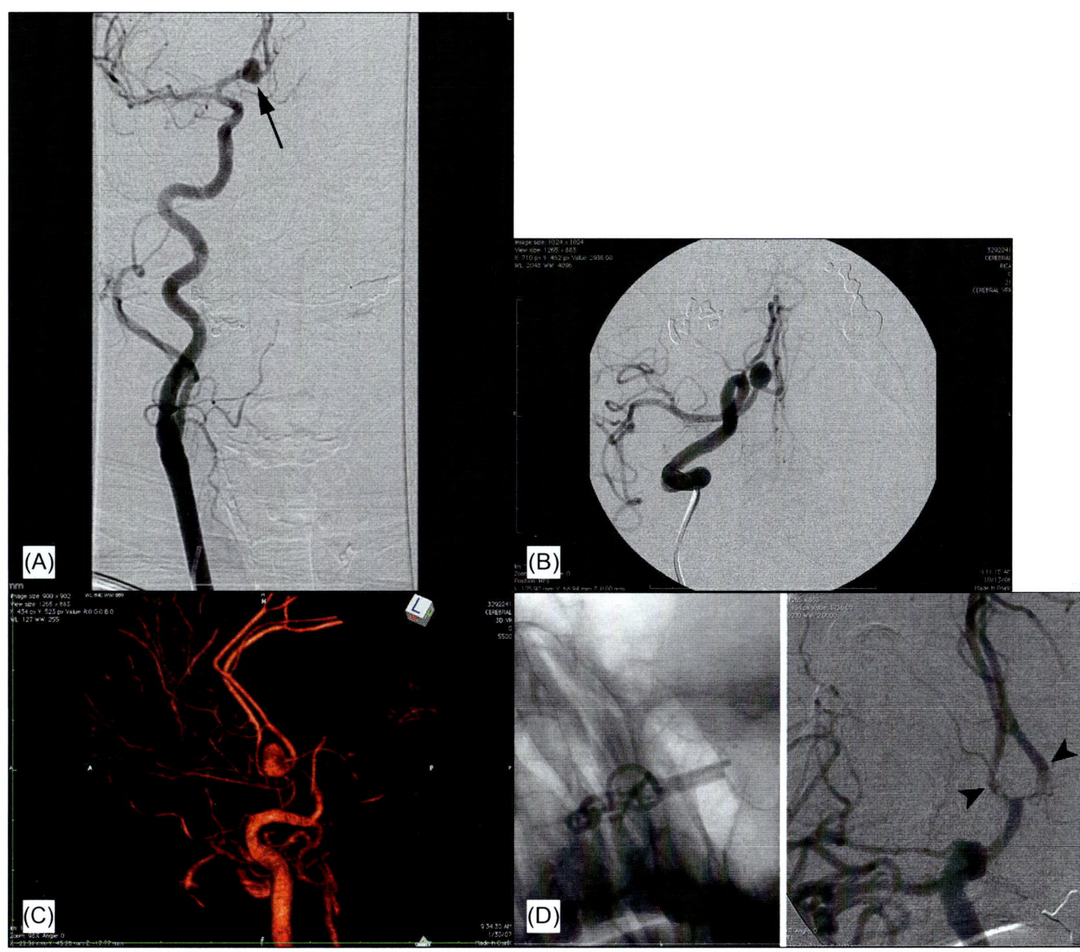

2.14 Conventional cerebral angiography of aneurysm evaluation and treatment. An A-Comm aneurysm shown on conventional angiography: (A) right ICA injection, with the lesion (arrow); (B) a submental, pre-operative view (i.e., image obtained by shooting from below the jawline upwards); (C) three-dimensional rotational angiographic study, oblique view, demonstrating the A2 segments coursing laterally from the sides of the IA; and (D) intra-operative study showing the surgical clip (unsubtracted view, left); and then a subtracted view demonstrating where the aneurysm existed previously (right) (arrowheads point at the A2 segments that are directly adjacent to the clipped aneurysm).

Management

Medical and neurological treatments

Excellent overviews of general medical and neurological management of non-traumatic aneurysmal SAH have been published (*Table 2.2*).[2,23,24]

- Nimodipine, a calcium channel antagonist, provides a modest but significant improvement in clinical outcomes and is thus a standard part of early medical treatment.[2,25]
- 'Triple-H therapy' (hypervolemia, hypertension, and hemodilution) is commonly used to prevent vasospasm that can lead to cerebral ischemia,[5] although there is little efficacy data demonstrating improved outcomes.

Recent therapeutic trials have evaluated hypothermia,[26] tranexamic acid (an antifibrinolytic agent to reduce rebleeding rates),[27] neuroprotective agents, intravenous magnesium sulfate, and statin agents.[5] Other interventions reported to prevent or treat complications and ensure accurate aneurysm clipping include intra-operative and postoperative angiography, microsurgical fenestration of the third ventricle (to reduce the need for ventriculoperitoneal shunting), and decompressive craniectomy for intracranial hypertension.[5,28]

Table 2.2 Treatment guidelines for subarachnoid hemorrhage*

Management	Recommendations
(A) Neurologic areas and related medical complications	
Aneurysm treatment	
Surgical clipping	Procedure within first 72 hours
Endovascular coiling	Procedure within first 72 hours
Common complications	
Seizures	Administer lorazepam (0.1 mg/kg, at rate of 2 mg/min), followed by phenytoin loading (20 mg/kg IV bolus at <50 mg/min)
Hydrocephalus	Insert external ventricular (or lumbar) drain
Rebleeding	Provide supportive care and emergency treatment of aneurysm
Cerebral vasospasm	Maintain hypervolemia or induced hypertension with pressors; provide endovascular treatment (transluminal angioplasty or direct vasodilators); monitor for daily or qod with bedside transcranial Doppler ultrasonography
Calcium antagonist	Administer nimodipine orally, 60 mg q 4 hour for 21 days
Hyponatremia	With SIADH, restrict fluids. With cerebral salt-wasting syndrome, replace fluids with 0.9% or hypertonic saline solution
Myocardial injury	Administer metoprolol; evaluate ventricular function; arrhythmias treat arrhythmias
Pulmonary edema	Provide ventilatory support if necessary; monitor PCWP and ventricular function; distinguish cardiogenic versus neurogenic pulmonary edema
(B) General management	
Airways and cardiovascular	Monitor in ICU, preferably neurologic critical care unit
Environment	Reduce noise level and limit visitors until aneurysm is treated
Pain	Administer morphine sulfate, or codeine
Gastrointestinal	Administer ranitidine or lansoprazole prophylaxis
Deep venous thrombosis	Use thigh-high stockings and sequential compression pneumatic devices; administer subcutaneous heparin after aneurysm treatment
Blood pressure	Keep systolic blood pressure 90–140 mmHg before aneurysm treatment; then allow hypertension to keep systolic blood pressure <200 mmHg
Serum glucose	Maintain level at 80–120 mg/dl; use continuous glucose infusion or insulin drip as needed
Core body temperature	Maintain ≤37.2°C; administer acetaminophen or cooling devices
Fluids and hydration	Maintain euvolume (CVP, 5–8 mmHg); if vasospasm is present, maintain hypervolemia (CVP, 8–12 mmHg)
Nutrition	Oral route after swallow evaluation, depending upon level of consciousness. Otherwise, enteral feeding
(C) Long-term care	
Rehabilitation	Physical, occupational, and speech therapy
Neuropsychologic	Global and domain-specific neuropsychologic testing; provide cognitive rehabilitation
Depression	Administer antidepressant medications; consider psychotherapy
Chronic headaches	Consider preventive agents, such as tricyclic antidepressants; administer abortive agents, such as non-steroidal anti-inflammatory drugs

*Adapted from Suarez *et al.*[2]

CVP, central venous pressure; PCWP, pulmonary capillary wedge pressure; qod, every other day; SIADH, syndrome of inappropriate antidiuretic hormone secretion.

The major neurologic complications of SAH are vasospasm with delayed cerebral ischemia (46%), hydrocephalus (20%), and aneurysm rebleeding (7%).[2]

Vasospasm (see case study 1)

Vasospasm develops within 3 days post-SAH, with maximal risk from days 4 to 14 and peak symptoms from 5 to 7 days. It accounts for one-third of poor outcomes,[2,5,23] and gradually resolves between 2 and 4 weeks post-SAH. Thus, routine monitoring for vasospasm with daily transcranial Doppler ultrasound is recommended during the first 2 weeks following SAH.[2,29,30] Predictors for vasospasm are: advanced age (>60 years), large amount of subarachnoid blood on CT scan, and depressed level of consciousness on admission.[5] Despite many trials with pharmacologic agents, such as intra-arterial nicardipine, balloon angioplasty remains the standard treatment for vasospasm, with >90% success rates and complication rates of <5%.[31]

Hydrocephalus

This occurs acutely in 15–20% of patients with SAH, but may occur later at 3–21 days. Overall, 20% of patients with SAH require shunting for chronic hydrocephalus.

Rebleeding

This carries a very high mortality rate of ~50% (**2.15**).[2,32] It occurs in at least 4% of patients with SAH over the first 24 hours and in 1–2%/day over the first 2 weeks. The cumulative risk of rebleeding is 20% at 2 weeks, 30% at 1 month, and 40% at 6 months. Rebleeding is associated with the clinical severity of SAH and larger aneurysm size.[33]

Aneurysm ablation

The major treatments for IA before or after rupture are open *neurosurgical clipping* and *endovascular coiling*. The approach needs to be tailored to the individual patient, and critical issues relate to age and general health, location of the aneurysm, and the neurovascular morphology of the lesion. The trend has been toward early intervention to secure a ruptured aneurysm by clipping or coiling within the first 24–72 hours, because early rehemorrhage mortality rates are high and also, presumably, triple-H therapy increases the risk of rehemorrhage from an unsecured aneurysm.[2,5,11]

Neurosurgical clipping (2.16)

For decades, the standard of care for aneurysm management has been neurosurgical clipping. Blood flow into the IA is arrested by temporarily clipping more proximal feeding arteries and/or also exiting branches, a technique called aneurysm trapping.[11] This approach makes the IA more malleable and less pulsatile for permanent clip placement, and controls bleeding that may result from premature, intra-operative rupture. One critical concern with clipping is not to compromise perforator arteries originating from the circle of Willis. Perforator infarcts from aggressive clipping and artery manipulation can contribute greatly to poor outcomes, particularly resulting in cognitive deficits due to ischemia of deep subcortical structures, the thalamus, and the brainstem (**2.17**).

Endovascular coiling (case study 2)[21]

This technique began with technologic advances in catheters and detachable metallic coils during the early 1990s. The first aneurysm coil received US Food and Drug Administration (FDA) approval in 1996.[2,34] The modern era of clinical trials for the evaluation of treatment for aneurysmal SAH began with the landmark study, the International Subarachnoid Aneurysm Trial (ISAT) published in 2002.[35,36] This study randomized 2143 patients with primarily good grade ruptured aneurysms (mostly small, anterior circulation lesions) to surgical clipping versus endovascular coiling.[35] At 1 year post-treatment, no difference between fatality rates was found between clipping and coiling, but combined death and dependency rates were significantly reduced in the coiling group. Catheter-based coiling is less invasive than neurosurgical clipping and thus associated with lower morbidity, particularly in older patients. Endovascular treatment had already been the standard approach to surgically difficult vertebrobasilar lesions, particularly at the basilar artery apex (**2.18**). Therefore, the chief impact of the ISAT study may be to increase the application of endovascular approaches to anterior circulation lesions.[5]

Lesion sites that are usually not amenable to neurosurgery include those encased in bone, such as the skull base, cavernous sinus, and orbit (e.g., para-ophthalmic internal carotid or ophthalmic artery), and within the vertebrobasilar circulation. Other aneurysm characteristics, such as brittle intramural calcification (**2.9**), may make open surgical clipping more difficult. Patients with multiple aneurysms and previous unilateral surgical clipping have a risk for cognitive impairment if contralateral lesions are later treated with open surgery; endovascular coiling is then preferred to avoid bilateral craniotomies (**2.19**).

Lesions with wider necks, in which the ratio of neck diameter to the largest dome diameter is >0.5, are less favorable for endovascular coiling, as are lesions with normal branches arising from the lesions' base or dome.[2,8] In these cases, neurosurgical clipping may be preferable so as not to compromise exiting arteries beyond the lesion. A common location where clipping is often preferred is at the bifurcation of the MCA (**2.8**). Newer technologies, such as the Neuroform™ Microdelivery Stent System (to prevent coil prolapse into the parent vessel of wider neck lesions) and polymeric-coated coils (to stimulate aneurysm thrombosis) should continue to reduce the morbidity and widen the application of endovascular coiling (**2.18**).

Potential drawbacks of endovascular coiling (**2.17**) include:

- Thromboembolic and hemorrhagic complications of this procedure. One study found up to a 42% rate of ischemic lesions on diffusion-weighted MRI in patients who had unruptured aneurysms coiled.[37] In addition, hemorrhage may occur due to the aggressive periprocedural use of antithrombotic agents.

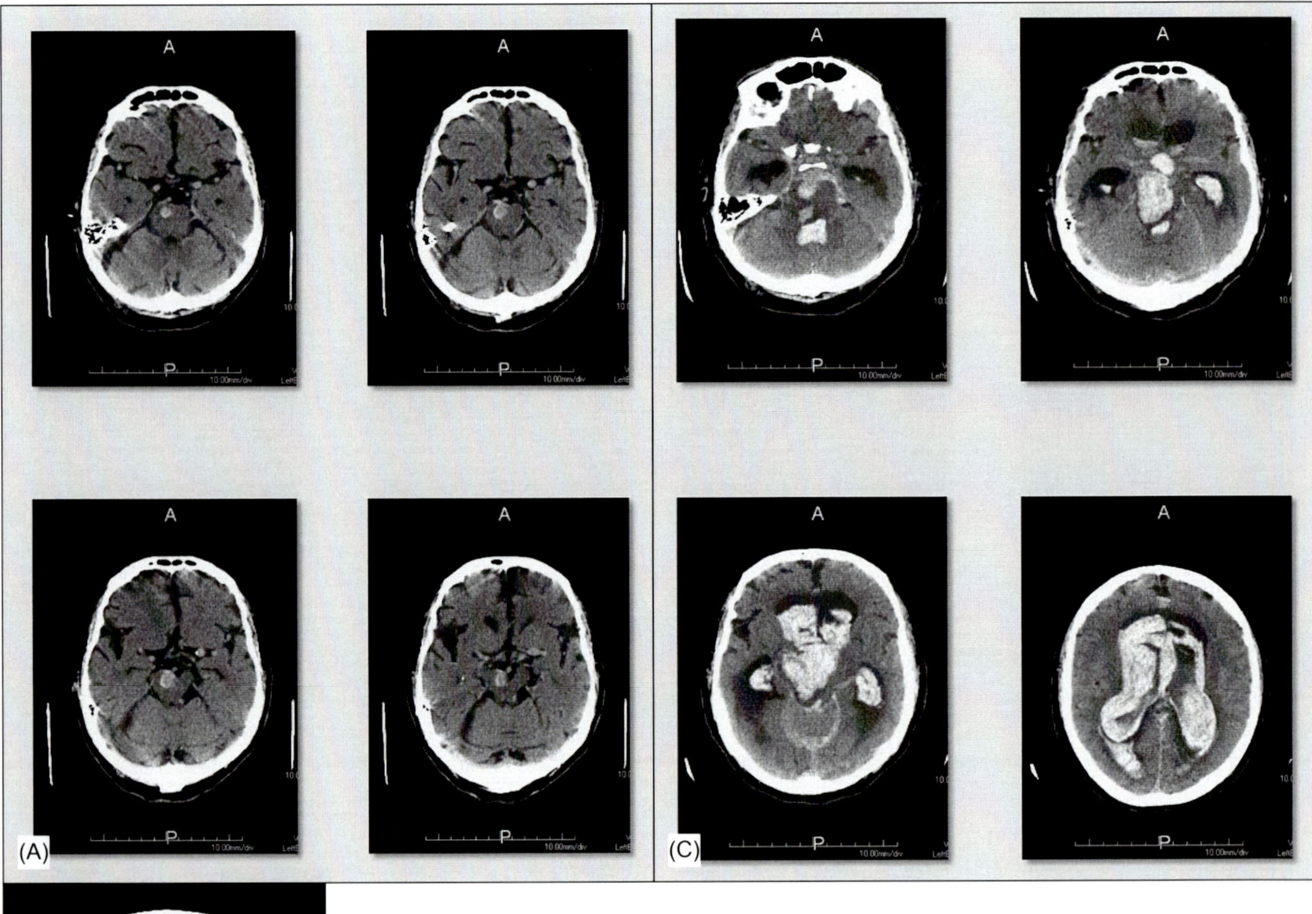

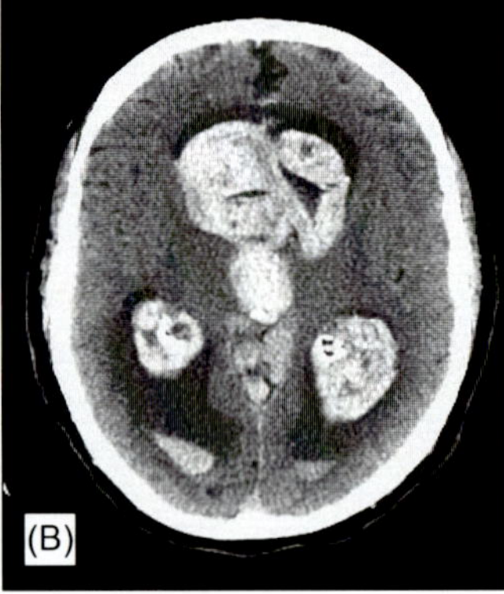

2.15 Rebleeding from a posterior cerebral artery (PCA) aneurysm. This patient presented with diplopia from a partial third-nerve palsy due to localized expansion from a small right pontomesencephalic lesion, a 12.8-mm aneurysm of the right PCA (A, composite of the initial CT scan). The aneurysm invaginates from the P1 segment into the right midbrain. Within hours, as treatment for the IA was being prepared, the patient's mental status rapidly deteriorated. The second head CT scan (B,C) documented fulminant growth of the hemorrhage, expanding up through the third ventricle, almost completely filling the ventricular system. This massive ICH likely resulted from rebleeding of the PCA IA.

- Incomplete aneurysm obliteration and the related need to monitor radiographically (with skull films and/or repeated conventional angiograms). The duration of follow-up angiography after aneurysm coiling remains unresolved, but aneurysm neck remnants (that may occur after coil compaction, or after incomplete surgical obliteration[38]) may be treated with endovascular coiling.
- Risk of increased radiation exposure from repeated conventional angiography studies.[5,39]
- The impact of coiling upon vasospasm is unclear.
- Some patients with acute SAH may still also need emergent neurosurgical evacuation an associated parenchymal or subdural clot, before subsequent coiling (**2.19**).

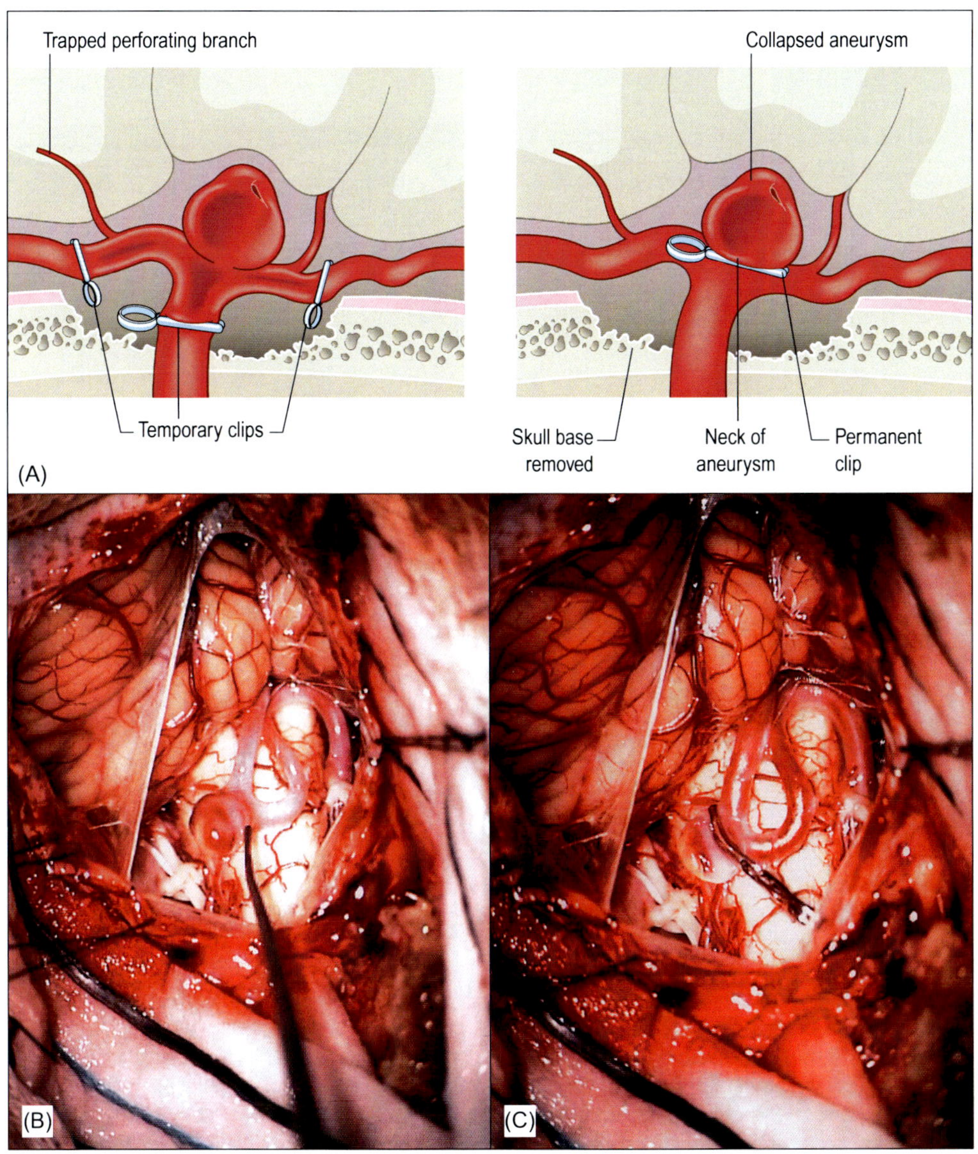

2.16 Neurosurgical clipping of intracranial aneurysms. A ruptured IA is shown relative to the adjacent subarachnoid space, with temporal clips that 'trap' the lesion. During surgical repair (A, left), surgical clips are placed on the proximal feeding artery alone, or on both the proximal and distal arteries to secure the lesion. Trapping causes ischemia and the potential for infarction. A permanent clip is placed (A, right), to exclude the IA from the circulation. The skull base may be partly removed to enhance operative exposure. The adjacent branches around the lesion are assessed visually and with Doppler ultrasound to ensure that their arterial flow is preserved (image adapted from Ellegala and Day[11]).

Clipping of an unruptured aneurysm. This IA, on the tonsillar loop of the posterior inferior cerebellar artery, was exposed via a midline suboccipital craniotomy and C1 vertebroplasty (B); the cerebellum is located directly superior and left, relative to the aneurysm. The second image is following placement of a surgical clip (C) (intra-operative photographs courtesy of Inam Kureshi, MD).

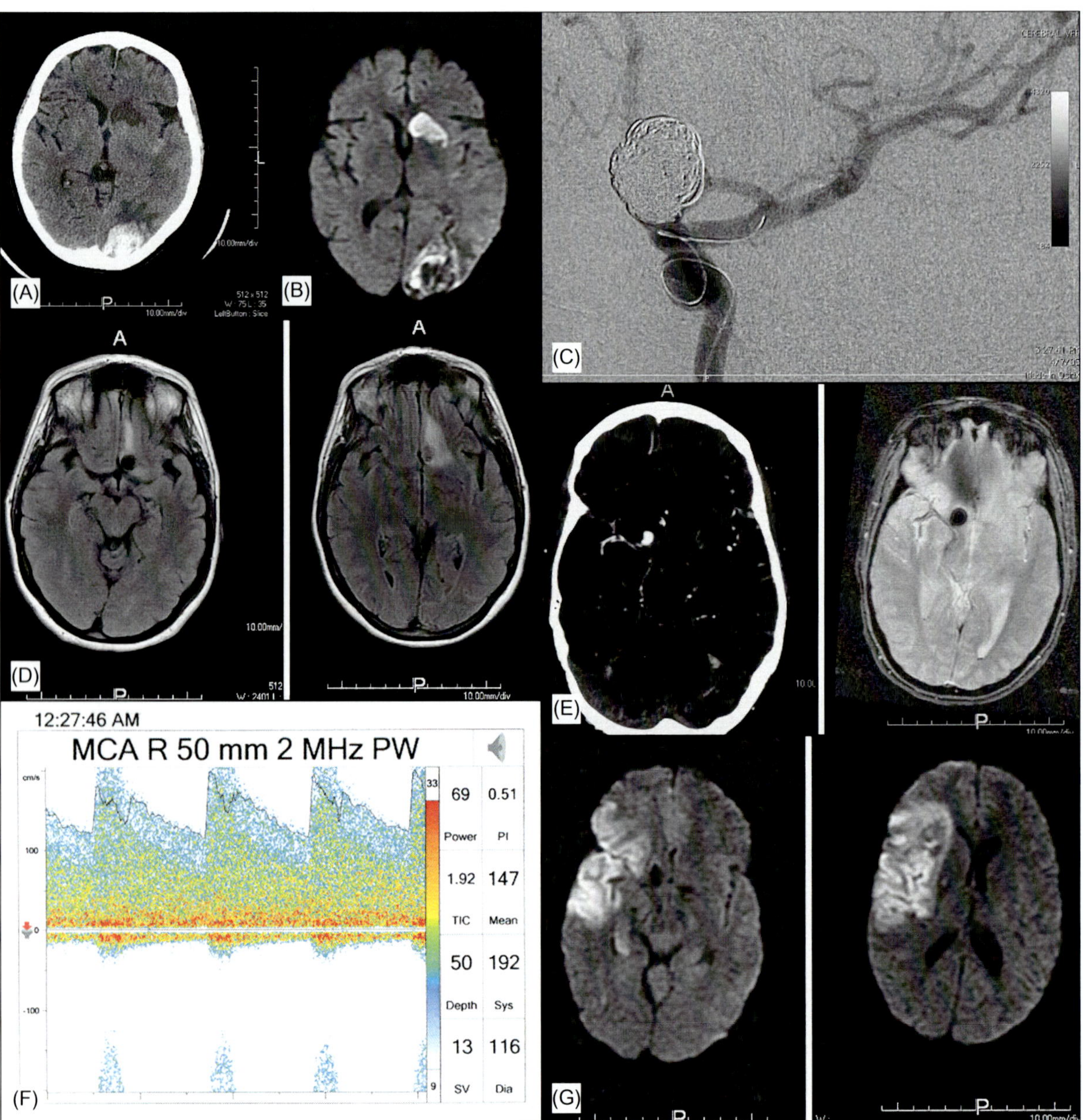

2.17 Complications of aneurysm ablation procedures.

(1) Perforator infarction and intraparenchymal hemorrhage (A, B). An infarct developed in the head of the caudate nucleus where the left A1 segment was sacrificed via endovascular coiling of a large A-Comm IA (shown in **case study 2**). The same CT scan (A) shows a concurrent lobar hemorrhage in the left parieto-occipital region, attributed to exposure to anticoagulation (IV unfractionated heparin peri-procedurally), clopidogrel, and relative hypertension. The lesions are also shown on a diffusion-weighted-MRI sequence (B).

(2) Parenchymal edema (C, D). A 13-mm left para-ophthalmic aneurysm, discovered incidentally during a diagnostic work-up for headache, was treated with endovascular coiling, as shown on conventional angiography, left ICA injection (C), with a microcatheter tip located just before the parent vessel's bifurcation into the ACA and MCA (C). Edema, presumably a local inflammatory response to the coiling of this aneurysm, caused a mild expressive aphasia that resolved over several weeks. The area of heightened signal intensity on this FLAIR MR sequence (D) is directly anterior and above the coiled IA.

(3) Vasospasm and associated ischemic infarct (E–G). A third patient underwent coiling of a ruptured right ICA bifurcation aneurysm 6 days after presenting to another hospital with headache and vomiting, with SAH in the right hemisphere and basal cisterns. She was transferred to a tertiary care center when left hemiparesis developed. The IA is shown on CTA (left) and GE-MRI sequence (right) (E). Bilateral MCA vasospasm developed; a transcranial Doppler (TCD) ultrasound study insonating the right MCA (F) shows severe vasospasm, with an elevated peak systolic velocity of 192 cm/s. Despite triple-H therapy, as well as angioplasty, a large right MCA ischemic infarct developed, shown on diffusion-weighted-MRI (G).

- Uncertain longevity. Given the relative infancy of the endovascular field, long-term outcomes data are limited, with low re-rupture rates at up to 9 years.[40,41]

Formal guidelines for the management of IA and SAH recommend experienced, high-volume tertiary care centers that offer both surgical and endovascular procedures and track outcomes data.[11,42,43] At such centers, the benefits and risks for clipping versus coiling can be considered for each patient by a multidisciplinary team. Large volume neurovascular programs also typically have access to modern neuroimaging and neurocritical care for periprocedural management.

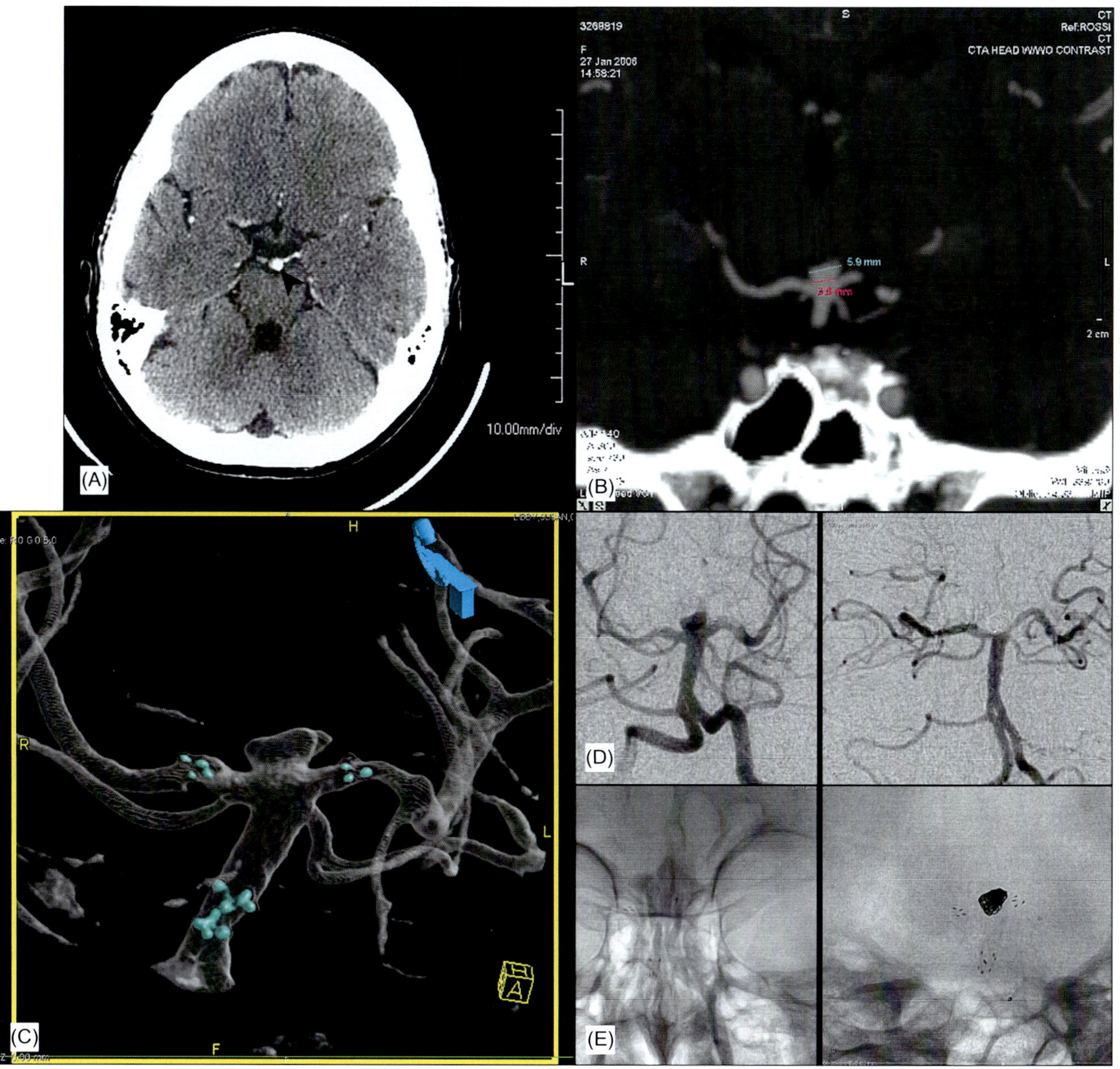

2.18 Stent-assisted coiling of basilar tip aneurysm. The 52-year-old woman had an IA at the top of the basilar artery (BA), a difficult lesion to treat with open surgical clipping. The lesion is seen as a dilated hyperdensity on the contrast-enhanced CT scan (arrowhead), <1 cm per the ruler along the left-hand margin (A). The aneurysm is measured on CTA (B) to have a relatively wide neck of 3.8 mm and diameter of 5.9 mm. Because of the concern that endovascular coils would prolapse out of this with neck into the distal BA, the Y-stent technique is first performed. In this technique, one stent is passed through the interstices of another, in the Y-configuration that remodels the basilar tip. Note in the three-dimensional rendering of the conventional angiography (C) the two sets of stents evidenced by their green end-markers of this stent. These two stents each originate within the mid-basilar segment and branch into each of the proximal PCA (P1) segments. In the subsequent figure (D), the conventional angiogram is shown after Y-stent placement (left) and following the BA aneurysm coiling (right). The final images (E) are an unsubtracted X-ray, AP view, without IV contrast dye, to show the relative location of the aneurysm treatments, before (left; note the orbits) and after (right) coiling.

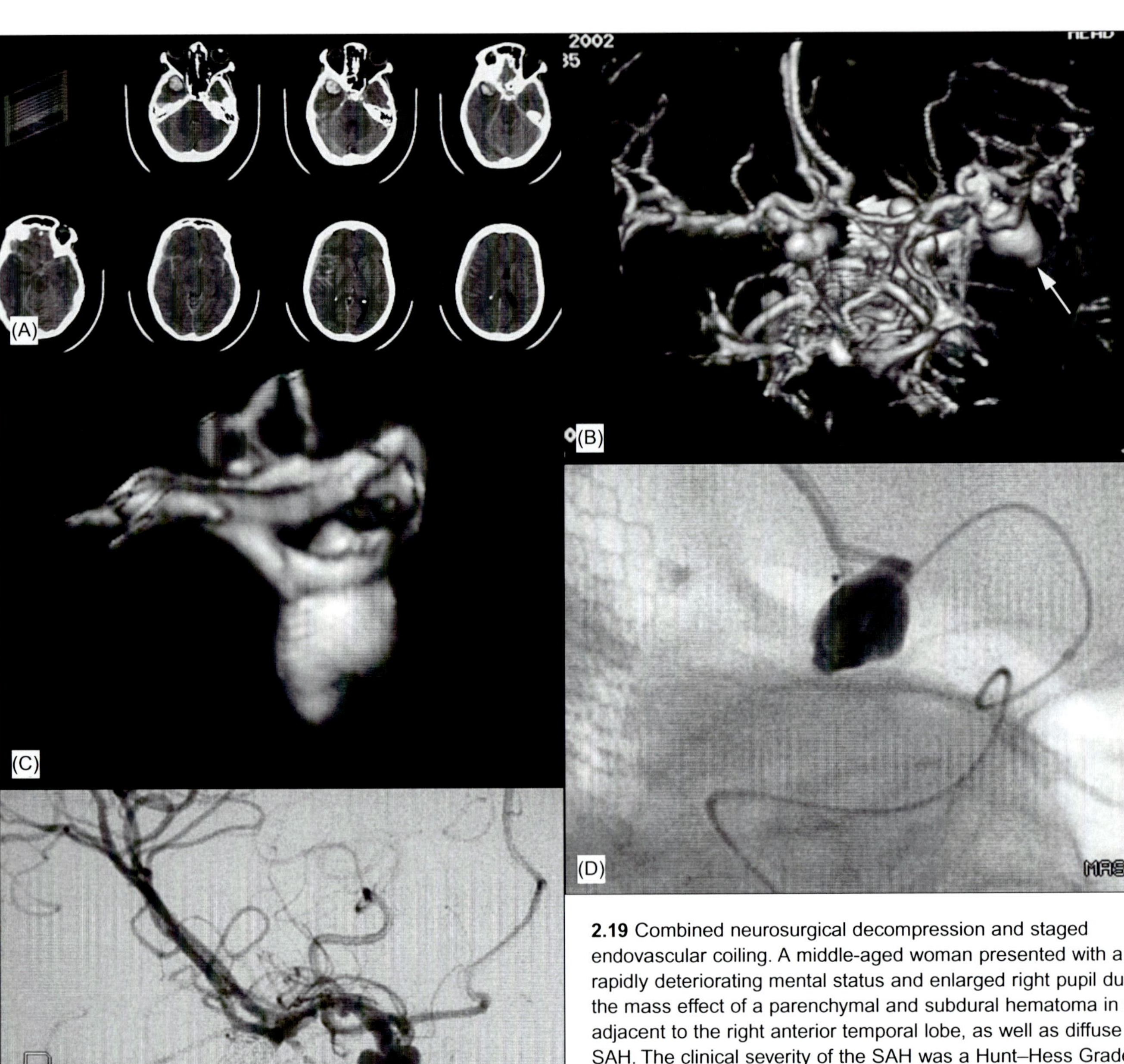

2.19 Combined neurosurgical decompression and staged endovascular coiling. A middle-aged woman presented with a rapidly deteriorating mental status and enlarged right pupil due to the mass effect of a parenchymal and subdural hematoma in and adjacent to the right anterior temporal lobe, as well as diffuse SAH. The clinical severity of the SAH was a Hunt–Hess Grade 5.

A composite of the admission head CT scan is shown (A), just before an emergent, life-saving neurosurgical decompression of the subdural hematoma. The CTA study (left and right sides are reversed in this rendering) shows the likely cause of the initial hemorrhage, a complex, 10 mm, inferiorly pointing right MCA (M2-origin) IA (arrow) (B). This lesion is isolated on CTA (C) and on a microcatheter injection (D). The lesion was treated with GDC® coils (arrowheads), as shown on conventional angiography, a subtracted right ICA injection (E). The patient's other aneurysms (not well-visualized in B) were also 5-mm lesions of the right ophthalmic origin of the ICA and the right P-Comm, as well as a 6-mm IA of the left P-Comm. These were treated during later endovascular procedures.

Prognosis and outcomes

The annual risk of rupture of an asymptomatic aneurysm is 0.7%/year; however, previously ruptured aneurysms have a significantly higher annual risk of rupture beyond 6 months of 2–4%/year.[44,45] Thus, ruptured aneurysms responsible for SAH represent a different disease in that the immediate risk for re-rupture, and the associated morbidity and mortality from rebleeding, are much greater than for unruptured IAs.

Aneurysm size and location play major roles in determining the risk of rupture. Larger size and posterior circulation lesions hold higher risk.[44,45] For 5-year cumulative rates of rupture see *Table 2.3*.[44,45] Based upon these data, one threshold for treatment with neurosurgical clipping or endovascular coiling of anterior circulation lesions is to monitor the IA until its size is approximately ≥7 mm. However, aneurysm rupture at smaller sizes is not uncommon given their greater prevalence (than larger lesions) in the general population. Finally, for some elderly patients, particularly with higher-risk lesions, the periprocedural risk of IA ablation may outweigh the relative risk of the lesion's natural history (**2.20**).

Prognostic factors associated with poor outcomes from SAH are greater patient age, decreased level of consciousness on admission, and the amount of blood present on the initial head CT scan.[2]

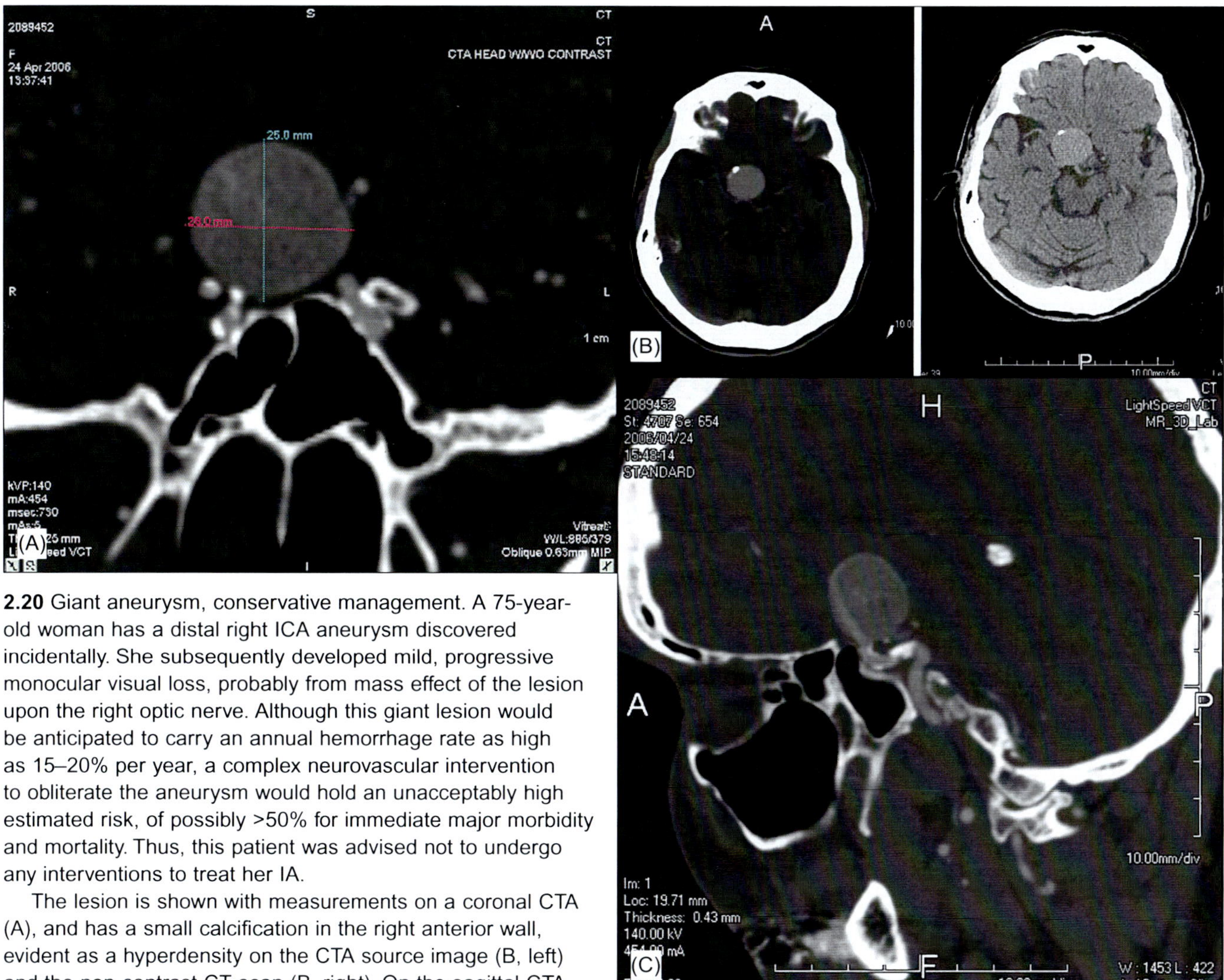

2.20 Giant aneurysm, conservative management. A 75-year-old woman has a distal right ICA aneurysm discovered incidentally. She subsequently developed mild, progressive monocular visual loss, probably from mass effect of the lesion upon the right optic nerve. Although this giant lesion would be anticipated to carry an annual hemorrhage rate as high as 15–20% per year, a complex neurovascular intervention to obliterate the aneurysm would hold an unacceptably high estimated risk, of possibly >50% for immediate major morbidity and mortality. Thus, this patient was advised not to undergo any interventions to treat her IA.

The lesion is shown with measurements on a coronal CTA (A), and has a small calcification in the right anterior wall, evident as a hyperdensity on the CTA source image (B, left) and the non-contrast CT scan (B, right). On the sagittal CTA (C), the distal right ICA appears to wrap around the anterior surface of the aneurysm.

Table 2.3 Five-year cumulative rates of rupture for intracranial aneurysms

	Anterior circulation IA	Posterior circulation IA
<7 mm	0%	2.5%
7–12 mm	2.6%	14.5%
13–24 mm	14.5%	18.4%
>25 mm	40%	50%

The average acute case fatality rate for SAH is quite high. More than half of all patients (51%) die acutely, with most mortality occurring during the first 2 weeks, 10% die before reaching medical care, and 25% die during the first 24 hours after the event.[2] Early mortality is due to cerebral herniation from rapid, diffusely increased intracranial pressure.[46] About 70% of all patients with aneurysmal SAH have poor outcomes of either death or dependency.[5] In addition to early herniation, the neurologic and medical complications that accumulate during the initial several weeks following SAH contribute to the poor outcome (*Table 2.2*).

For survivors of SAH, long-term cognitive impairment is very common, with >50% reporting difficulties with memory, mood, or neuropsychologic function.[47] Still, one-half to two-thirds of those survivors are able to return to the workplace within 1 year following SAH.[48]

Other related lesions

Mycotic aneurysms

This lesion occurs when a blood-borne infection, typically bacterial, seeds the walls of intracranial arteries. The most common etiology is bacterial endocarditis, and the most common locations, in contrast to atherosclerotic aneurysms around the circle of Willis, are the distal MCA branches (**2.21**; see **case study 3**). The aneurysmal wall may become friable, such that vessel ligation (rather than aneurysm clipping) is frequently the treatment of choice. Given their peripheral location within the vasculature, mycotic aneurysms may be difficult to detect without conventional angiography (**2.21, 2.22**).

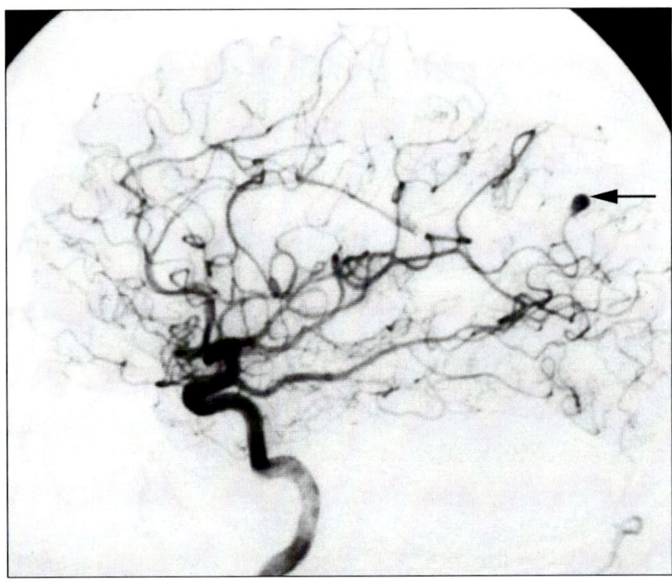

2.21 Mycotic aneurysm, untreated. Angiography (lateral view) of a 45-year-old woman who developed headache, fever and SAH within several days of a dental procedure. A classic mycotic aneurysm is visualized in a typical location, a distal MCA branch (arrow).

Non-aneurysmal perimesencephalic subarachnoid hemorrhage

In this benign cause of SAH, hemorrhage is localized initially in the region of the perimesencephalic cistern, anterior to the brainstem (**2.23**). Conventional and CTA studies in these patients reveal no IA as the etiology for SAH; CTA alone was the best diagnostic strategy in a decision analysis study.[49] The source of hemorrhage is believed to be rupture of a deep vein.[4] Patients with perimesencephalic SAH have a normal life expectancy and are not at risk for rebleeding.[50]

Non-aneurysmal convexity subarachnoid hemorrhage

The second type of non-aneurysmal SAH occurs in an entirely different location, in the periphery of the cerebral hemispheres (**2.24**). The etiology in such cases is not always clear. The differential diagnosis includes isolated cortical vein thrombosis, hypertension, postpartum eclampsia, and CAA. In one study, conventional angiography did not identify any aneurysms to cause this type of SAH.[51]

Aneurysm-to-artery embolism

This rare cause of acute ischemic stroke is usually associated with giant aneurysms. With larger lesions, local intra-aneurysmal (*in situ*) clot is more likely to develop over time and may eventually embolize to distal intracranial

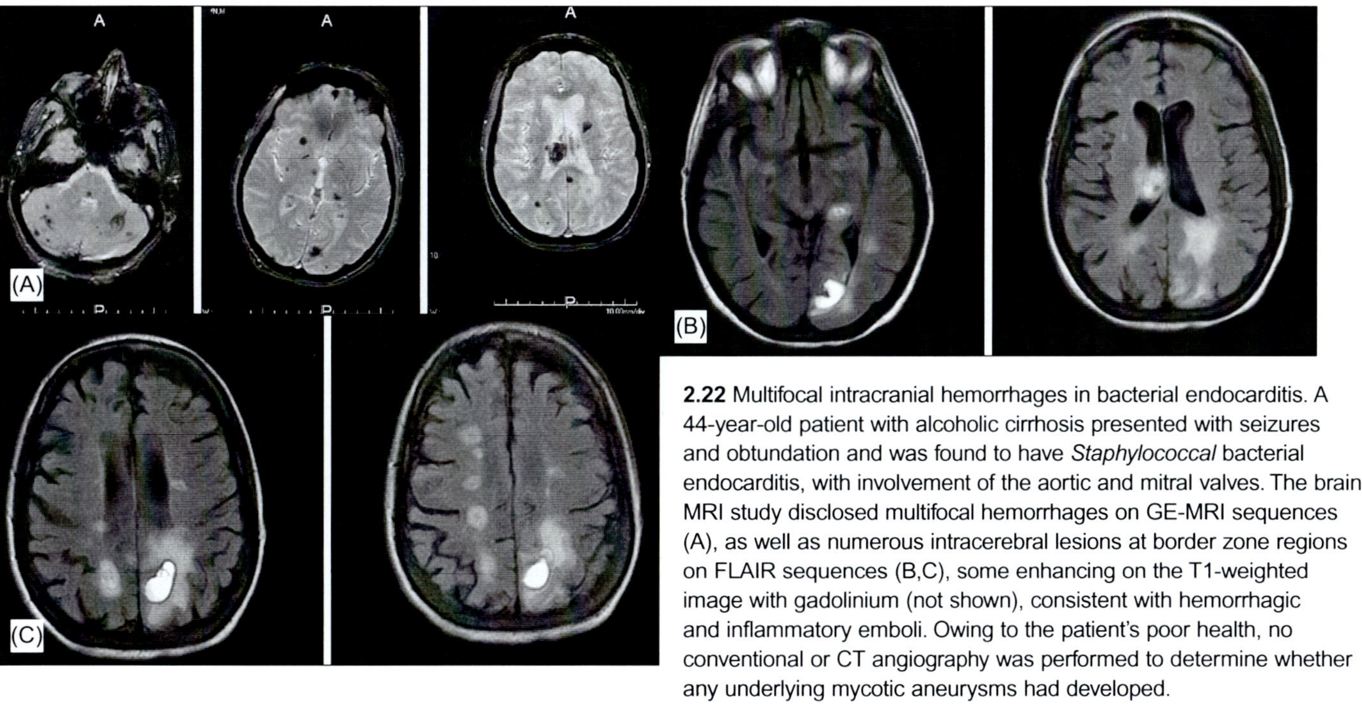

2.22 Multifocal intracranial hemorrhages in bacterial endocarditis. A 44-year-old patient with alcoholic cirrhosis presented with seizures and obtundation and was found to have *Staphylococcal* bacterial endocarditis, with involvement of the aortic and mitral valves. The brain MRI study disclosed multifocal hemorrhages on GE-MRI sequences (A), as well as numerous intracerebral lesions at border zone regions on FLAIR sequences (B,C), some enhancing on the T1-weighted image with gadolinium (not shown), consistent with hemorrhagic and inflammatory emboli. Owing to the patient's poor health, no conventional or CT angiography was performed to determine whether any underlying mycotic aneurysms had developed.

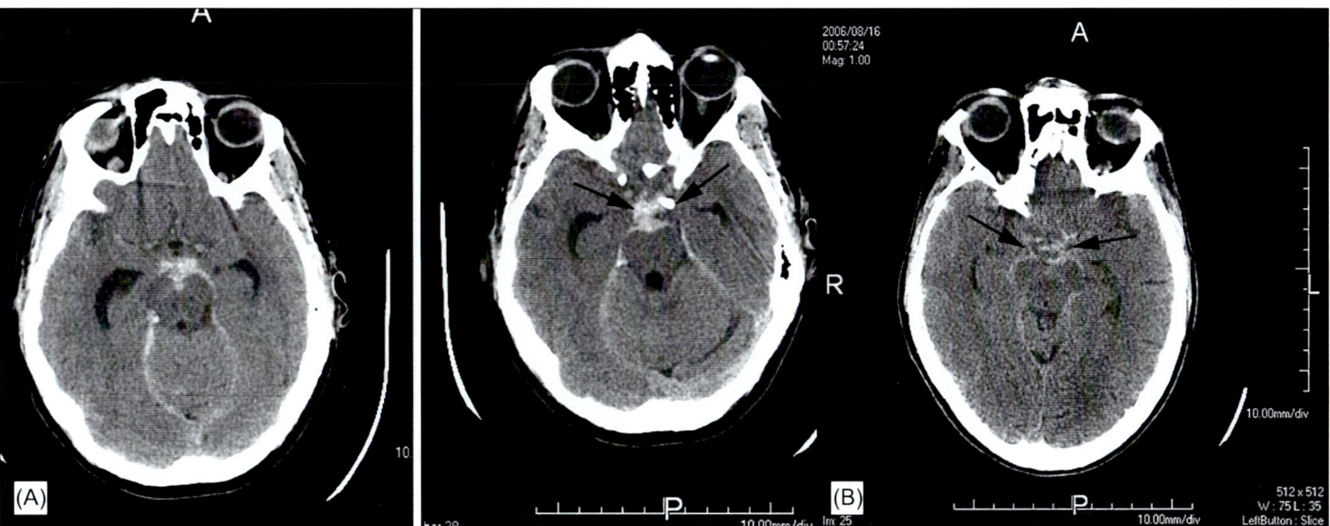

2.23 Non-aneurysmal perimesencephalic SAH. Head CT scans of two patients (A,B) are shown, which demonstrate that subarachnoid blood diffuses widely through the basal cisterns and along the cerebellar tentorium but is initially based in the region of the perimesencephalic cistern, anterior to the brainstem (arrows). Temporal horns consistent with hydrocephalus are more prominent in the first case (A). Conventional and CT angiography studies in these patients revealed no aneurysms.

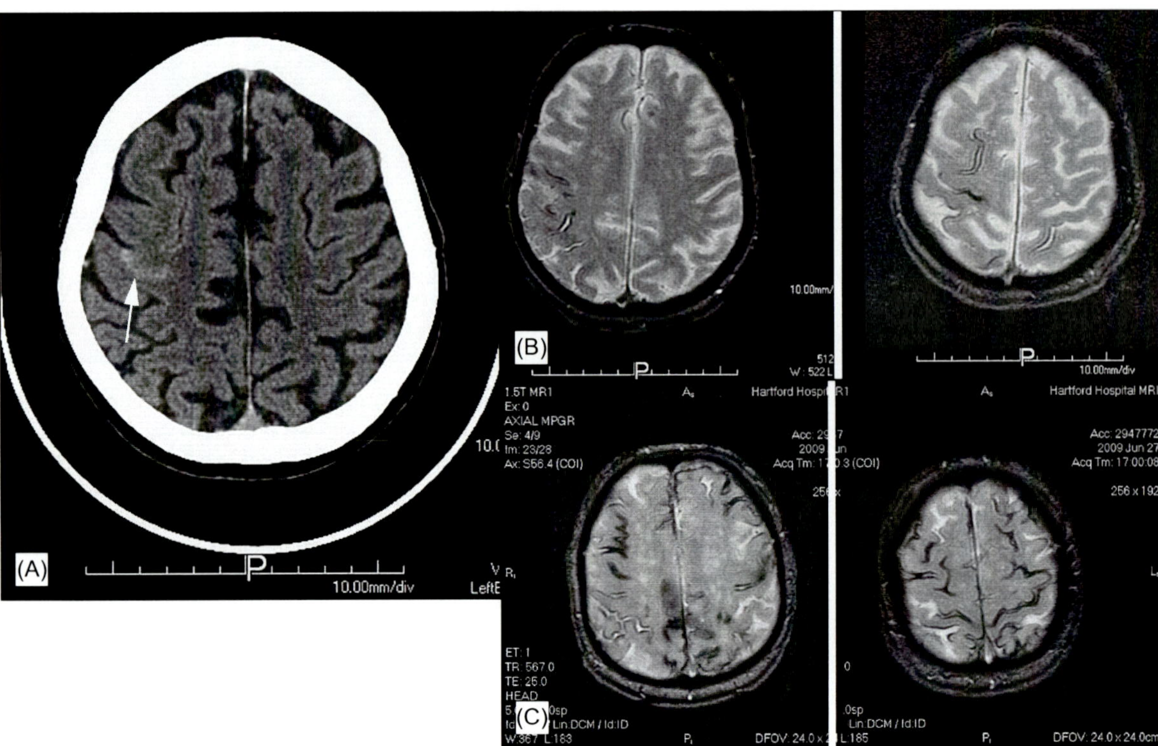

2.24 Non-aneurysmal convexity SAH. Two cases are shown of multifocal hemispheric SAH. The first is shown on a non-contrast CT scan (arrow) (A) and then, demonstrating its greater sensitivity, a GE-MRI sequence (B).

The second demonstrates diffuse chronic layering of blood throughout the subarachnoid spaces of the hemispheres, as shown on the GE-MR sequence (C). This 80-year-old patient with vascular dementia presented on two separate occasions, with lobar hemorrhages (not shown) in the left parietal and right temporal lobes, and also had multifocal microhemorrhages. In this case, the etiology for SAH and ICH is likely CAA.

arterial territories.[52] Etiology may be difficult to document with certainty, but occasionally, neuroimaging provides compelling evidence (**case study 4**).

Case studies

Case study 1. Vasospasm causing delayed ischemia

A 42-year-old woman presented with a Hunt–Hess grade 3 SAH, due to a ruptured IA of the right internal carotid/posterior communication artery (**CS 1.1**). Part of the aneurysm is visualized as a hyperdense lesion on the non-contrast head CT scan obtained on admission (**CS 1.1**A, left, arrowhead). This lesion was emergently treated by placement of a right frontal external ventricular drain; the catheter tip appears as a hyperdensity in the left frontal horn (**CS 1.1**A, right). Next, the complex 10 mm lesion was treated with open neurosurgical clipping; the aneurysm clip (arrow) is seen on an X-ray (lateral view) relative to the skull base (**CS 1.1**B).

Six days postoperatively, the patient worsened, clinically, from vasospasm (**CS 1.2**). Part of the transcranial Doppler (TCD) study is shown (**CS 1.2**A); insonation of the left MCA and right MCA at 54 mm (the upper and lower right corner waveforms respectively) shows waveforms with markedly elevated peak systolic velocities of approximately 200 cm/s. Treatment of this vasospasm with balloon angioplasty of the right distal ICA, A1 and M1 segments as well as the left A1 and A2 segments was attempted. Conventional angiogram is shown (anteroposterior (AP) view, right ICA injection; **CS 1.2**B). During evaluation of the right M1 and A1, distal stenosis from vasospasm of this A1 segment is evident (arrowhead; left); the microcatheter for balloon angioplasty is threaded up into the right A1 segment for balloon angioplasty of this stenosis (right).

The patient was treated again 4 days later (**CS 1.3**) with an endovascular intervention for vasospasm with a total

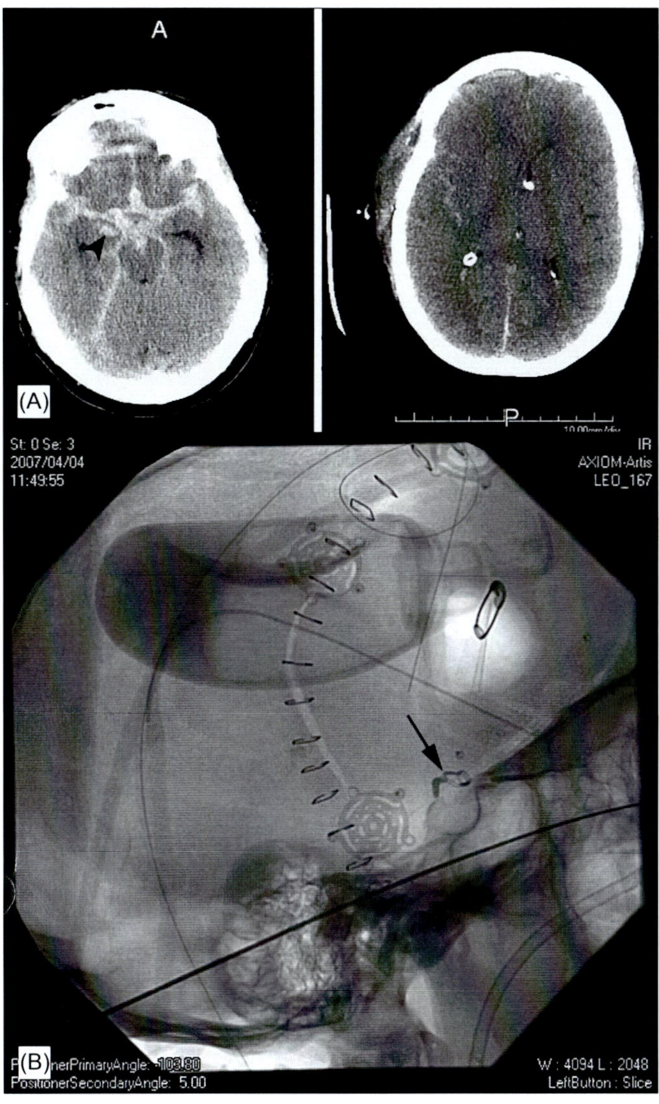

CS 1.1

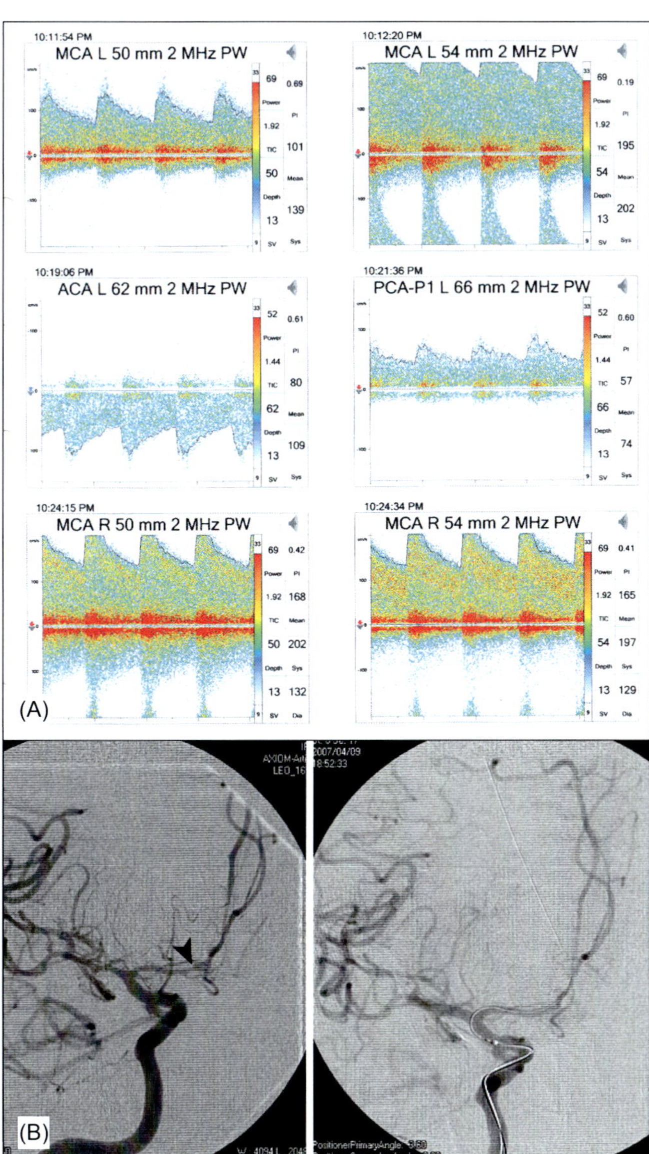

CS 1.2

of 0.7 mg of intra-arterial nicardipine, for severe, diffuse narrowing of the left A1 and A2 segments (seen here on a left ICA injection, AP view; **CS 1.3**A). Compare the pretreatment lumens of the A1 and A2 segments with the adjacent M1 segment (left); the other image (right) shows a guidewire entering the M1 segment. The transcranial Doppler waveform insonating the left anterior cerebral artery (ACA) at 64 mm (the lower right-hand corner) was estimated at 150 cm/s (**CS 1.3**B). A post-treatment left ICA injection (unsubtracted AP view; **CS 1.3**C) demonstrates improved flow in the left A1 and A2 segments.

A patchy right MCA-territory acute ischemic stroke, shown on diffusion-weighted MRI sequence (**CS 1.4**), occurred due to the earlier vasospasm.

Comments

This case study demonstrates the unpredictable nature of vasospasm associated with SAH. Any major vessel around the circle of Willis is susceptible to vasospasm from aneurysmal SAH. In addition, earlier treatment of vasospasm, as shown here, may not prevent a later recurrence and subsequent ischemic stroke. Transcranial Doppler sonography is helpful in demonstrating clinical and subclinical vasospasm of the proximal intracranial arteries,[29,30] enabling the neurointerventionalist to identify which arteries to target with catheter-based treatments.

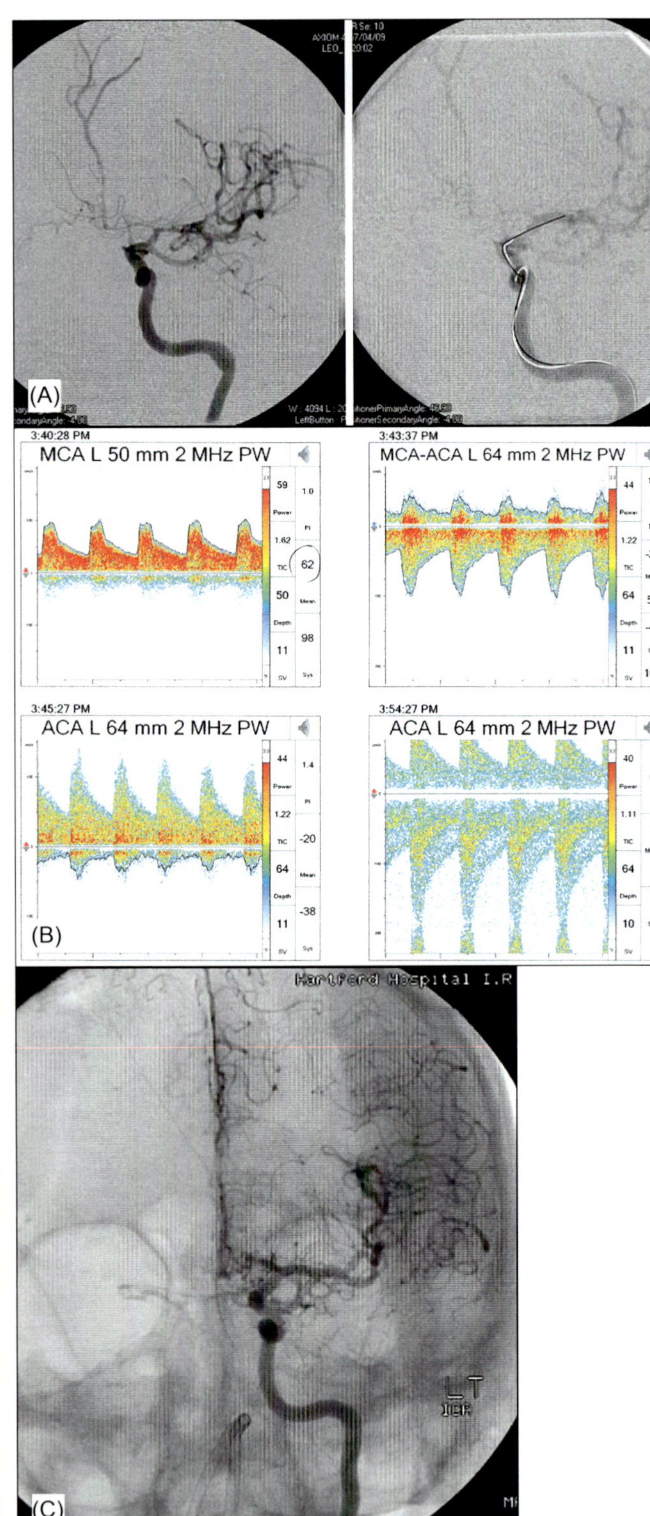

CS 1.3

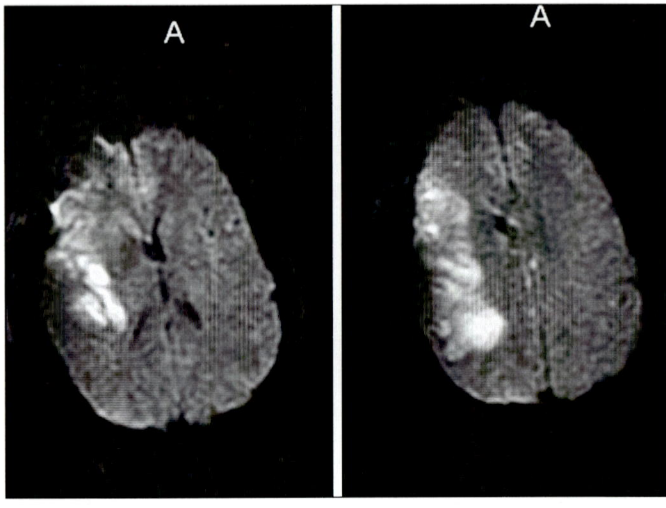

CS 1.4

Case study 2. Coiling an unruptured A-Comm aneurysm

A 21-mm A-Comm aneurysm (**CS 2.1**) is observed on a sagittal CT (**CS 2.1**A) and CTA (**CS 2.1**B). The lesion is supplied predominantly by the left A1 segment, as measured on the CTA study (**CS 2.1**B). Of concern is the very wide neck within this A1 segment, making preservation of the parent vessel technically challenging. A microballoon system that enabled intermittent occlusion of selected intracranial arteries around the circle of Willis (not shown) suggested that, due to cross-filling into the left A2 segment via the anterior communicating artery, the parent left A1 segment could be sacrificed safely in order to completely coil this IA.

Progressive endovascular coiling is shown on the subsequent images (**CS 2.2**). The first view (**CS 2.2**A, left) is a lateral image, at the entry site with a guidewire or coil into the lesion. Several of these demonstrate flow predominantly into the left MCA: left ICA injection, AP views, subtracted (**CS 2.2**B, left) and unsubtracted (**CS 2.2**A, right; B, right; C,D). A total length of 268 cm in endovascular detachable coils (GDC®, Matrix®, and HydroCoil Embolization System) were inserted to tightly pack the lesion.

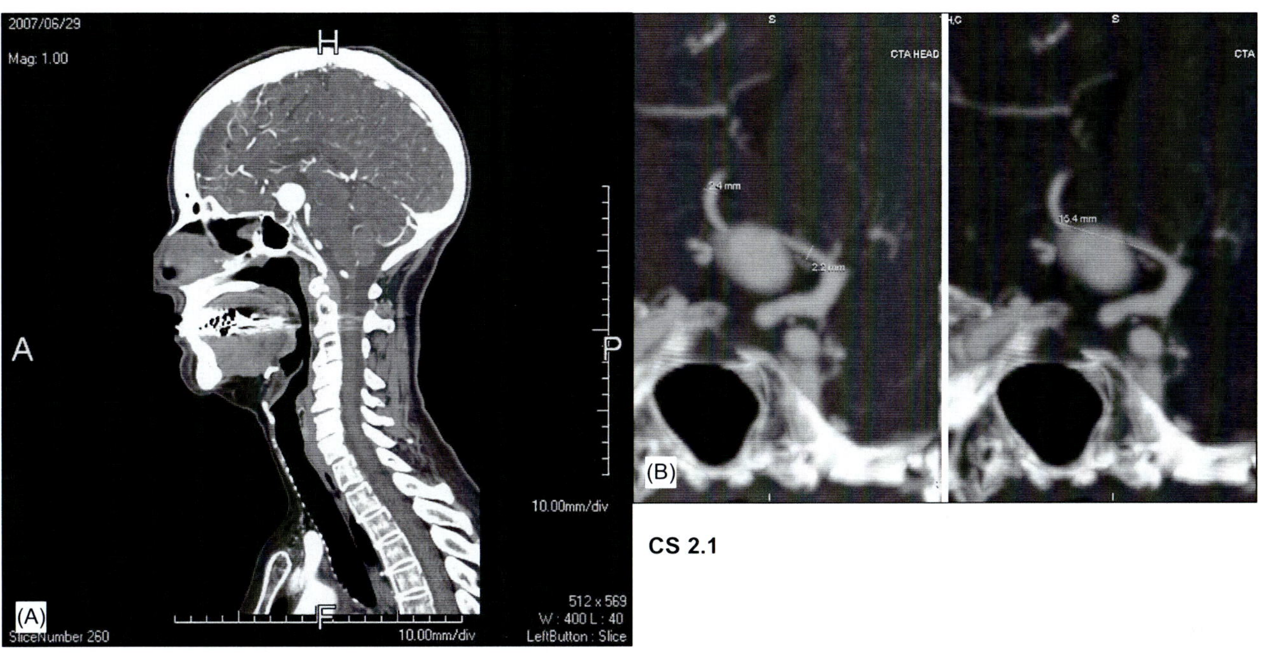
2007/06/29
Mag: 1.00
H
A
P
F
10.00mm/div
512 x 569
W : 400 L : 40
LeftButton : Slice
SliceNumber 260
(A)
CTA HEAD
CTA
(B)

CS 2.1

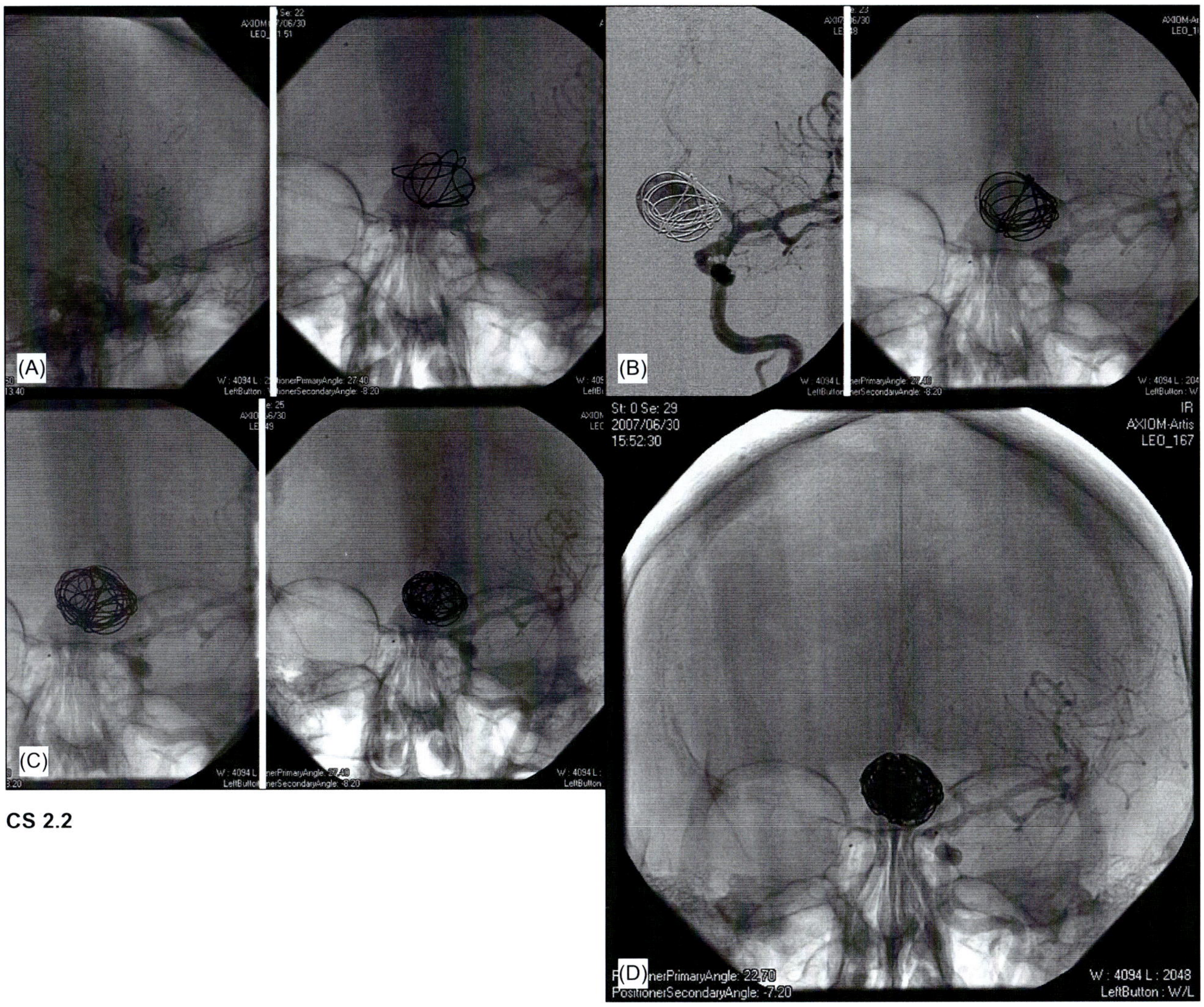

CS 2.2

Comments

This angiographic series demonstrates the careful coiling of a large IA. Such a procedure typically takes many hours, and the amount and type of embolic material required may be great and diverse. A standard frequency for follow-up (post-treatment) angiography and the duration for follow-up studies, to assess the status of endovascular coils within a treated aneurysm, has not been established. If the intra-aneurysmal coils shift, such that the IA becomes incompletely packed, current clinical practice is to add new material into the lesion in order to effectively remove any new spaces or residual aneurysm neck.[34,39]

Case study 3. Treatment of a mycotic aneurysm

This patient (**CS 3.1**) with bacterial endocarditis presented with a large subdural hematoma on CT scan (**CS 3.1**A, left). Significant edema within the left frontoparietal region, shown on a FLAIR (fluid attenuated inversion recovery) MRI sequence (**CS 3.1**A, right), was caused by an inflammatory mycotic aneurysm.

The mycotic aneurysm at a peripheral MCA (M3) bifurcation was identified. Surgical clipping did not obliterate the lesion; dye filling the aneurysm is still evident on the conventional angiogram (lateral view; **CS 3.1**B). This 8.3-mm lesion is shown measured on a 3D rendering of the angiogram (**CS 3.1**C), as well as on a microcatheter injection directly into the lesion (**CS 3.1**D); the catheter tip (arrowhead) is just proximal to the aneurysm.

This aneurysm was then treated with an embolic mixture of N-butyl cyanoacrylate (NBCA) acrylic glue via a microcatheter infusion. The radio-opaque glue (immediately adjacent to the aneurysm clip on this X-ray, a lateral view of the skull; **CS 3.1**E) is observed to create a cast of the aneurysm and its more distal MCA branch (arrow) as well as a feeding pedicle (arrowhead).

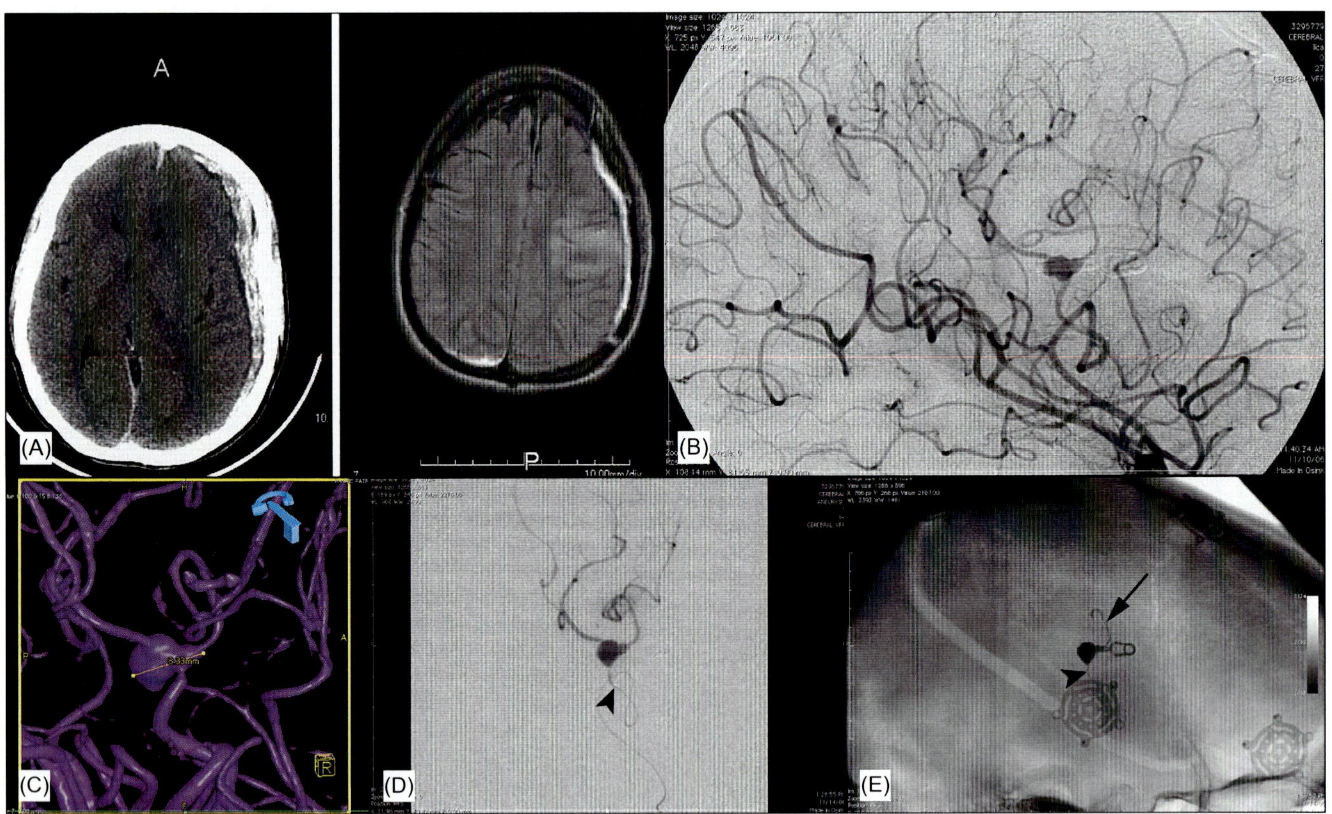

CS 3.1

Case study 4. Aneurysm-to-artery thromboembolic stroke

An 85-year-old woman was evaluated in the emergency room for a possible seizure; however, she later developed right hemispheric stroke syndrome. The head CT scans (**CS 4.1**) initially compare the admission study (**CS 4.1**A, left) to one following the onset of stroke symptoms (**CS 4.1**A, right), with an 8-hour interval between studies. Note the hyperdensity (**CS 4.1**A, right, arrowhead), consistent with an acute thrombus, situated in a dilated component at the MCA bifurcation. Subsequent CT perfusion imaging (**CS 4.1**B) showed diminished cerebral blood flow (left) and prolonged mean transit time (right), consistent with the evolution of a large ischemic infarction involving the entire right MCA territory.

The lesion responsible for this MCA stroke (**CS 4.2**) is visualized on CTA (**CS 4.2**A); there is an abrupt stump-like truncation at the level of MCA bifurcation (arrowhead), with a complete lack of flow into the inferior division, the M2 segment. The next image (**CS 4.2**B) shows an AP view of the conventional angiography; note the same occlusion (arrowhead; B, left). A microcatheter tip (arrowhead), infusing 20 mg of intra-arterial tissue plasminogen activator, begins to reveal the underlying thrombosed aneurysm (**CS 4.2**B, right). The IA, situated at the MCA bifurcation, is also shown on a 3D rendering of the angiogram (**CS 4.2**C).

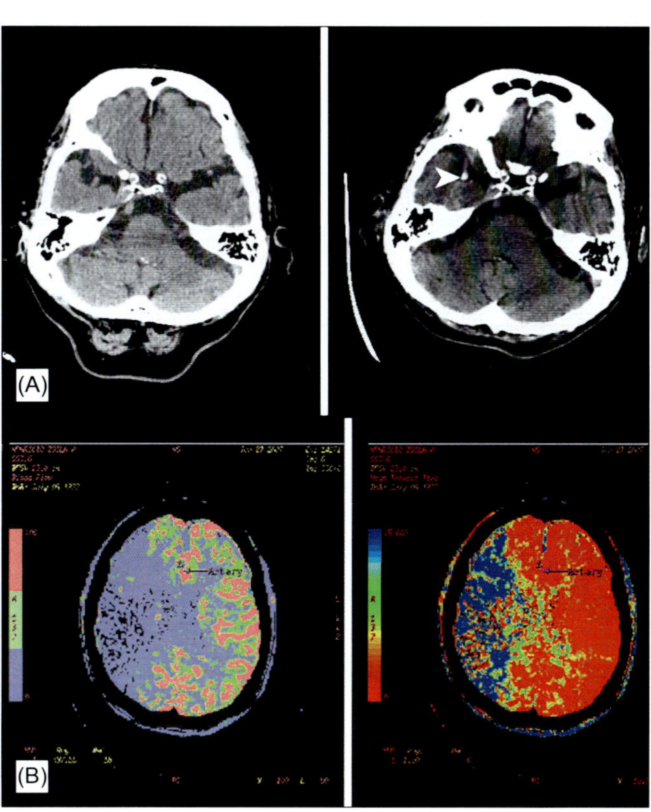

CS 4.1

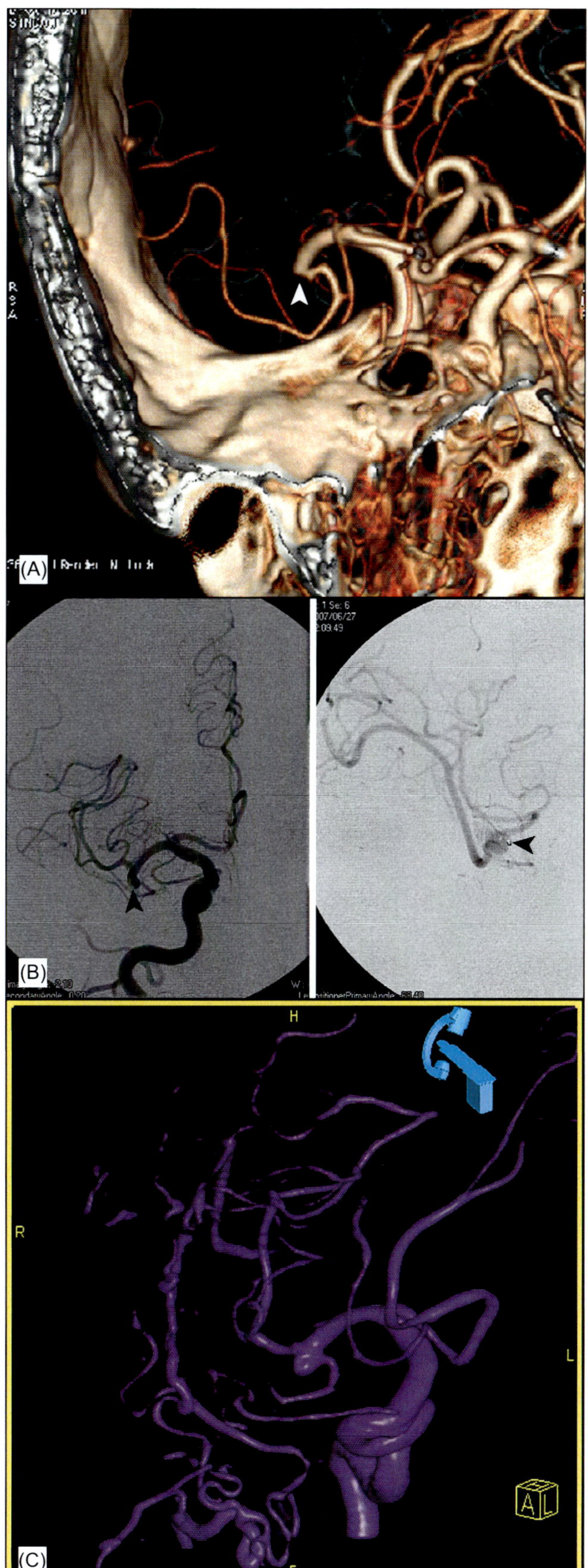

CS 4.2

Post-treatment (CS 4.3)

A final view of the three-dimensional rendering (**CS 4.3**A) isolates the aneurysm to measure the diameter of its dome at 3.4 mm (right). Following the intra-arterial tissue plasminogen activator infusion, the aneurysm is evident on a right ICA injection (AP view) and flow is restored to the inferior MCA branch (arrows) (**CS 4.3**B). Unfortunately, a large MCA stroke, encompassing much of the temporoparietal region on a FLAIR sequence (**CS 4.3**C), occurred despite this restoration of blood flow.

Comments

Neurovascular imaging identified that spontaneous thrombosis of this MCA bifurcation IA appeared to cause this stroke syndrome by occluding the aneurysm and the adjacent M2 branch. Angiography cannot readily visualize the true extent of a thrombus within an IA, because thrombus prevents penetration of contrast dye. However, when the thrombus was dissolved by the local infusion of tissue plasminogen activator, the source of clot, the aneurysm, became evident. In this case study, rapid recanalization of an occlusive intracranial lesion was unsuccessful in averting an acute ischemic stroke.

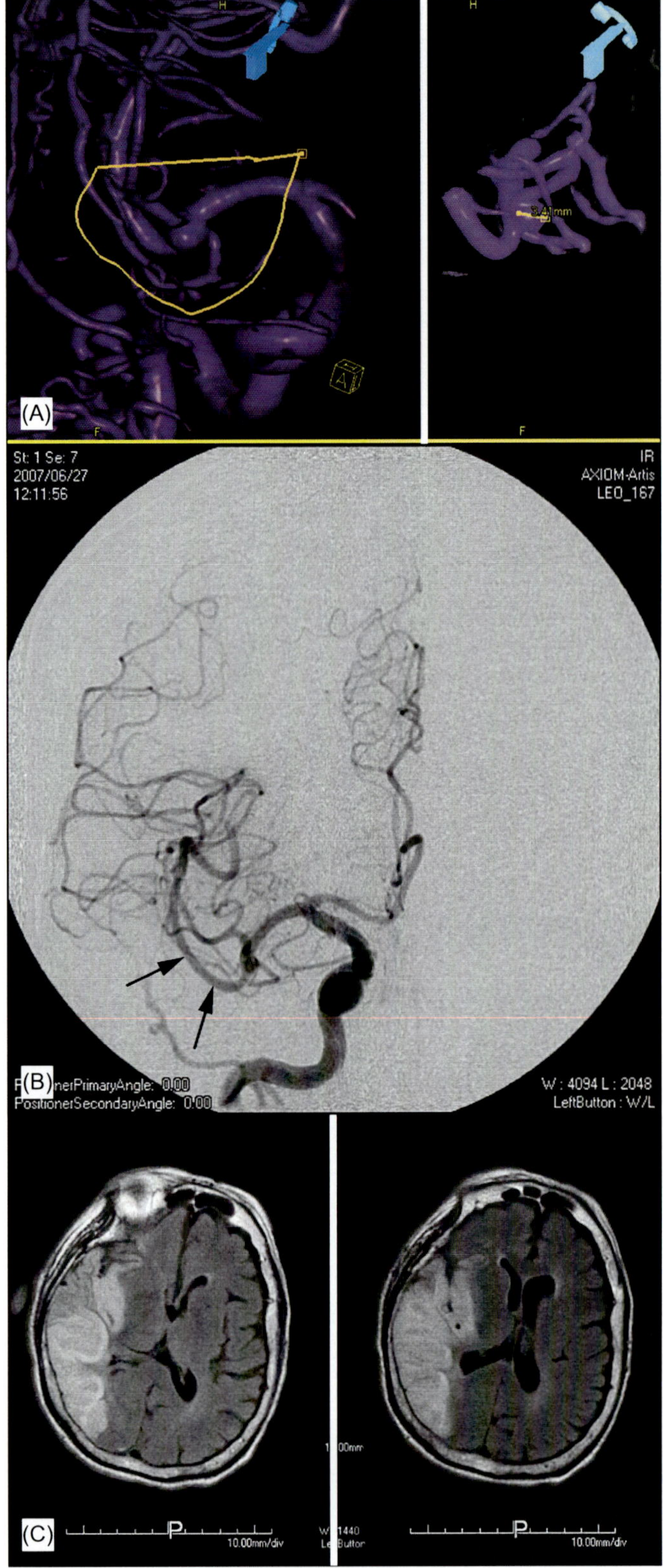

CS 4.3

References

1. Schievink WI, Michels V, Piepgras DG. Neurovascular manifestations of heritable connective tissue disorders: a review. *Stroke* 1994; **25**: 889–903.
2. Suarez J, Tarr R, Selman W. Aneurysmal subarachnoid hemorrhage. *N Engl J Med* 2006; **352**: 387–96.
3. van Gijn J, van Dongen KJ, Vermeulen M, Hijdra A. Perimesencephalic hemorrhage: a nonaneurysmal and benign form of subarachnoid hemorrhage. *Stroke* 1985; **35**: 493–7.
4. van der Schaaf IC, Velthuis BK, Gouw A, Rinkel GJE. Venous drainage in perimesencephalic hemorrhage. *Stroke* 2004; **35**: 1614–18.
5. Feigin V, Findlay M. Advances in subarachnoid hemorrhage. *Stroke* 2006; **37**: 305–8.
6. Johnston S, Selvin S, Gress D. The burden, trends, and demographics of mortality from subarachnoid hemorrhage. *Neurology* 1998; **50**: 1413–18.
7. Broderick J, Brott T, Tomsick T, Huster G, Miller R. The risk of subarachnoid and intracerebral hemorrhages in blacks as compared with whites. *N Engl J Med* 1992; **326**: 733–6.
8. Schievink W. Intracranial aneurysms. *N Engl J Med* 1997; **336**: 28–40.
9. ter Berg HW, Dippel DW, Limburg M, Schievink WI, van Gijn J. Familial intracranial aneurysms. A review. *Stroke* 1992; **23**: 1024–30.
10. Wermer MJH, Rinkel GJE, van Gijn J. Repeated screening for intracranial aneurysms in familial subarachnoid hemorrhage. *Stroke* 2003; **34**: 2788–91.
11. Ellegala D, Day A. Ruptured cerebral aneurysms [Editorial]. *N Engl J Med* 2005; **352**: 121–4.
12. Edlow J, Caplan L. Avoiding pitfalls in the diagnosis of subarachnoid hemorrhage. *N Engl J Med* 2000; **342**: 29–36.
13. Report of Worlds Federation of Neurological Surgeons committee on a universal subarachnoid hemorrhage grading scale. *J Neurosurg* 1988; **68**: 985–6.
14. Hunt W, Hess R. Surgical risk as related to time of intervention in the repair of intracranial aneurysms. *J Neurosurg* 1968; **28**: 14–20.
15. Edlow J. Diagnosis of subarachnoid hemorrhage: are we doing better? *Stroke* 2007; **38**: 1129–31.
16. Butler W, Barker F, Crowell R. Patients with polycystic kidney disease would benefit from routine magnetic resonance angiographic screening for intracerebral aneurysms: a decision analysis. *Neurosurgery* 1996; **38**: 506–16.
17. The Magnetic Resonance Angiography in Relatives of Patients with Subarachnoid Hemorrhage Study. Risks and benefits of screening for intracranial aneurysms in first-degree relatives of patients with sporadic subarachnoid hemorrhage. *N Engl J Med* 1999; **341**: 1344–50.
18. Wiebers D, Torres V. Screening for unruptured intracranial aneurysms in autosomal dominant polycystic kidney disease. *N Engl J Med* 1992; **327**: 953–5.
19. Wintermark M, Uske A, Chalaron M, *et al.* Multislice computerized tomography angiography in the evaluation of intracranial aneurysms: a comparison with intraarterial digital subtraction angiography. *J Neurosurg* 2003; **98**: 828–36.
20. Thai Q-A, Raza S, Pradilla G, Tamargo R. Aneurysmal rupture without subarachnoid hemorrhage: case series and literature review. *Neurosurgery* 2005; **57**: 225–9.
21. Meyers PM, Schumacher HC, Higashida RT, *et al.* Indications for the performance of intracranial endovascular neurointerventional procedures. *Circulation* 2009; **119**: 2235–49.
22. Dion J, Gates P, Fox A, Barnett H, Blom R. Clinical events following neuroangiography: a prospective study. *Stroke* 1987; **18**: 997–1004.
23. Bederson JB, Awad IA, Wiebers DO, *et al.* Recommendations for the management of patients with unruptured intracranial aneurysms: a statement for healthcare professionals from the Stroke Council of the American Heart Association. *Stroke* 2000; **31**: 2742–50.
24. Bederson JB, Connolly ES, Batjer HH, *et al.* Guidelines for the management of aneurysmal subarachnoid hemorrhage: a statement for healthcare professionals from a special writing group of the Stroke Council, American Heart Association. *Stroke* 2009; **40**: 994–1025.
25. Rinkel G, Feigin V, Algra A, van den Berg W, Vermeulen M, van Gijn J. Calcium antagonists for aneurysmal subarachnoid hemorrhage. Cochrane Database of Systematic Reviews 2005:CD000277.
26. Todd M, Hindman B, Clarke W, Torner J. Mild intraoperative hypothermia during surgery for intracranial aneurysm. *N Engl J Med* 2005; **352**: 135–45.

27. Hillman J, Fridrikssojn S, Nilsson L, Ua A, Saveland H, Jakobsson K-E. Immediate administration of tranexamic acid and reduced incidence of early rebleeding after aneurysmal subarachnoid hemorrhage: a prospective randomized study. *J Neurosurg* 2002; **97**: 771–8.
28. Schirmer C, Hoit D, Malek A. Decompressive hemicraniectomy for the treatment of intractable intracranial hypertension after aneurysmal subarachnoid hemorrhage. *Stroke* 2007; **38**: 987–92.
29. Sloan M, Alexandrov A, Tegeler C, *et al.* Assessment: transcranial Doppler ultrasonography: Report of the Therapeutics and Technology Assessment Subcommittee of the American Academy of Neurology. *Neurology* 2004; **62**: 1468–81.
30. Vora Y, Suarez-Almazor M, Steinke D, Martin M, Findlay J. Role of transcranial Doppler monitoring in the diagnosis of cerebral vasospasm after subarachnoid hemorrhage. *Neurosurgery* 1999; **44**: 1237–48.
31. Pelz D, Levy E, Hopkins L. Advances in Interventional Neuroradiology 2006. *Stroke* 2007; **38**: 232–4.
32. Kassell N, Torner J. Aneurysmal rebleeding: a preliminary report from the Cooperative Aneurysm Study. *Neurosurgery* 1983; **13**: 479–81.
33. Naidech A, Janjua N, Kreiter K, *et al.* Predictors and impact of aneurysm rebleeding after subarachnoid hemorrhage. *Arch Neurol* 2005; **62**: 410–16.
34. Lanzino G, Kanaan Y, Perrini P, Dayoub H, Fraser K. Emerging concepts in the treatment of intracranial aneurysms: stents, coated coils, and liquid embolic agents. *Neurosurgery* 2005; **57**: 449–59.
35. Molyneux A, Kerr R, Stratton I, *et al.* International Subarachnoid Aneurysm Trial (ISAT) of neurosurgical clipping versus endovascular coiling in 2143 patients with ruptured intracranial aneurysms: a randomised trial. *Lancet* 2002; **360**: 1267–74.
36. Molyneux A, Kerr R, Yu L-M, *et al.* International Subarachnoid Aneurysm Trial (ISAT) of neurosurgical clipping versus endovascular coiling in 2143 patients with ruptured intracranial aneurysms: a randomised comparison of effects on survival, dependency, seizures, rebleeding, subgroups, and aneurysm occlusion. *Lancet* 2005; **366**: 809–17.
37. Grunwald I, Papanagiotou P, Politi M, Struffert T, Roth C, Reith W. Endovascular treatment of unruptured intracranial aneurysms: occurrence of thromboembolic events. *Neurosurgery* 2006; **58**: 612–18.
38. Rabinstein AA, Nichols DA. Endovascular coil embolization of cerebral aneurysm remnants after incomplete surgical obliteration. *Stroke* 2002; **33**: 1809–15.
39. Murayama Y, Nien Y, Duckwiler G, *et al.* Guglielmi detachable coil embolization of cerebral aneurysms: 11 years' experience. *J Neurosurg* 2003; **98**: 959–66.
40. Pelz D, Andersson T, Soderman M, Lylyk P, Negoro M. Advances in interventional neuroradiology 2005. *Stroke* 2006; **37**: 309–11.
41. CARAT Investigators. Rates of delayed rebleeding from intracranial aneurysms are low after surgical and endovascular treatment. *Stroke* 2006; **37**: 1437–42.
42. Johnston SC, Zhao S, Dudley RA, *et al.* Treatment of unruptured cerebral aneurysms in California. *Stroke* 2001; **32**: 597–605.
43. Bederson JB, Connolly ES, Batjer HH, *et al.* Guidelines for the management of aneurismal subarachnoid hemorrhage: a statement for healthcare professionals from a special writing group of the Stroke Council, American Heart Association. *Stroke* 2009; **40**: 994–1025.
44. The International Study of Unruptured Intracranial Aneurysms I. Unruptured intracranial aneurysms – risk of rupture and risks of surgical intervention. *N Engl J Med* 1998; **339**: 1725–33.
45. Wiebers D, Whisnant J, Huston J, III, *et al.* Unruptured intracranial aneurysms: natural history, clinical outcome, and risks of surgical and endovascular treatment. *Lancet* 2003; **362**: 103–10.
46. Hop J, Rinkel G, Algra A, van Gijn J. Case-fatality rates and functional outcome and subarachnoid hemorrhage: a systematic review. *Stroke* 1997; **28**: 660–4.
47. Mayer S, Kreieter K, Copeland D, *et al.* Global and domain-specific cognitive impairment and outcome after subarachnoid hemorrhage. *Neurology* 2002; **59**: 1750–8.
48. Hackett M, Anderson C. Health outcomes 1 year after subarachnoid hemorrhage: an international population-based study. *Neurology* 2000; **55**: 658–62.
49. Ruigrok Y, Rinkel G, Buskens E, Velthuis B, van Gijn J. Perimesencephalic hemorrhage and CT angiography: a decision analysis. *Stroke* 2000; **31**: 2976–83.
50. Greebe P, Rinkel G. Life expectancy after perimesencephalic subarachnoid hemorrhage. *Stroke* 2007; **38**: 1222–4.

51. Patel K, Finelli P. Nonaneurysmal convexity subarachnoid hemorrhage. *Neurocrit Care* 2006; **4**: 229–33.
52. Blecic S, Bogousslavsky J. Other uncommon angiopathies. In: Bougousslavksy J, Caplan L, eds. *Uncommon Causes of Stroke*. New York: Cambridge University Press; 2001: 355–68.
53. Osborn A. Intracranial aneurysms. In: *Diagnostic Cerebral Angiography*, 2nd edn. Philadelphia, PA: Lippincott Williams & Wilkins; 1999: 241–76.

Further reading

Bederson JB, Connolly ES, Batjer HH, *et al.* Guidelines for the management of aneurysmal subarachnoid hemorrhage: a statement for healthcare professionals from a special writing group of the Stroke Council, American Heart Association. *Stroke* 2009; **40**: 994–1025.

Edlow J, Caplan L. Avoiding pitfalls in the diagnosis of subarachnoid hemorrhage. *N Engl J Med* 2000; **342**: 29–36.

Ellegala D, Day A. Ruptured cerebral aneurysms [editorial]. *N Engl J Med* 2005; **352**: 121–4.

Molyneux A, Kerr R, Stratton I, *et al.* International Subarachnoid Aneurysm Trial (ISAT) of neurosurgical clipping versus endovascular coiling in 2143 patients with ruptured intracranial aneurysms: a randomised trial. *Lancet* 2002; **360**: 1267–74.

Schievink W. Intracranial aneurysms. *N Engl J Med* 1997; **336**: 28–40.

Resources for patients

American Stroke Association (www.strokeassociation.org)

Aneurysm and AVM Support (www.brain-aneurysm.com/related.html)

National Stroke Association (www.stroke.org)

The Aneurysm and AVM Foundation (www.aneurysmfoundation.org/resources.html)

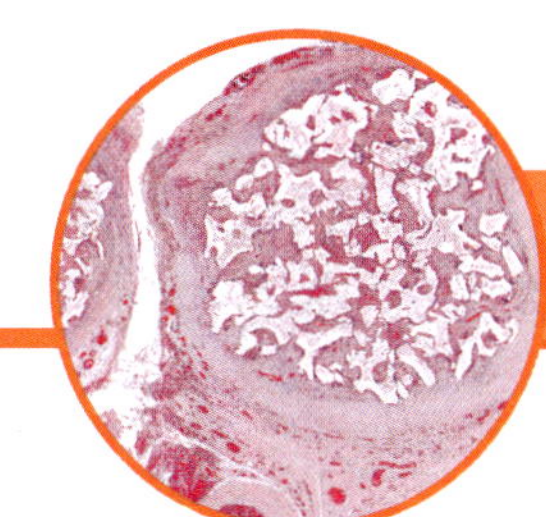

Chapter 3

Arteriovenous Malformations

Introduction

Vascular malformations vary widely in pathology, clinical presentation, and prognosis. In the modern era of increased access to neuroimaging, these lesions are frequently identified as incidental findings in patients with non-specific symptoms. Although some vascular malformations remain benign and asymptomatic, others may cause major neurologic morbidity and mortality, usually from hemorrhage and seizures. The vast majority of malformations are congenital. When symptomatic, they usually present during childhood or young adulthood. A common classification scheme is provided (*Table 3.1*). This chapter will discuss the most complex of vascular malformations, arteriovenous malformations (AVMs), while Chapter 4 will review the other major types.

Table 3.1 Cerebral vascular malformations: classification

A. Cerebral vascular malformations with AV shunting
   1. AVM (Chapter 3)
      a. Plexiform nidus
      b. Mixed (plexiform-fistulous) nidus
   2. AV fistula (Chapter 5)
      a. Single or multiple fistulae
      b. Mono- or multipedicular
      c. Cerebral vascular malformations without AV shunting
B. Cavernous malformations (cavernoma) (Chapter 4)
C. Venous malformations (Chapter 4)
   1. Developmental venous anomaly
   2. Venous varix (without associated AVM or AVF)
D. Capillary malformations (capillary telangiectasias) (Chapter 4)

Adapted with permission from Chaloupka and Huddle.[22]

Definition, angioarchitecture, and pathology

The defining characteristic of an AVM is a large vessel lesion through which direct shunting from the arterial to the venous circulation occurs, without an intervening capillary bed to dissipate the high arterial pressure (**3.1**). This arteriovenous (AV) shunting is not found in any of the other types of vascular malformations (*Table 3.1*).[1,2] The developmental abnormality responsible for AVM formation may occur at the embryonic stage of vessel formation, at the fetal stage, or after birth.

The vascular walls within an AVM are abnormal.[2,3] The small arteries are deficient in the smooth muscle layer. The veins, subject to high-pressure blood flow, may have an incompetent elastic lamina and fibromuscular thickening, and are at risk of rupturing (**3.1**). Both arteries and veins frequently enlarge and develop areas of vasculopathic stenoses.

The two major types of AV shunting depend upon whether or not there is any underlying local abnormal brain tissue.[1,3]

- AVMs consist of a web of small, tangled vessels (plexiform), with or without single or multiple fistulae (mixed plexiform fistula) associated with a nidus of gliomatous, abnormal brain parenchyma (**3.1–3.3**).
- AV fistulas (AVF) are direct single or multiple AV connections without underlying abnormal brain tissue (**3.1, 3.4**).

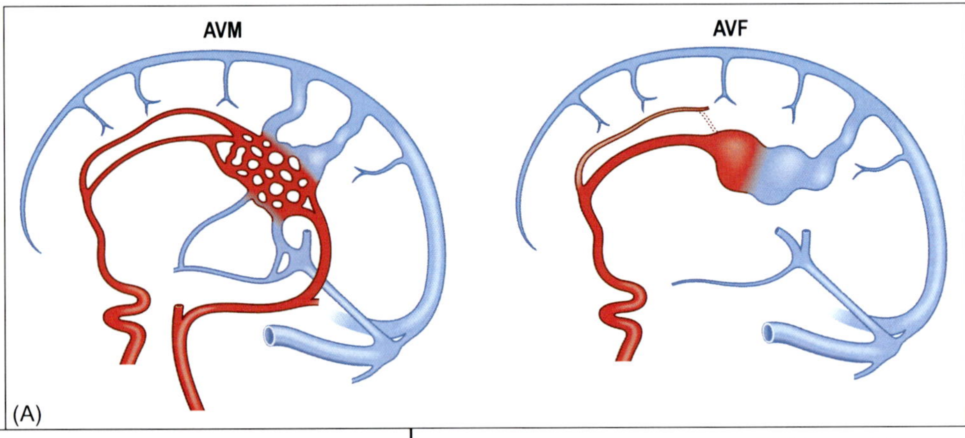

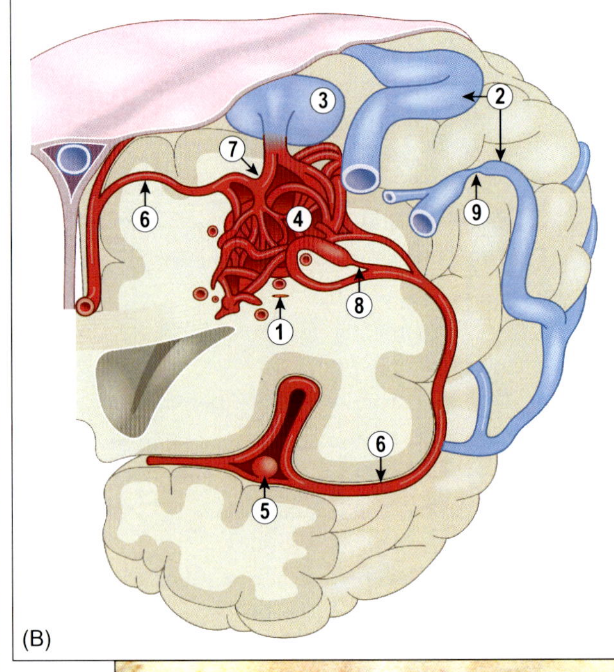

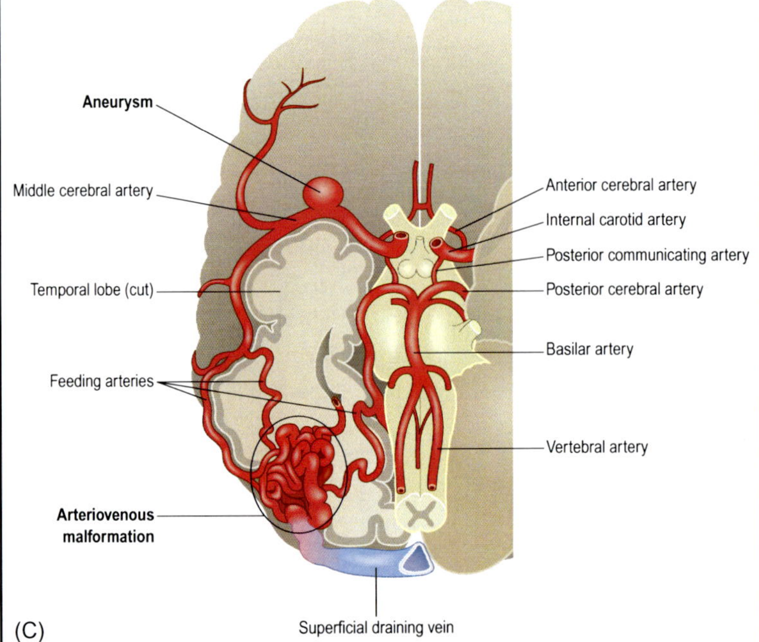

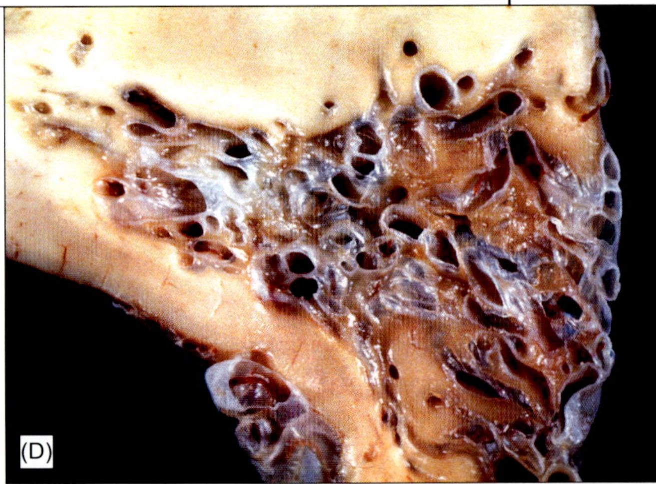

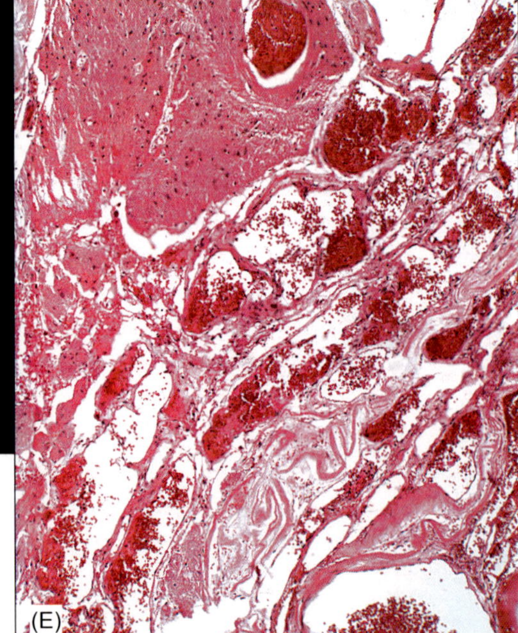

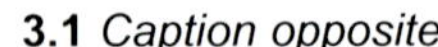
3.1 *Caption opposite*

3.1 (*opposite*) Morphology and pathology of AVM. Illustration (A) of an AVM (left) and cerebral, or pial, arteriovenous fistula (AVF) (right). An AVM is comprised of single or multiple arterial feeders (red) and dilated draining veins (blue), with a plexiform nidus. An AVF consists of a direct communication between an enlarged artery into a dilated cortical vein.

Common features of AVMs (B) include: AVM nidus (entire red mass) (1); enlarged cortical draining veins (2); venous varix (3); location of an intranidal aneurysm (4); flow-related aneurysm on a feeding (*en passage*) artery (5); enlarged anterior cerebral artery (ACA) and MCA branches (6); AV fistula (7); high-flow vasculopathy with focal stenosis of arteries (8); and vasculopathic change in draining vein (9).

A drawing (C) shows a lobar temporo-occipital AVM. (A and B adapted with permission from Osborn[1]; C from Friedlander,[3] with permission).

Gross pathology of an AVM (D) shows a honeycomb-like tangle of large vessels (arteries and veins), within abnormal gliotic brain tissue. Micropathology (E) shows several dysmorphic, irregular arterial and venous walls, of varied calibers (H&E stain, 40×).

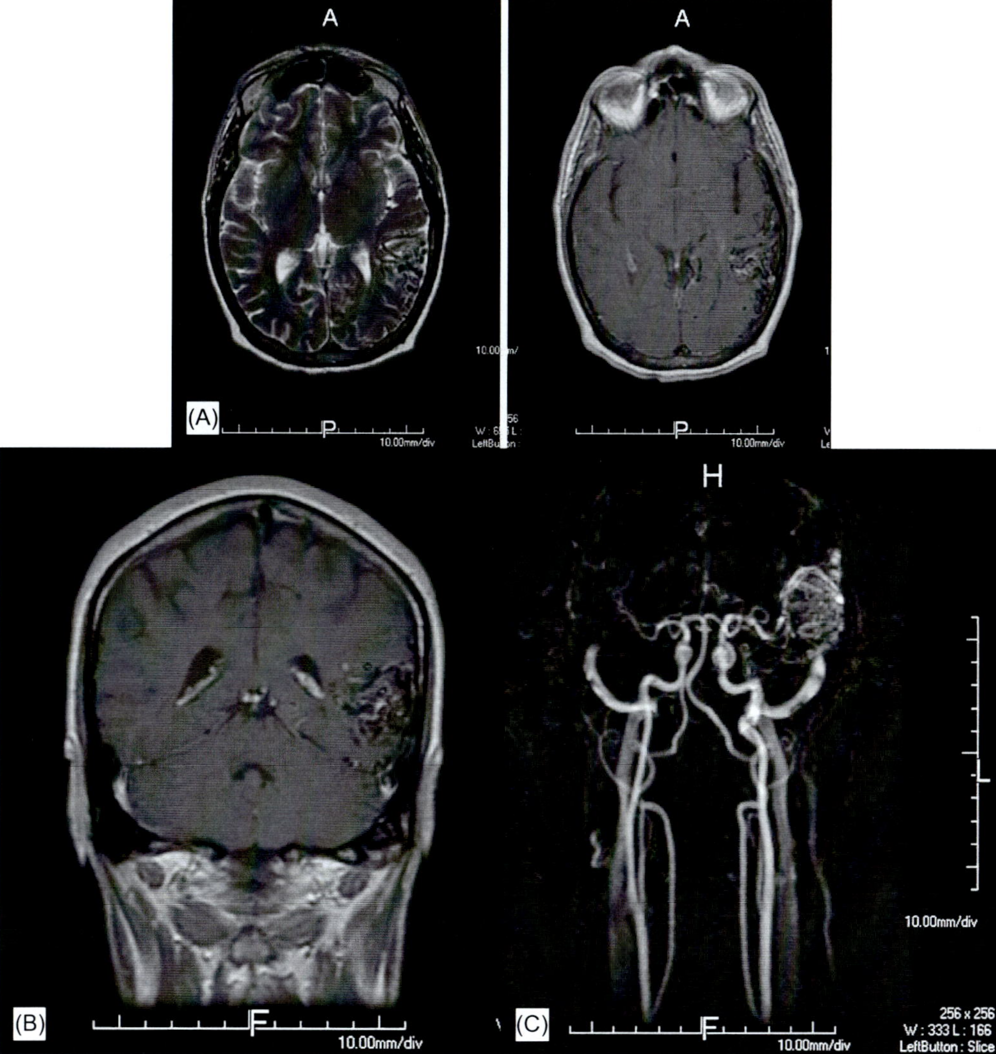

3.2 Lobar AVM. This patient had a longstanding history of complex partial seizures, with an aura of auditory and déjà-vu sensations. The classic appearance of a 'bag of worms' in the left temporo-occipital region is evident on transaxial non-contrast images (A), T2-weighted image (left) and T1-weighted image (right), as well as a gadolinium-enhanced coronal image (B). Finally, a coronal MR angiography (C) suggests a prominent region of abnormal large vessels in the left MCA territory.

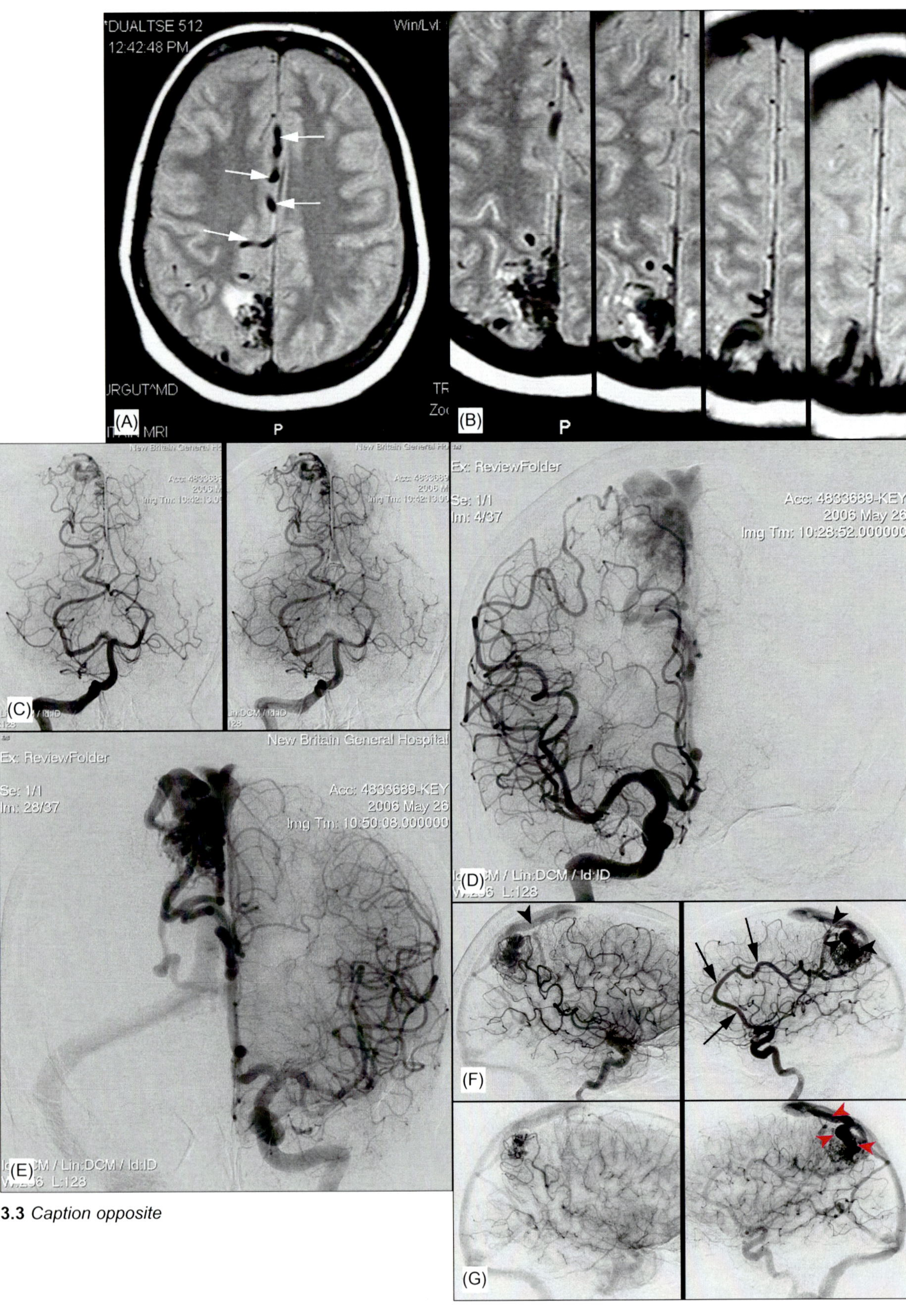

3.3 *Caption opposite*

3.3 (*opposite*) Parasagittal AVM. A 55-year-old woman was evaluated for an episode of headache and left facial numbness. The initial brain MRI scan is consistent with an unruptured AVM. The transaxial turbo spin echo (A) shows a tangle of enlarged vessels in the right posterior parasagittal region, with flow voids anterior to the AVM, suggestive of a large feeding artery or draining vein (arrows). A composite of adjacent transaxial slices (B) suggests multiple arteries at lower cuts, and prominent posterior draining veins at higher cuts.

Part of the AVM in the posterior right occipital lobe is evident on a Townes' projection of a conventional angiogram, right vertebral artery injection (C); at left is an early phase of the study, and on the right a later phase, with some early venous drainage. A right ICA injection (D), mid-arterial phase, AP view, shows little direct supply to the AVM from either the right MCA or ACA. Conversely, a left ICA injection (E), late arterial phase, AP view, shows that the AVM nidus is extensively supplied by the left hemispheric blood supply. Note the extensive venous ectasia, predominantly posterior and above the AVM nidus.

Contrasting views of lateral injections, the right ICA (left) and left ICA (right) are shown: mid-arterial (F) and late arterial (G) phases. The impressive findings are the massively dilated left ACA, the predominant arterial supply to the AVM (F, right (arrows), and the venous ectasia (F, right and G, right (arrowheads)) draining into the superior sagittal sinus.

The Spetzler–Martin Scale grading for this lesion is a total of 2 points = 1 (eloquent tissue, specifically the right occipital lobe) + 1 (nidus size, <3 cm) + 0 (superficial venous drainage).

Further classification of AVM and AVF depends on whether the AV connectivity occurs in the meninges (i.e., dural AVM/AVF) or within the brain parenchyma (i.e., pial AVM/AVF). Dural-based lesions are discussed at the beginning of Chapter 5.

Intracranial AVMs have other unique anatomical components (**3.1**B):[1,2]

- Aneurysms, found in 10–58% of AVMs, may be located at any point along the course of feeding arteries, and also within the nidus of brain tissue (**3.5**; **case study 1**). As intranidal aneurysms are associated with a higher risk of rupture, they should often be treated with embolization earlier than other components of an AVM.[2–4]
- Draining veins of AVMs are frequently abnormal, with kinking, reflux (flow reversal), venous sinus thrombosis (**3.6**), and occlusion, as well as venous aneurysms and, most commonly, venous ectasia (**3.3, 3.5**; **case study 1**).
- Arteries that supply the AVM and normal adjacent brain tissue, so-called *en passage* feeders, must be left intact during treatment or risk ischemic stroke. Irregular stenoses indicative of an associated high-flow angiopathy comparable with that found in moyamoya disease are also common (**3.7**). Often, feeding arteries are substantially enlarged (e.g., **3.3**F).

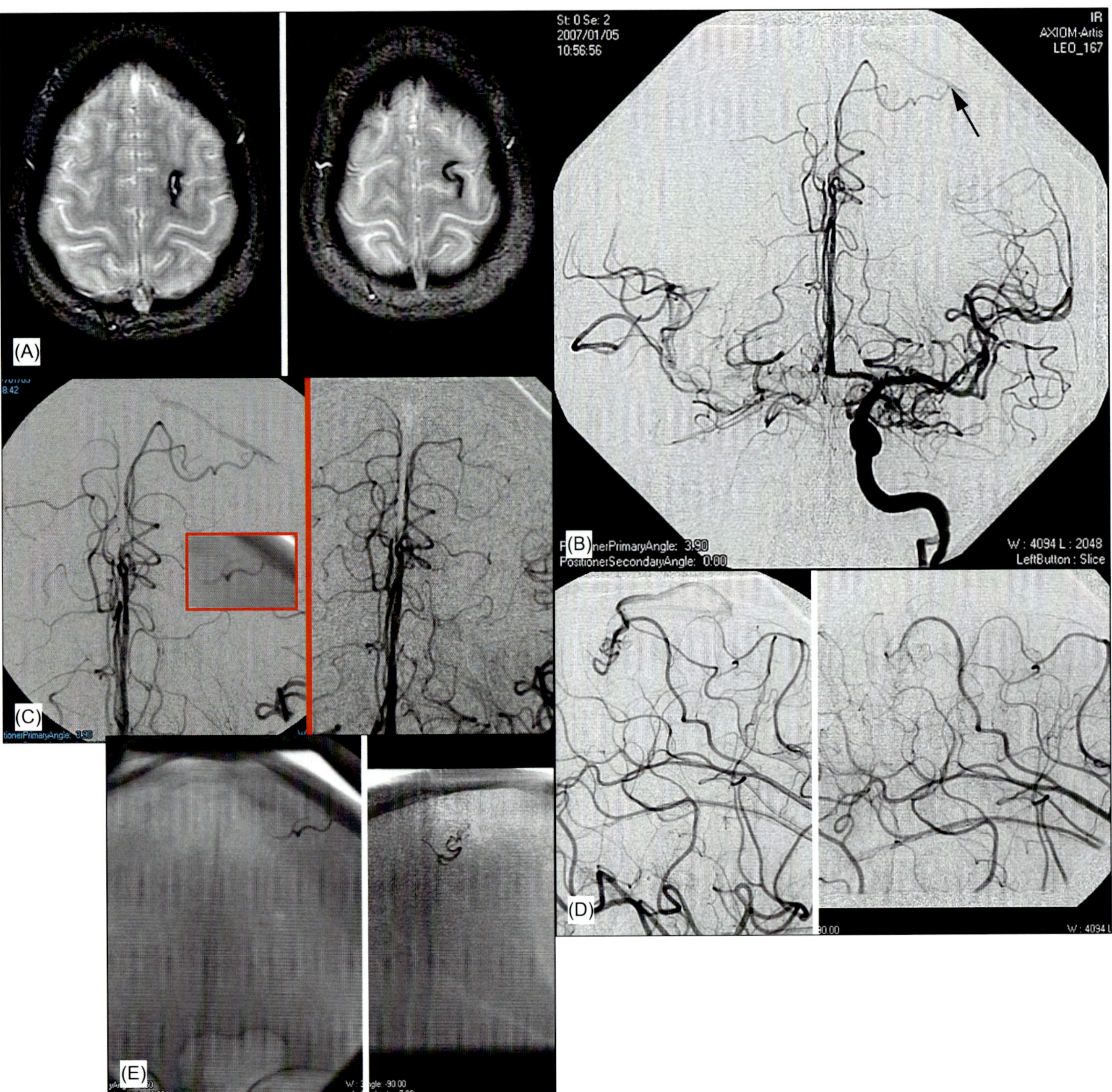

3.4 Pial AV fistula, treated with embolization. A 42-year-old patient presented with recurrent partial seizures involving the right hemibody, starting from the arm and subsequently spreading to involve the right face and leg. The episodes resolved with an anticonvulsant medication. The cause of seizures, a left frontoparietal hemorrhage, is shown on transaxial gradient-echo (GE)-MRI sequence (A).

Conventional angiography, left ICA injection (B), shows the fistula as a point of early venous filling from a distal callosal marginal branch of the left ACA (arrow); this artery is the sole feeder of this small lesion. The occlusion of this single pedicle was accomplished with only 0.2 ml of Onyx® embolic material. The next two images show pre- and post-treatment views (left versus right) of the lesion, on AP (C) and lateral (D) views, respectively. The inset, outlined in red (C), shows a cast of the embolized branch on an unsubtracted film. Note how the draining vein of this lesion is absent on the right, post-treatment images (C,D). Finally, the location of the casted material (E) is shown relative to the skull on unsubtracted AP (left) and lateral (right) views. This intervention is considered curative for preventing recurrent hemorrhage.

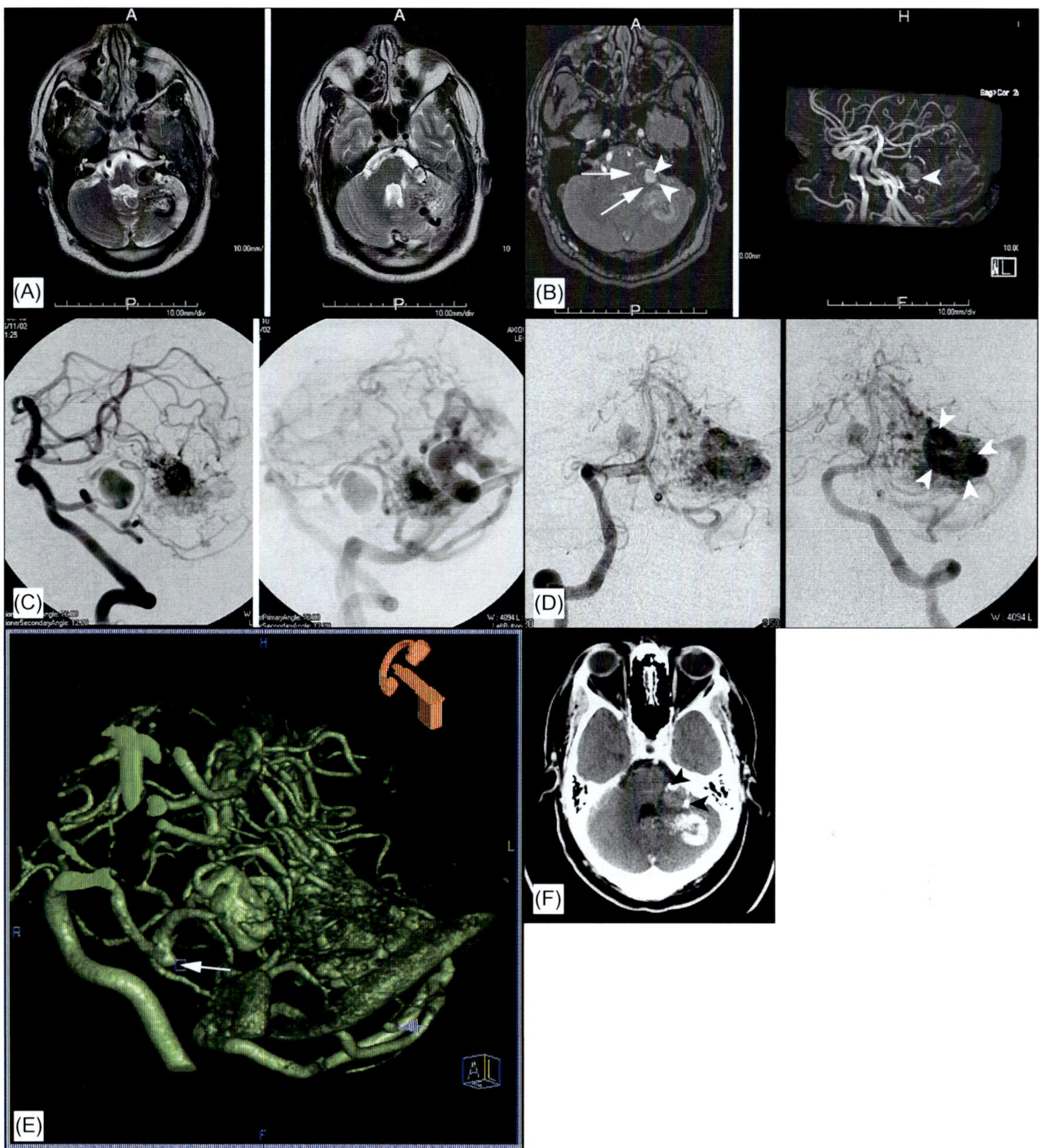

3.5 Posterior fossa AVM, with associated aneurysms. A large anterior inferior cerebellar artery (AICA) aneurysm produces mass effect upon the medulla, seen here on T2-weighted image sequences (A), and appears partially thrombosed on MRA source images (B, left); there is a rim of gray tissue (thrombus) between the bright area of blood flowing into the aneurysm (arrowheads) and the aneurysm outer wall (arrows). The aneurysm is also appreciated on an intracranial MR angiography study (arrowhead) (B, right). Situated posterior to this aneurysm is an AVM, with an apparent large draining vein, encompassing much of the left cerebellar hemisphere (A).

Conventional angiography delineates the lesion from lateral (C) and AP (D) views, respectively. The lateral views (C) show a late arterial phase (left) and a venous phase (right). The AP views (D) show right and left vertebral artery injections side-by-side at mid-late arterial phase. The three major discernible structures are the large AICA aneurysm, the plexiform AVM nidus, and a massive venous ectasia (arrowheads), immediately posterior to the AVM. A three-dimensional rendering of the angiography (E) shows also an additional <4-mm aneurysm (white arrow) along the left AICA–posterior inferior cerebellar artery (PICA) trunk to the AVM nidus.

A contrast-enhanced CT scan (F) shows the lesion the day after the first treatment of several separate embolization procedures. First, embolization of the AICA pedicle with Onyx® beyond the thrombosed aneurysm was performed, which resulted in a 50% reduction in flow into the AVM, and reduction of the nidus size by 25%. Some hyperdense, embolic material (arrowheads) is observed immediately adjacent and anterior to the venous varix (F).

The Spetzler–Martin grading for this lesion is a total of 4 points = 1 (eloquent, involving cerebellar peduncle) + 2 (nidus size, ≥3 cm) + 1 (deep venous drainage).

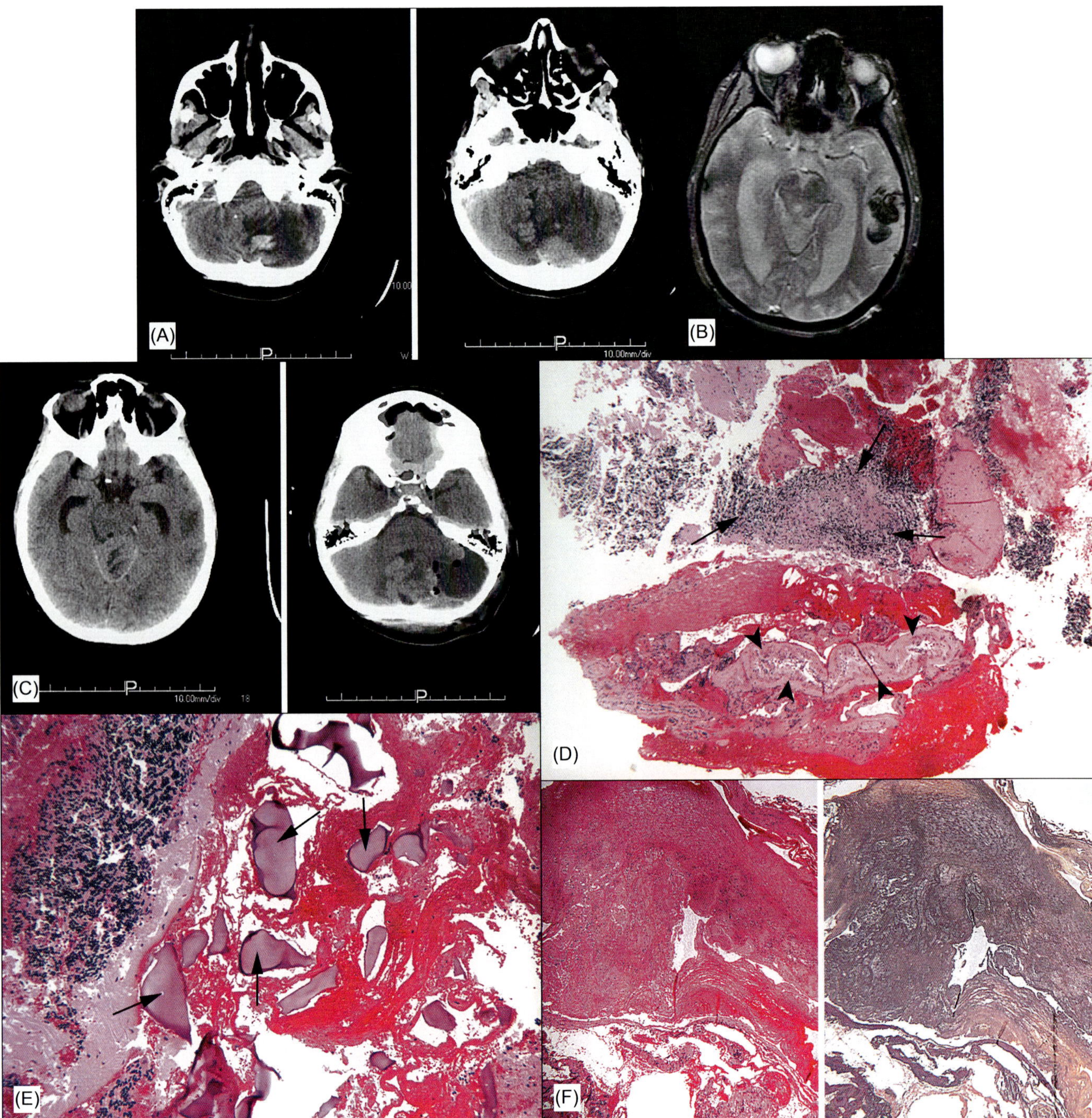

3.6 An AVM mimicking venous sinus thrombosis. A young woman presented with diminished sensorium and lesions in the left temporal lobe and cerebellar hemisphere, initially attributed to venous thrombosis of the adjacent transverse sinus. The admission CT scans show severe edema, with patchy hemorrhage, in the left cerebellar hemisphere and effacement of the basal cisterns (A), and a GE-MRI sequence (B) documents the hemorrhagic component within the left temporal lobe. Owing to the tumoral mass effect in the left cerebellum, with obstructive hydrocephalus, the patient underwent an emergent craniotomy. Next (C), the initial CT scan, demonstrating early hydrocephalus (left), is compared with a postoperative view of the posterior fossa following decompressive left cerebellectomy (right).

The micropathology of the resected segment shows hemorrhage into a cerebellar AVM: (D) dysmorphic arterial walls (arrowheads) below a region of granular cell tissue of the cerebellum (arrows) and free hemorrhage (red blood cells) at the bottom of the image (H&E, 40×); (E) granular cell layers, the dark cell bodies in the left third of this image, along with hemorrhage and multiple foreign bodies, likely fragments of Gelfoam® inserted during the surgical procedure, staining pink-purple (arrows) (H&E, 100×); and (F) markedly thickened arterial walls, shown on an H&E stain (left) juxtaposed with an elastin stain (right), low-power views. Normally, the elastin stains the internal elastic lamina layer a dark purple, but here, there is little intact, dark staining within this arterial wall (pathology courtesy of Dean Uphoff, MD; compare with **CS 2.3**B).

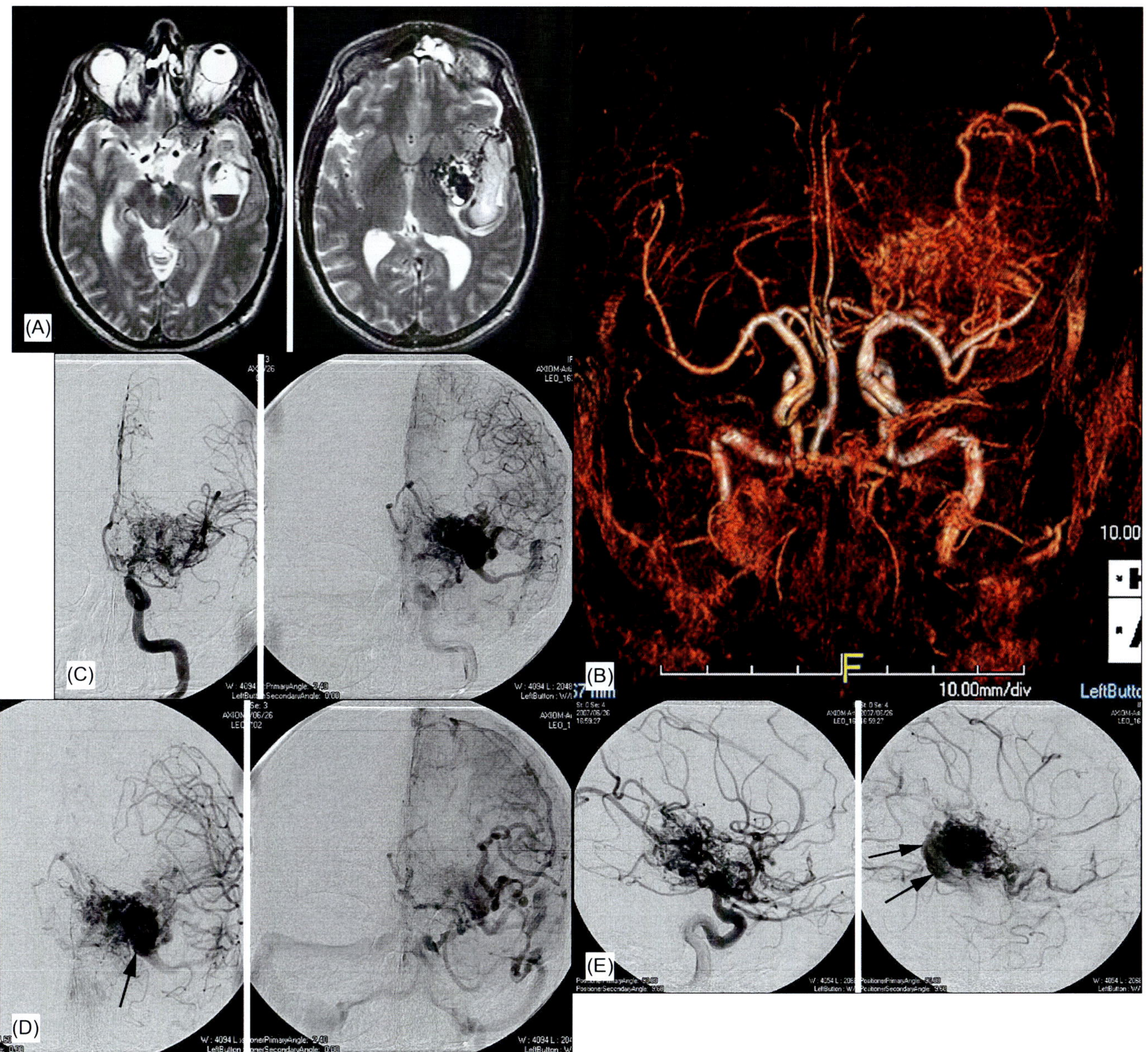

3.7 Deep AVM based in the basal ganglia. A 42-year-old man presented to another hospital with a large, left subcortical hemorrhage, causing an expressive aphasia and right hemiparesis. The initial MRI scan raised the concern of a large AVM based in the basal ganglia (A, turbo spin echo sequence). An intracranial MR angiography documented a dense tangle of arteries in the deep left hemisphere (B).

Conventional angiography, obtained on the day of transfer, showed a large AVM based in the subinsular cortex and basal ganglia, predominantly fed by numerous left MCA branches. The images (C,D) are parts of a sequence from an AP injection of the left ICA, from arterial into venous phase, while the next image (E) is a lateral view. The branches were too numerous to count, consistent with a tight nidus. Venous drainage exits from both superficial and deep venous systems, with no clear aneurysms or focal vascular ectasia. A large ectatic pouch immediately adjacent to AVM nidus, situated in the posterior aspect of the nidus (arrows) and draining into both superficial and deep venous systems, was appreciated (D, left; E, right).

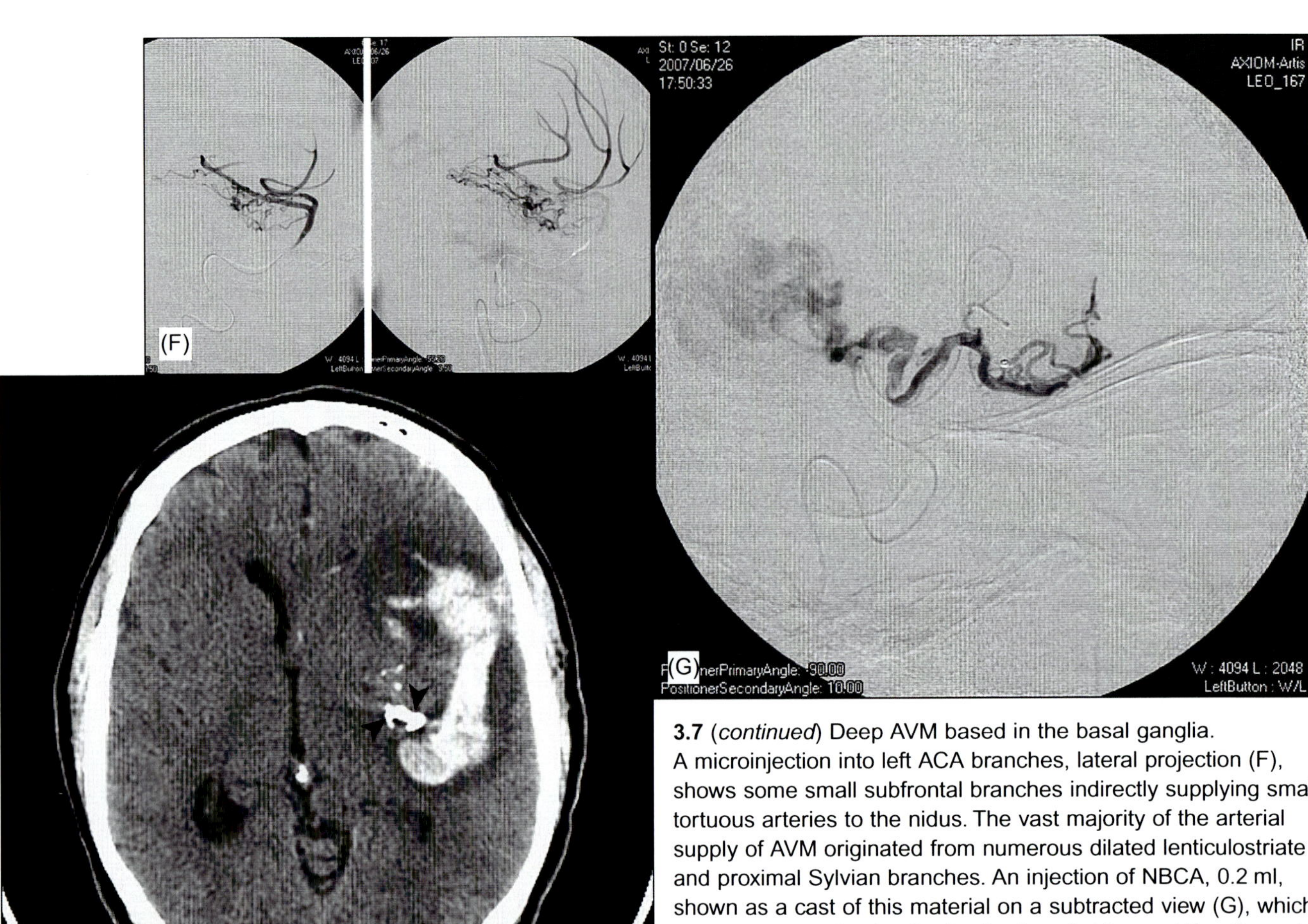

3.7 (*continued*) Deep AVM based in the basal ganglia. A microinjection into left ACA branches, lateral projection (F), shows some small subfrontal branches indirectly supplying small, tortuous arteries to the nidus. The vast majority of the arterial supply of AVM originated from numerous dilated lenticulostriate and proximal Sylvian branches. An injection of NBCA, 0.2 ml, shown as a cast of this material on a subtracted view (G), which caused only minimal reduction in size of nidus and flow through the AVM. At least six separate arterial feeders were defined, but they were too attenuated and tortuous to otherwise successfully embolize; none had any aneurysmal dilatation.

A postprocedural CT scan (H) shows a postcontrast view of the hemorrhage and its associated edema, located lateral to the deeper area of hyperdense, embolic material (arrowheads) in the region of the putamen and posterior limb of the internal capsule.

The Spetzler–Martin Scale grading for this lesion, consistent with a high surgical risk, is a total of 4 points = 1 point (eloquent tissue) + 1 (deep as well as superficial venous drainage) + 2 (nidus size, 3–6 cm). He did not undergo neurosurgical decompression, and the right hemiparesis recovered in the leg more than in the arm.

Natural history

Incidence and prevalence

Prevalence data indicate that up to 0.1% of the US population (300 000) may harbor an AVM. Overall, intracranial AVMs account for <2% of all intracerebral hemorrhages.[2,5] A detection rate for AVMs ranges from 0.5 cases per 100 000 adults per year with first-ever hemorrhage versus 0.9 of 100 000 discovered before hemorrhage.[6,7]

A large Scottish study of AVM found a median age at presentation of 46 years.[6] In the New York Islands AVM study, patients <21 years of age were diagnosed with 20% of all AVMs, including 8% in children ≤10 years of age.[8] Approximately half of all strokes in childhood are hemorrhagic, and the majority of these hemorrhages are attributable to cerebral AVMs.[9]

Hemorrhage risk

Most epidemiologic studies suggest that intracranial AVMs usually become symptomatic during the patient's lifetime, with a single hemorrhage being the most common event.[10] However, many of the contributing studies are not population-based and suffer from selection bias. A generally accepted annual hemorrhage risk for unruptured AVMs is 1.5–4.1%.[3,11]

Previous hemorrhage from an AVM is the most important predictor of future hemorrhage.[2,5] An early study that largely pre-dated the era of modern neuroimaging, with over 24 years of follow-up, reported annual rates of hemorrhage of 18% when there had been previous hemorrhage versus 2% when there was no previous hemorrhage.[12] A more recent prospective study of 622 patients with a mean follow-up of 2.3 years found that an annual hemorrhage risk with conservative treatment was 5.9% with previous hemorrhage versus 1.3% without.[5]

Prospective studies have also shown a particularly high rehemorrhage rate during the initial year following a first hemorrhage.[13] A review of these studies cites a 6% risk of hemorrhage during the first year post-hemorrhage.[3] Thus, the best time to treat a patient's AVM that has bled is probably as soon as this patient is stabilized.

Hemorrhage risk for an AVM in a given patient with previous hemorrhage is often informally calculated, based upon one long-term follow-up study, using the equation:

{100-(85-age in years)} =
% likelihood for recurrent hemorrhage.[12]

For example, a 25-year-old patient (e.g., **case study 2**) diagnosed with a brain AVM that has already bled would carry a lifetime 40% {100-(85-25)%} risk for recurrent hemorrhage.

Spontaneous hemorrhage may be increased in patients with certain characteristics:[3,4,11]

- small AVM size;
- deep location (i.e., basal ganglia, internal capsule, thalamus, corpus callosum);
- deep venous drainage pattern;
- associated arterial aneurysms; the larger the aneurysm, the higher the risk;
- high intranidal pressure.

A recent study identified three features as the critical independent predictors of hemorrhage: previous hemorrhage, deep venous drainage, and deep nidus location.[5] In this population, the following annual risks for hemorrhage, respectively, were found for unruptured versus previously ruptured AVMs, respectively: 1% versus 5% if none of the other two risk factors (i.e., deep drainage, deep location) were present; 3% versus 11–15% if one other risk factor was present; and 8% versus 35% if both risk factors were present.

Clinical presentation[2,3]

- *Intracerebral hemorrhage* is the most common presenting cause of symptoms in AVMs (30–82%) (**3.7**; **case studies 1 and 2**).
- The clinical deficits depend upon the location of the underlying AVM. For example, an occipital AVM may cause visual seizures, resembling a migrainous aura (**case study 3**).[14]
- *Seizures* not caused by hemorrhage are also a common initial symptom (16–53%). Peripheral hemorrhage into cortical tissue may also incite seizures.
- *Headache* is the presenting complaint in 7–48% of patients, but has no unique or distinctive presenting features (**case study 4**).
- *Focal deficits* not related to hemorrhage are uncommon, although it has been postulated that steal phenomena (from an AVM diverting normal vascular supply to itself), venous hypertension, and mass effect may all potentially cause symptoms.

Diagnosis

Brain magnetic resonance imaging (MRI) with contrast is sensitive in identifying the classic 'bag of worms' appearance of an intracerebral AVM (**3.2**, **3.3**, **3.5**), but cannot resolve the complex anatomy of individual arteries and veins within the malformation. In addition, MRI may not detect small, dural-based or parenchymal lesions, particularly an AVF that involves little or no abnormal brain parenchyma (**3.4; CS** 4). Although a non-contrast head computed tomography (CT) scan is not nearly as sensitive as MRI in identifying AVMs, a contrast-enhanced CT scan can sometimes help delineate a complex underlying lesion (**3.8; CS 1.1**A), and CT angiography can delineate some of the large vessel anatomy (**3.9**D,E; **CS 1.1**B,C and **4.1**B).

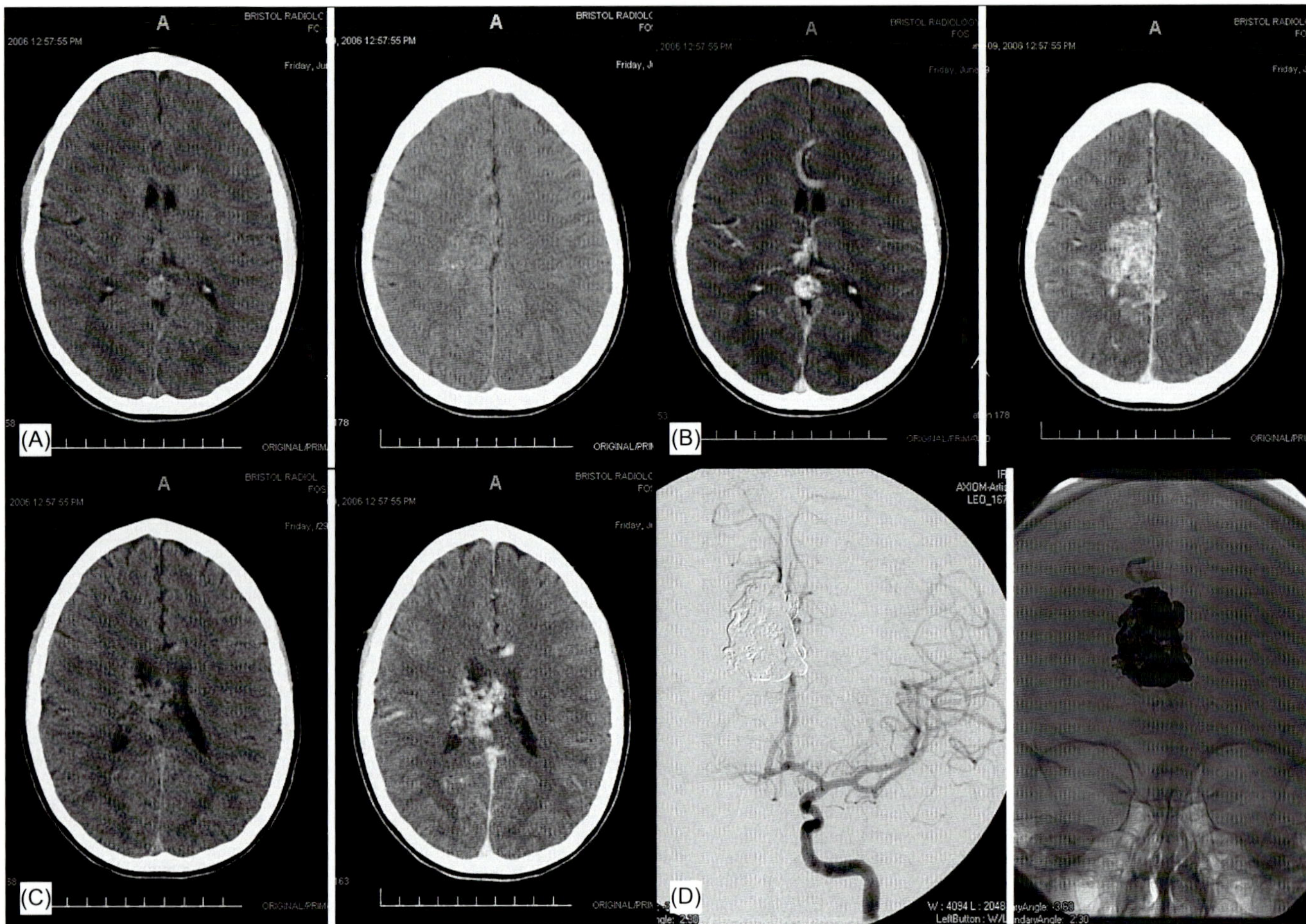

3.8 Large hemispheric AVM, with deep venous drainage. This lesion was initially identified during a work-up for tension headache and non-specific dizziness. The CT scans show a marked difference comparing non-contrast (A and C, left) with contrast-enhanced (B and C, right) studies, demonstrating a midline hemispheric lesion, predominantly involving the right parasagittal region.

Conventional angiography (D) obtained after embolization of the frontal AVM with NBCA and Onyx® depositions show the nidus in a subtracted AP view, on a left ICA injection (left) and also the unsubtracted view of the embolized nidus (right). Note how the lesion straddles the midline, but the larger component of the nidus, as seen on the CT with contrast, is situated within the right hemisphere.

Only conventional cerebral angiography can fully define the flow dynamics of an AVM and all its components (e.g., **3.3–3.5, 3.7, 3.8; case studies 1, 3, and 4**).

- Selective angiography defines feeding arteries and the total arterial territories affected by the lesion, its nidus, draining veins, and venous drainage of the entire brain.
- Superselective (microcatheter) angiography delineates the distal segments of feeding arteries, arterionidal junction, nidus angioarchitecture, and proximal segments of draining veins (e.g., stenosis, outlet obstruction, ectasias, and varices). Microcatheter angiography can also assess the high pressure in feeding arteries or restriction of venous outflow.[1]

Management

Intracranial AVMs are unique lesions for which treatment must be individually tailored. Decisions regarding treatment modalities must consider: patient age, lesion morphology and location, associated aneurysms, the pattern of venous drainage, and previous hemorrhage.[3,15,16]

Lesion location is critical in determining the safest management strategy for an AVM:

- Peripheral, superficial cortical-based AVMs usually drain through superficial cortical veins, and are the easiest to resect or embolize (**case studies 3 and 4**).

- Deeper, non-cortical lesions of the hemispheres are often wedge-shaped in the periventricular region or in border zone territories, with the potential to hemorrhage into the ventricular system, resulting in hydrocephalus (**case study 2**).
- Deep AVMs may have both superficial and deep arterial supplies, and often deep venous drainage, making neurosurgical interventions higher risk (**3.7**). For example, lesions of the basal ganglia, brainstem, and thalamus are typically supplied by the small, deep lenticulostriate and thalamostriate perforating arteries from the circle of Willis.

Treatment modalities consist of three types of interventions: vascular neurosurgery; endovascular neurosurgery; and radiosurgery.

Vascular neurosurgery

Surgery serves to ligate feeding arteries, obliterate draining veins, resect the nidus, and, occasionally, clip associated aneurysms (**3.6**; **case studies 1 and 3**).[2] Care must be taken to preserve normal blood supply to adjacent intact brain tissue. Functional MRI neuroimaging, Wada testing and intraoperative studies (i.e., electrophysiologic cortical mapping and cerebral angiography) intra-operative electrophysiologic cortical mapping, and intra-operative angiography are critical to identify eloquent brain tissue adjacent to an AVM that must be preserved during elective surgery. In the setting of emergent decompressive surgery to remove an associated hematoma, the pathway to this clot may provide a surgical corridor to simultaneously remove the underlying AVM (**2.12**, **3.6**; **case study 2**).

The Spetzler–Martin Grading Scale (*Table 3.2*) is used to estimate the risk of surgery for intracranial AVMs.[17] Patients with lower total scores (1–3) are at lower perioperative risk (0–15%) for major morbidity (permanent paralysis, aphasia, and/or hemianopsia), than those with higher scores (4–5).[3] The American Stroke Association guidelines recommend the consideration of surgery for lesions of Spetzler–Martin grades 1 and 2.[16] Patients with scores of 3 are a controversial group, for which embolization is usually recommended before surgery. Patients with the highest grades (>3) may instead be candidates for endovascular and/or radiosurgical approaches, or no interventional treatments (conservative management).[3,16]

Table 3.2 The Spetzler–Martin Scale for evaluating the surgical risk for patients with AVM[17]

A. Size	
Small (maximum diameter, <3 cm)	1
Medium (3–6 cm)	2
Large (>6 cm)	3
B. Location	
Non-eloquent site	0
Sensorimotor, language, or visual; hypothalamus or thalamus; internal capsule; brainstem; cerebellar peduncles or nuclei	1
C. Venous drainage pattern	
Superficial only	0
Any deep	1

Grade (total score) of 4–5 associated with highest risk (20%) of persistent neurologic deficits after surgery, versus lower (<3%) for scores of 1, 2, or 3.

Endovascular neurosurgery

The endovascular, or neurointerventional approach is most often used to devascularize a lesion, and effectively reduce its size, prior to a later neurosurgical resection.[2,15] The reduction of blood flow to an AVM, especially from deep feeding arteries, reduces the risk associated with neurosurgery.[3] Such staged procedures of embolization followed by resection may generate excellent outcomes (e.g., 9% persistent deficits and 4% mortality in a series of 101 cases).[18] Catheters can deliver various occlusive agents, such as thrombosing coils, sclerosing drugs, quick-acting glues and other liquid embolic materials, such as n-butyl cyanoacrylate (NBCA) and the Onyx,[19] and permanent balloons (**3.7**, **3.9**, **3.10**; **case studies 1 and 4**), and can also deliver short-acting anesthetics to determine the functional impact of occluding the local arterial supply.

One common endovascular approach is the coiling of an AVM-associated aneurysm that may likely have been the source of incident hemorrhage followed by neurosurgery after reduction of cerebral edema.[3] It is typically recommended that larger aneurysms (e.g., >7 mm in diameter) be treated before additional embolization or surgical treatment of an AVM (**3.5**; **case study 1**).[3]

Endovascular occlusion is also used to eliminate smaller or surgically inaccessible deep pial or dural-based AVFs. In some cases, embolization is curative, and neurosurgery may be unnecessary (**3.4**, **case study 4**; see also Chapter 1, **case study 4**, and Chapter 5, **5.1–5.4**).

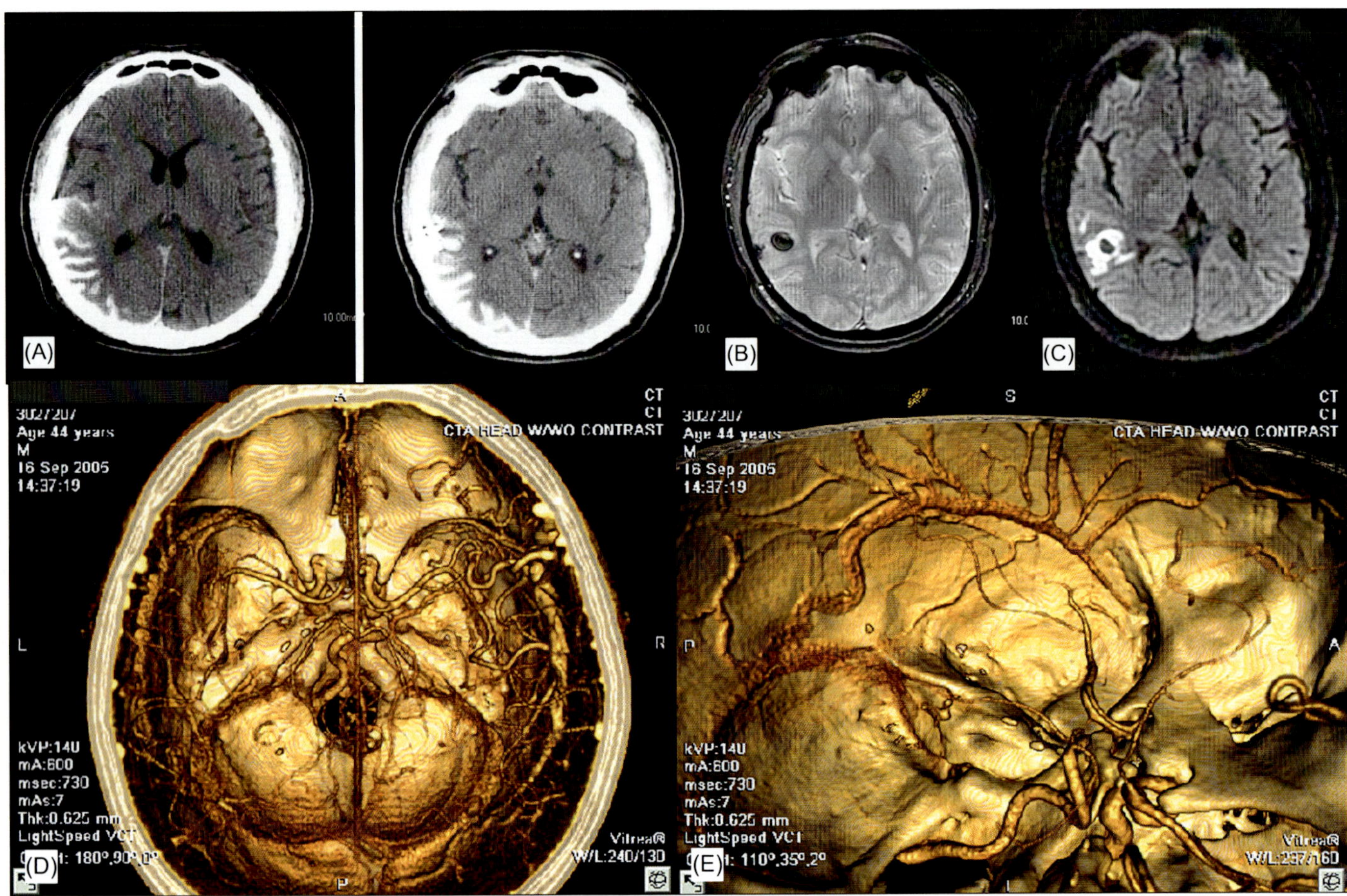

3.9 Contrast extravasation. In this patient with a pial dural AVM of the right Sylvian region, contrast extravasation occurring during an endovascular procedure is shown on a non-contrast CT scan (A). Two days later, a GE-MR sequence (B) demonstrates a 1 cm hematoma in the posterior right temporal lobe, surrounded by an area of restricted diffusion ≤3 cm in diameter on the DW-MR sequence (C). Months earlier, the AVM was suggested on CT angiography by an area of enlarged vessels in the right temporal lobe and Sylvian fissure; note the right and left sides are reversed (D). An internal window into the skull base surrounding the right cerebral convexity (E) shows multiple prominent venous channels, evidenced by bony grooves, which are a component of this AVM.

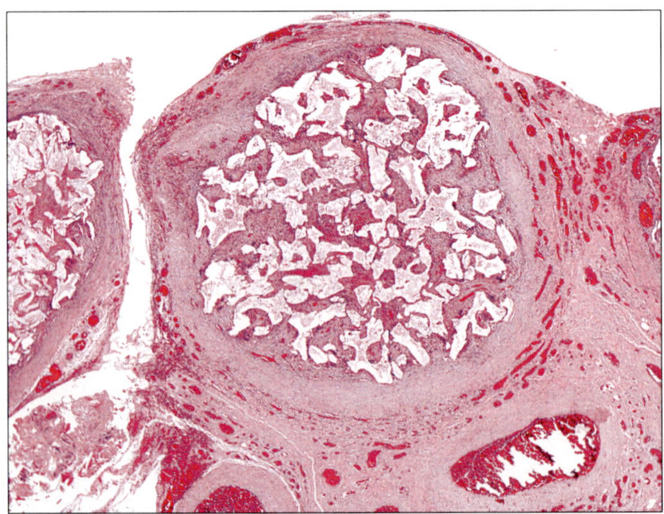

3.10 Embolic material, micropathology. The micropathology of a previously embolized AVM that was later resected is shown here as a transection through two arterioles, one centrally and part of a second to its left. Their lumens are completely filled with a crystallized material, which had been employed during an endovascular procedure (H&E stain, 100×).

Radiosurgery

Here, a gamma knife, proton beam, or a linear accelerator is used to shrink and obliterate AVMs. The success of radiosurgical obliteration is inversely proportional to lesion size. Those >3 cm are the most difficult to eradicate with radiotherapy alone.[2] It is a preferred modality for smaller lesions located in eloquent areas, where neurosurgery is likely to result in permanent neurologic deficits.[3] The mechanisms by which radiosurgery obliterates AVMs include: (1) progressive vascular (intimal layer) thickening within 3 years, decreasing the stress to vessel walls; (2) partial or complete thrombosis of irradiated vessels; and (3) the potential for occlusion of thickened endothelium, associated with stasis.[2]

An angiographic cure (obliteration) of an AVM for lesions <3 cm treated with radiosurgery occurs in 80–95% of patients.[2,3,20] However, this modality takes 1–3 years to completely obliterate an AVM.[3] A large prospective cohort study followed 500 patients with cerebral AVMs who had undergone gamma knife radiosurgery.[20] The report found a lower rate of hemorrhage both during the latency period (immediately after radiosurgery) and after angiographic obliteration. Though radiosurgery is non-invasive, the associated risk relates to radiation injury of adjacent brain parenchyma and can include seizures, hemorrhage, radionecrosis (with cognitive sequelae), progressive edema, and venous congestion.[3]

No clinical trials directly comparing the three treatment modalities for AVMs exist, and outcomes data are derived primarily from case series. Management at a medical center with a neurovascular program offering all modalities is recommended. The goal of treatment is complete AVM obliteration, as partial obliteration does not protect from hemorrhage.[3,4,20]

Outcomes

The outcomes from AVM hemorrhage are well appreciated. There is an initial neurologic morbidity of 20–30% and a mortality rate of 10–30% with each subsequent hemorrhage.[6,11,12] Poor outcomes from AVM-related hemorrhage are less common than for other intracerebral hemorrhages, such as primary intracerebral hemorrhage and subarachnoid hemorrhage (SAH). Patients with purely intraventricular hemorrhage or SAH from an AVM may have better prognoses than those that have primarily parenchymal involvement.[2]

While prevention of recurrent hemorrhages is the primary goal of AVM treatment, seizure reduction or eradication is another common positive outcome. In a series of 65 patients, 51% were seizure-free after stereotactic radiosurgery at 3-year follow-up.[21]

Case studies

Case study 1. Lobar AVM, presenting with ruptured intracranial aneurysm

A 51-year-old woman presented with SAH, attributed to an aneurysm of the anterior communicating artery (A-Comm), associated with a right frontotemporal AVM.

Initial neuroimaging (CS 1.1)

The initial CT scan (**CS 1.1**A) shows SAH involving the Sylvian fissures bilaterally, with diffuse cerebral edema (left). This study demonstrates that the frontal lesion is largely hidden before intravenous contrast dye is administered (right). The A-Comm aneurysm is shown on CT angiography, coronal (**CS 1.1**B) and transaxial (**CS 1.1**C, white arrow) images, measured at 8 mm × 9 mm × 6 mm, and also suggests a large draining vein in the temporal lobe (arrows).

Aneurysm treatment (CS 1.2)

The A-Comm aneurysm was first treated with five HydroSoft embolic coils, for a total length of 10 cm. A lateral view, unsubtracted, of the well-packed aneurysm is shown.

Angiography (CS 1.3)

A contrast between the left (**CS 1.3**A, right) versus the right (**CS 1.3**A, left) hemisphere is shown on internal carotid artery (ICA) injections (anteroposterior (AP) views) before embolization of the AVM. This peri-opercular AVM is supplied primarily by right middle cerebral artery (MCA) branches. The massive venous system (**CS 1.3**B), which drains superficially toward the superior sagittal sinus, is delineated on lateral views.

Endovascular treatments (CS 1.4)

The AVM was later treated with Onyx liquid embolization, beginning by casting the dominant feeding vessels. A total of 7 ml of Onyx material was injected into the nidus. Early and later views (**CS 1.4**A–C), comparing unsubtracted views (the left images) with subtracted views (the right images) are

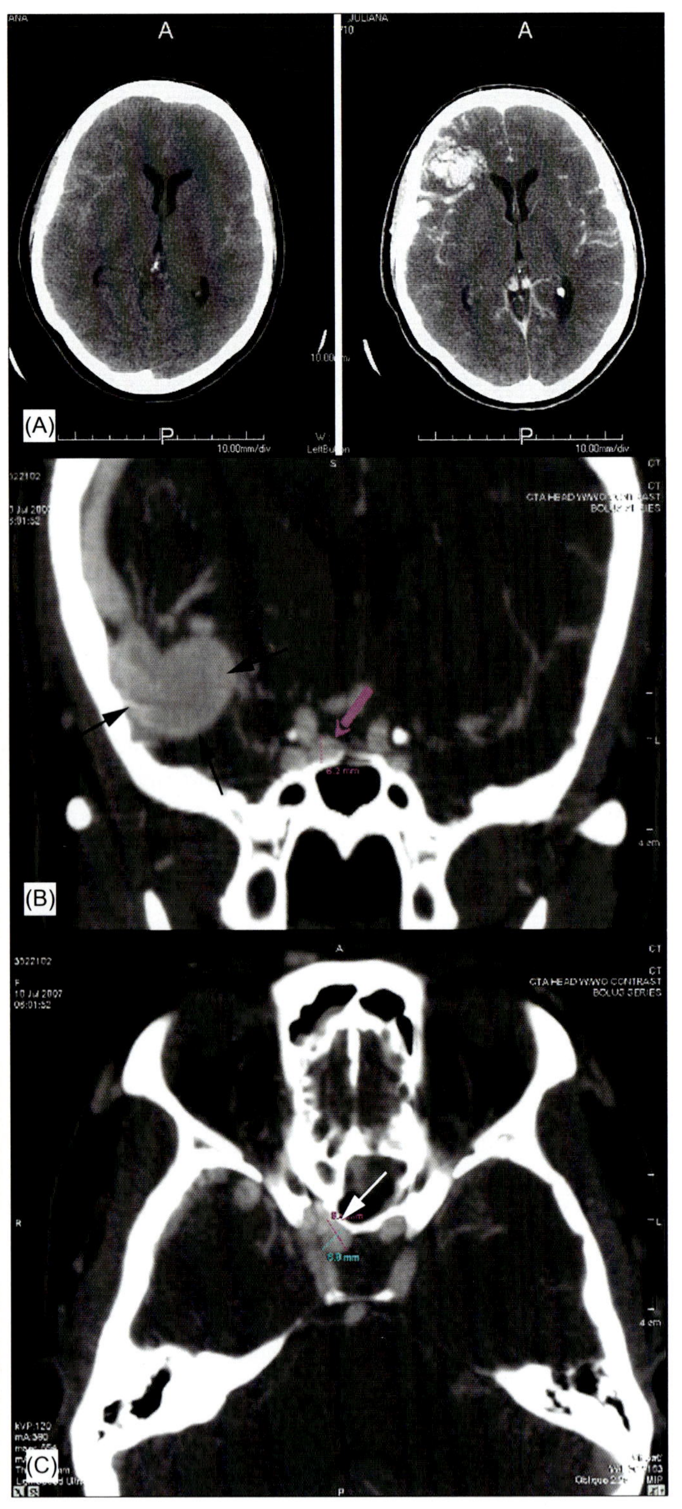

CS 1.1

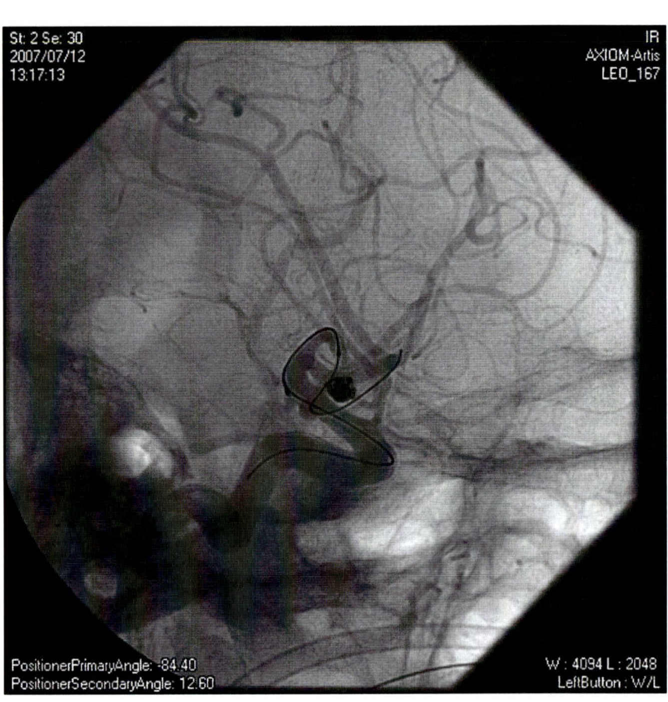

CS 1.2

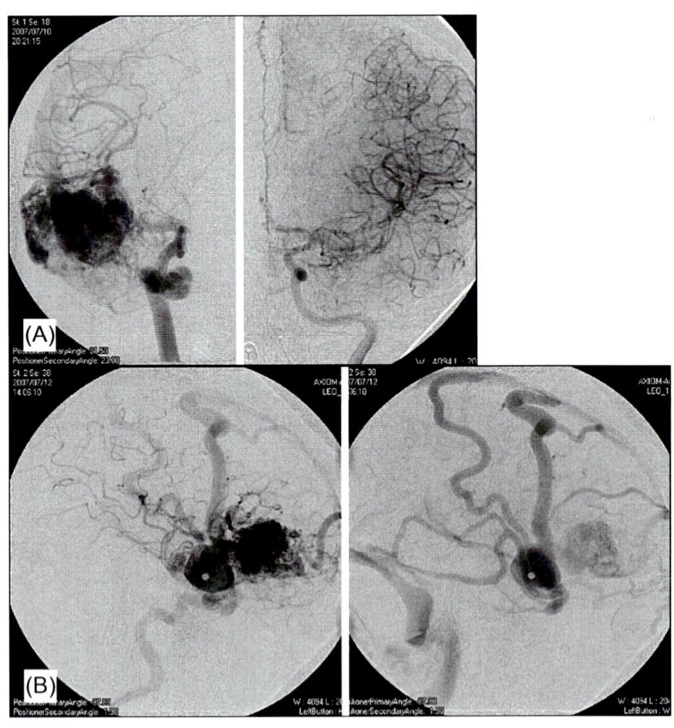

CS 1.3

shown, which demonstrate how the liquid material occludes individual arterial sections. The first two pairs (**CS 1.4**A,B) are AP views; note the orbit of the skull at the upper margin of the injected material. The third pair (**CS 1.4**C) is a lateral view. Approximately 80% of the arterial inflow to the AVM was occluded with this endovascular modality.

Neurosurgery

Subsequent neurosurgical resection of the AVM occurred the next day. A postoperative CT scan several days later (**CS 1.5**) shows hyperdense aneurysm coils at the midline (arrowhead), the hyperdense embolized material within the region of the AVM (arrows), and evidence of the right frontotemporal craniotomy, with extracranial swelling.

CS 1.4

Micropathology

The resected brain tissue (**CS 1.6**) is shown on elastin stains at low (40×; **CS 1.6**A) and high (100×; **CS 1.6**B) powers, and hematoxylin and eosin (H&E) stain (40×; **CS 1.6**C). The embolized Onyx material stains in a reticular, black pattern within the arterial lumens in all of these images (pathology courtesy of Dean Uphoff, MD).

Comments

This multidisciplinary approach is a typical treatment pattern for ruptured AVMs. First, endovascular treatments address the highest risk component (frequently a ruptured intracranial aneurysm) to prevent recurrent SAH, and then embolize arterial feeders to devascularize the AVM. Surgical extirpation follows at a later interval. Conventional angiography (not shown) would then later confirm that the AVM was effectively cured, without any residual, filling vascular structures.

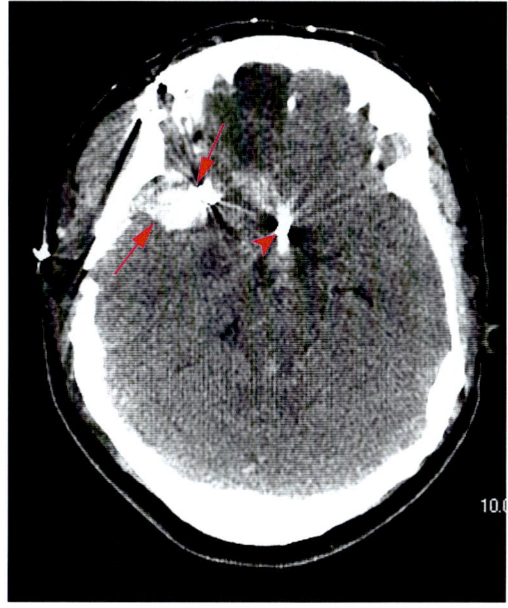

CS 1.5

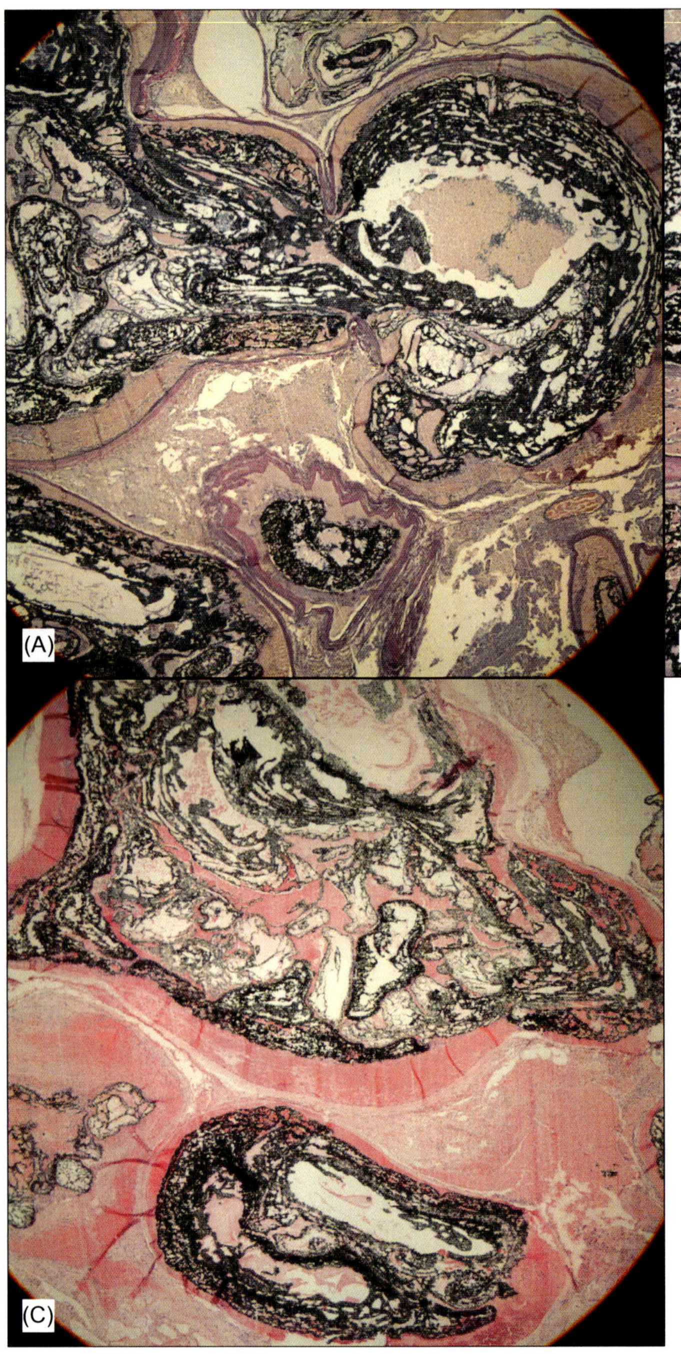

CS 1.6

Case study 2. Lobar hemorrhage due to AVM

A 25-year-old woman presented with severe deficits (diminished level of consciousness, dense aphasia, and right hemiparesis) due to an intracerebral hemorrhage, with significant ventricular involvement. The lesion is shown on admission head CT scan (**CS 2.1**), with contrast (left) and without (right).

Neurosurgery

The patient underwent emergent craniotomy on the day of admission, and postoperative studies are shown (**CS 2.2**): non-contrast head CT scan (**CS 2.2**A) at postoperative day 4 (left) and 9 (right) (the hyperdensity in the right frontal white matter is an external ventricular drain); and transaxial T2-weighted MRI with contrast at postoperative day 17 (**CS 2.2**B); and, finally, at 10 weeks following the initial hemorrhage (**CS 2.2**C). The eventual region of encephalomalacia is small, with mild enlargement of the lateral ventricle.

Micropathology (CS 2.3)

This shows severe arterial wall thickening on the H&E stain (**CS 2.3**A) and elastin stain (**CS 2.3**B) at high power (100×). The elastin stain, which normally stains the internal elastic lamina a dark purple, demonstrates abnormal fragmentation of this layer at multiple sites (arrowheads) (pathology courtesy of Dean Uphoff, MD).

Outcome

Follow-up cerebral angiography (not shown) demonstrated complete obliteration of the AVM. This patient made an excellent recovery, with only mild residual word-finding difficulty at 4 months following presentation and essentially no deficits at 1 year. The patient developed partial seizures that were controlled by a single anticonvulsant agent, levetiracetam.

Comments

The location of the hemorrhage, radiating outward from the periventricular region, is common for hemispheric AVMs. Appreciation of the underlying AVM on the admission head CT scan was initially obscured by the presenting hemorrhage. There was no opportunity to perform a pre-surgical conventional angiogram because of the emergent focus of treating the mass effect of this hemorrhage with a decompressive craniotomy. Fortunately, this single neurosurgical procedure alone was curative, with no residual large vessel lesion on subsequent angiography.

CS 2.1

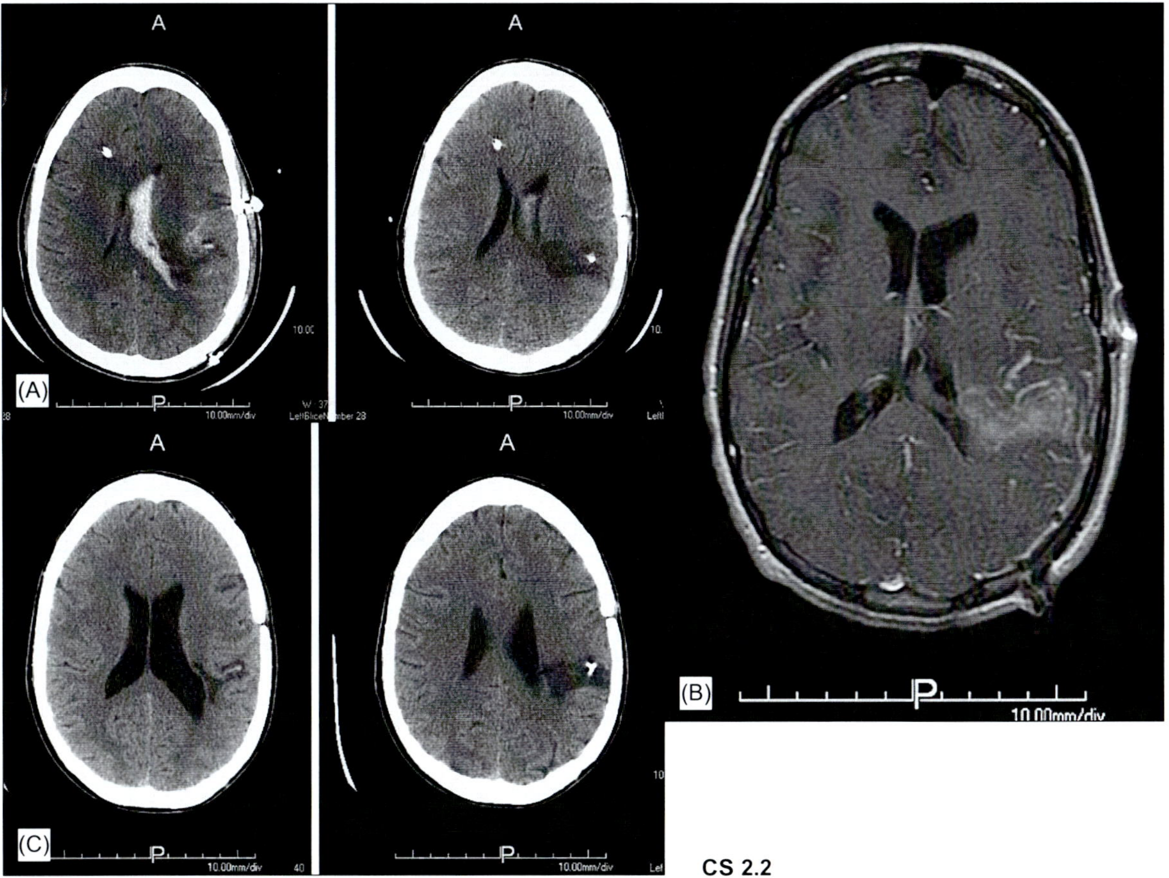

CS 2.2

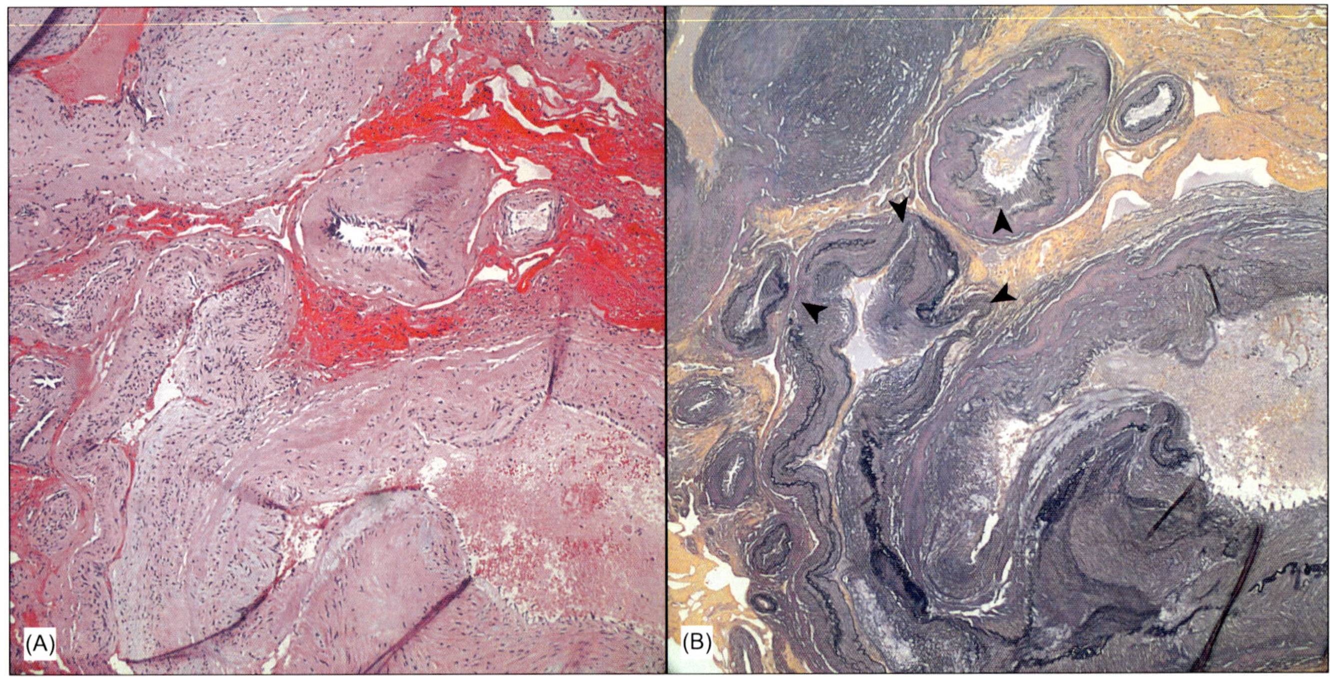

CS 2.3

Case study 3. Occipital AVM presenting with visual seizures

A 20-year-old college student presented with partial visual seizures (comprised of visual phenomena that she described as multicolored, poorly formed 'butterflies') due to an occipital AVM (**CS 3.1**). The initial MRI scan (**CS 3.1**A) showed a right occipital lesion on transaxial (left) and sagittal (right) images, involving predominantly the upper bank of the calcarine cortex, part of the primary visual cortex. Conventional angiography (**CS 3.1**B) shows the posterior cortical-based AVM supplied primarily by an enlarged right posterior cerebral artery (PCA) (arrowheads), on a mid-arterial phase. Early venous ectasia and drainage, during the late arterial phase (**CS 3.1**C), has been hand-marked with purple lines directly onto the X-ray film.

Treatment course (CS 3.2)

The lesion was initially embolized during an endovascular procedure (not shown), and, subsequently, vascular neurosurgery was prepared with three-dimensional brain mapping (**CS 3.2**A), isolating the AVM in various planes. Intra-operative images (**CS 3.2**B) are shown of the exposed, superficial lesion; note the abnormal, enlarged, gray–brown vessels on the surface of the operative bed in the occipitoparietal region; their appearance results from having been previously embolized. An image of the postoperative bed (**CS 3.2**C) is followed by one of the gross resected specimen in a Petri dish (**CS 3.2**D).

Outcome

Several years following surgery, the patient has required anticonvulsant therapy for visual seizures, but remains seizure-free on a single agent. She also has a patchy left inferior quadrantic visual field defect.

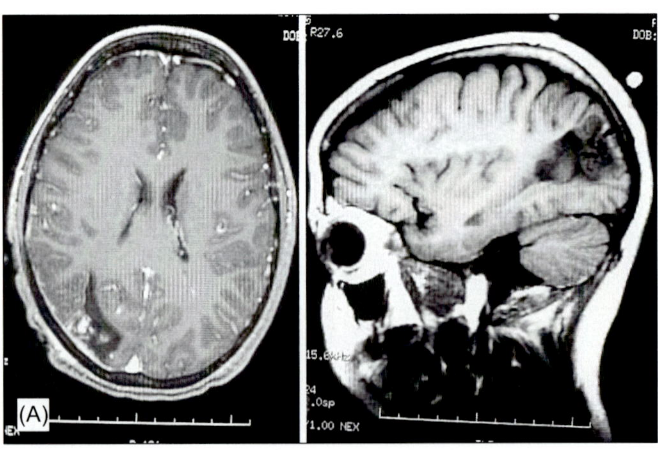

CS 3.1

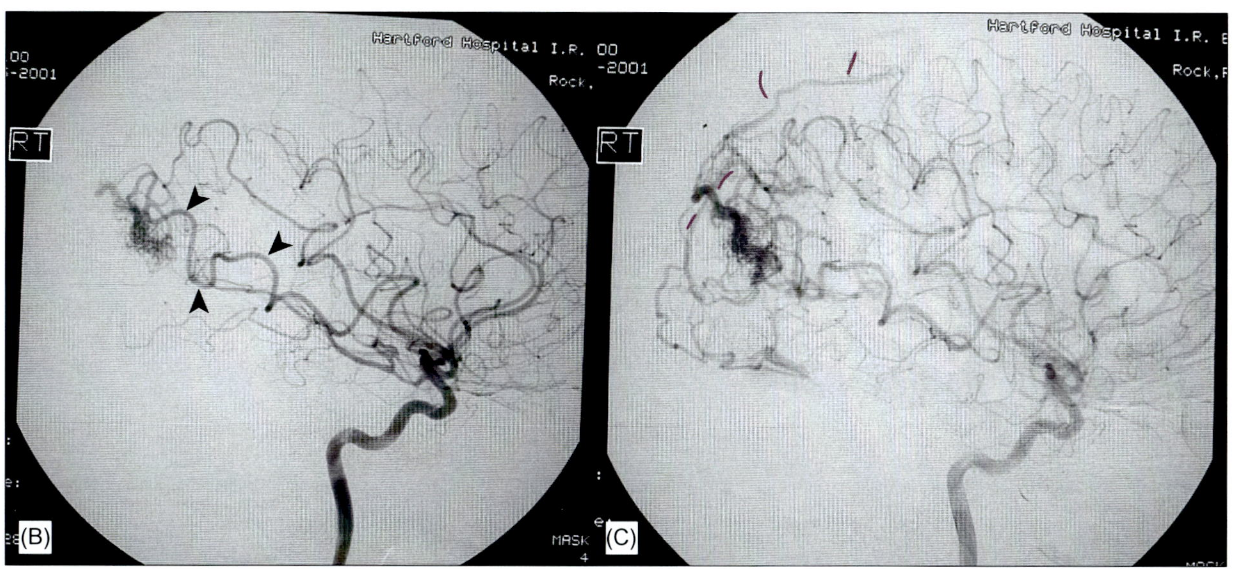

CS 3.1 (continued)

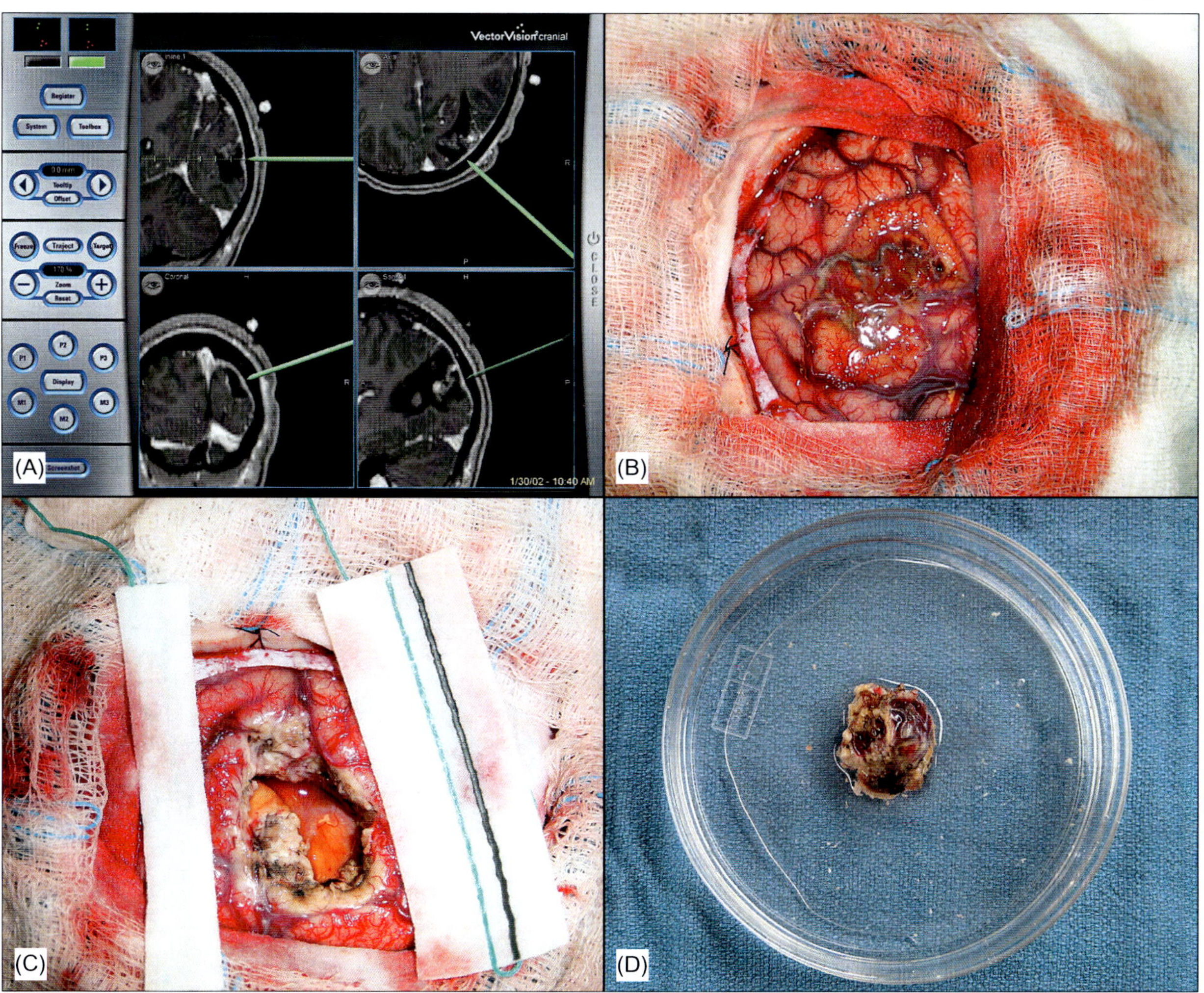

CS 3.2

Case study 4. Micro-AVF, with PCA and MCA supply

A healthy 27-year-old man presented with hemifield visual loss and headache while weight lifting. The onset specifically occurred during a Valsalva maneuver with bench-pressing. Admission head CT scan with contrast (**CS 4.1**) with contrast shows a small occipital hemorrhage with mild perihematomal edema (**CS 4.1**A). The CT angiography, sagittal image (**CS 4.1**B) readily demonstrates a yellow–orange hematoma within the posterior occipital lobe (arrows), but this study does not facilitate delineation of the arterial and venous supply to the region.

Angiography (CS 4.2)

An initial conventional angiogram (not shown) did not identify any clear arterial input responsible for this hemorrhage, but was obtained only days after the ictus. On a second angiogram obtained 5 weeks later by left vertebral injection (Townes projection; **CS 4.2**A), abnormal AV shunting in the left occipital polar region from the left PCA into a nearby cortical vein (arrowheads) is observed. A sequential view of this injection (**CS 4.2**B), from mid-arterial (far left) through to early venous (far right) phases, demonstrates the early venous filling into a cortical vein; this vein later ascends over the occipital convexity and drains into the superior sagittal sinus, but no discrete AVM nidus was observed.

Treatment (CS 4.3)

During a third angiogram, embolization of the left PCA arterial branch with NBCA was undertaken (not shown). An additional small distal MCA branch was identified on

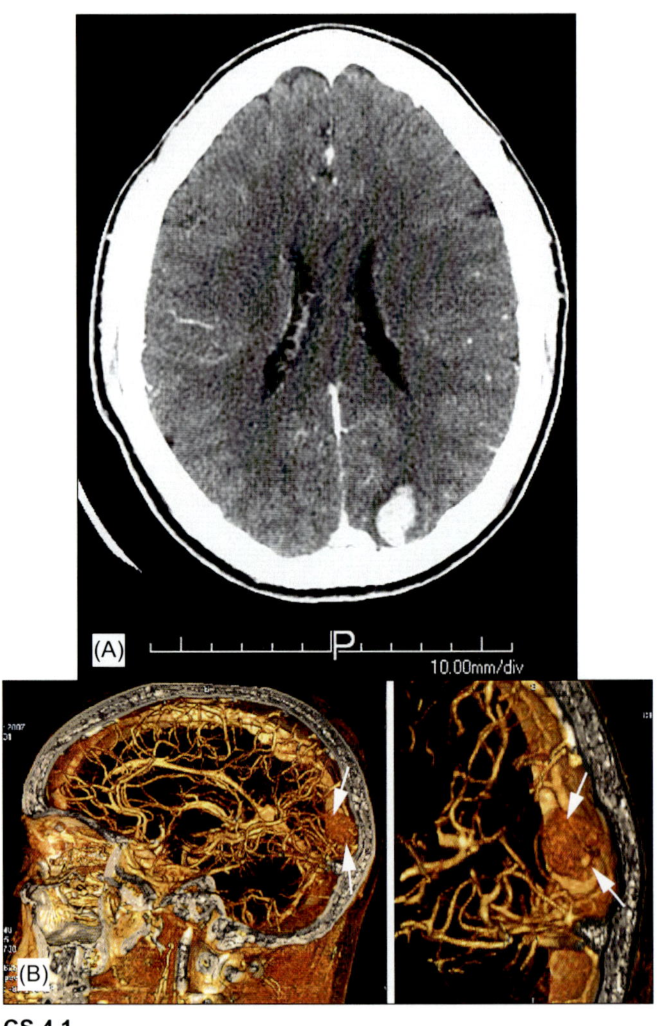

CS 4.1

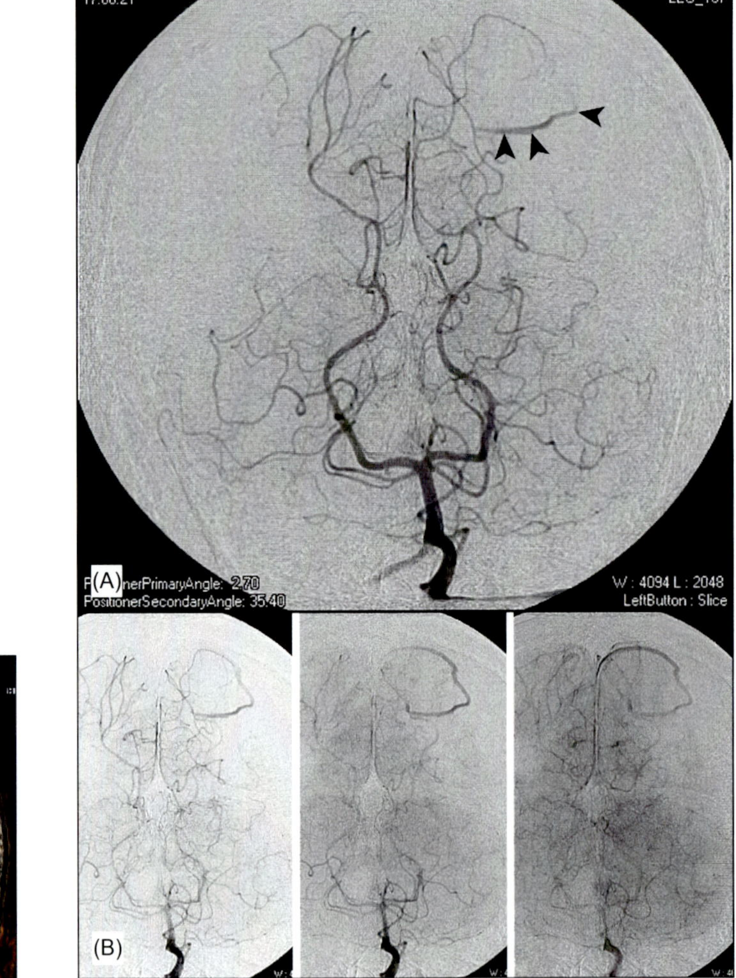

CS 4.2

left ICA injection (lateral view; **CS 4.3**A) with a single site of fistulization (arrow). A microinjection of its early filling into a cortical vein (arrows) is shown on two sequential images (**CS 4.3**B); the catheter tip is marked (arrowhead). This MCA branch was also embolized with NBCA.

Outcome

The patient developed mild worsening of the initial right visual field loss immediately after embolization of the PCA arterial feeder. An urgent MRI study documented a small acute ischemic stroke, an area of restricted diffusion on the diffusion-weighted imaging sequence (**CS 4.4**). Other than postprocedure complex partial seizures, controlled with oxcarbazepine, the patient has had a partial, right hemifield visual loss.

Comments

The initial angiography study probably failed to identify a vascular malformation because of local mass effect from the initial hemorrhage. The lack of a nidus on conventional angiography identified this lesion as a pial, or parenchymal-based, AV fistula. Embolization of the two major arterial branches (MCA and PCA) effectively cured the lesion so that it should not rebleed. This patient also suffered a small occipital stroke, a complication of the selective catheterization and embolization into the PCA branch of this lesion. The partial, residual, visual field loss has not prevented the patient from safely operating a motor vehicle.

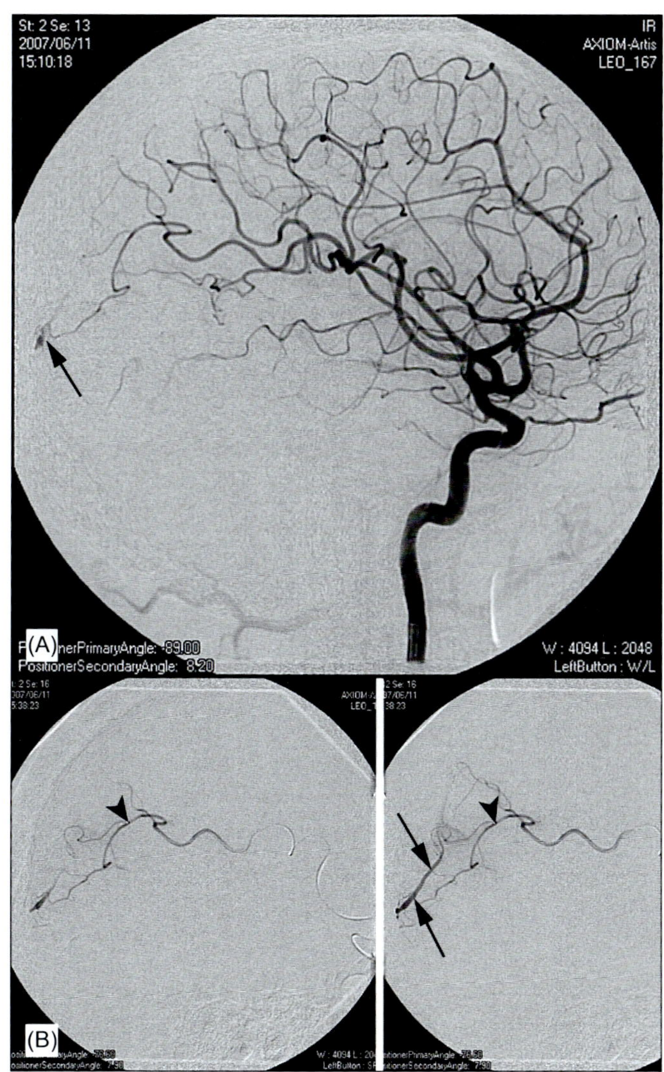

CS 4.3

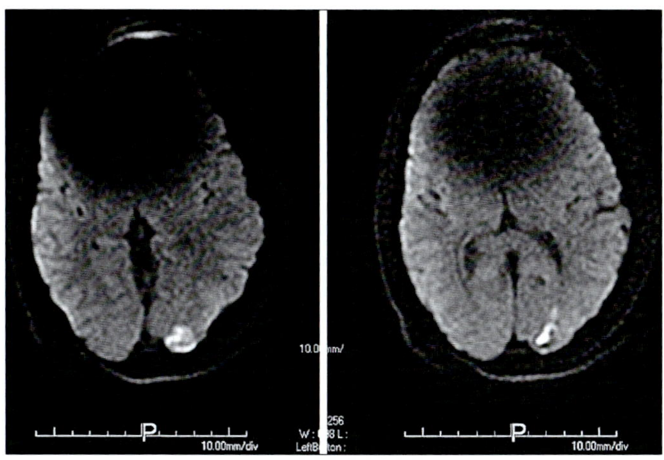

CS 4.4

References

1. Osborn A. Vascular malformations. In: *Diagnostic Cerebral Angiography*, 2nd edn. Philadelphia, PA: Lippincott Williams & Wilkins; 1999: 277–312.
2. The Arteriovenous Malformation Study Group. Arteriovenous malformations of the brain in adults. *N Engl J Med* 1999; **340**: 1812–18.
3. Friedlander R. Arteriovenous malformations of the brain. *N Engl J Med* 2007; **356**: 2704–12.
4. da Costa L, Wallace C, ter Brugge KG, O'Kelly C, Willinsky RA, Tymianski M. The natural history and predictive features of hemorrhage from brain arteriovenous malformations. *Stroke* 2009; **40**: 100–5.
5. Stapf C, Mast H, Sciacca RR, *et al.* Predictors of hemorrhage in patients with untreated brain arteriovenous malformation. *Neurology* 2006; **66**: 1350–5.

6. Al-Shahi R, Bhattacharya J, Currie D, *et al.* Prospective, population-based detection of intracranial vascular malformations in adults: the Scottish Intracranial Vascular Malformation Study (SIVMS). *Stroke* 2003; **34**: 1163–9.
7. Mast H, Young W, Koennecke H, *et al.* Risk of spontaneous haemorrhage after diagnosis of cerebral arteriovenous malformation. *Lancet* 1997; **350**: 1065–8.
8. Stapf C, Kham A, Sciacca R, *et al.* Effect of age on clinical and morphological characteristics in patients with brain arteriovenous malformation. *Stroke* 2003; **34**: 2664–9.
9. Fullerton H, Achrol A, Johnston S, *et al.* Long-term hemorrhage risk in children versus adults with brain arteriovenous malformations. *Stroke* 2005; **36**: 2099–104.
10. ApSimon H, Reef H, Phadke R, Popuvic E. A population-based study of brain arteriovenous malformation: long-term treatment outcomes. *Stroke* 2002; **33**: 2794–800.
11. Cockroft K. Unruptured cerebral arteriovenous malformations: to treat or not to treat [Editorial]. *Stroke* 2006; **37**: 1148–9.
12. Ondra S, Troupp H, George E, Schwab K. The natural history of symptomatic arteriovenous malformations of the brain: a 24-year follow-up assessment. *J Neurosurg* 1990; **73**: 387–91.
13. Halim A, Johnston S, Singh V, *et al.* Longitudinal risk of intracranial hemorrhage in patients with arteriovenous malformation of the brain within a defined population. *Stroke* 2004; **35**: 1697–702.
14. Kupersmith M, Berenstein A, Nelson P, ApSimon H, Setton A. Visual symptoms with dural arteriovenous malformations draining into occipital veins. *Neurology* 1999; **52**: 156–62.
15. Pelz D, Andersson T, Soderman M, Lylyk P, Negoro M. Advances in interventional neuroradiology 2005. *Stroke* 2006; **37**: 309–11.
16. Ogilvy C, Stieg P, Awad I, *et al.* Recommendations for the management of intracranial arteriovenous malformations: American Stroke Association. *Stroke* 2001; **32**: 1458–71.
17. Spetzler R, Martin N. A proposed grading system for arteriovenous malformations. *J Neurosurg* 1986; **65**: 476–83.
18. Vinuela F, Dion J, Duckwiler G, *et al.* Combined endovascular embolization and surgery in the management of cerebral arteriovenous malformations: experience with 101 cases. *J Neurosurg* 1991; **75**: 856–64.
19. Weber W, Kis B, Siekmann R, Kuehne D. Endovascular treatment of intracranial arteriovenous malformations with Onyx®: technical aspects. *AJNR* 2007; **28**: 371–7.
20. Maruyama K, Kawahara N, Shin M, *et al.* The risk of hemorrhage after radiosurgery for cerebral arteriovenous malformations. *N Engl J Med* 2005; **352**: 146–53.
21. Schauble B, Cascino G, Pollock B, *et al.* Seizure outcomes after stereotactic radiosurgery for cerebral arteriovenous malformations. *Neurology* 2004; **63**: 638–7.
22. Chaloupka J, Huddle D. Classification of vascular malformations of the central nervous system. *Neuroimaging Clin North Am* 1998; **8**: 295–321.

Further reading

Chaloupka J, Huddle D. Classification of vascular malformations of the central nervous system. *Neuroimaging Clin North Am* 1998; **8**: 295–321.

Friedlander R. Arteriovenous malformations of the brain. *N Engl J Med* 2007; **356**: 2704–12.

Ogilvy C, Stieg P, Awad I, *et al.* Recommendations for the management of intracranial arteriovenous malformations: American Stroke Association. *Stroke* 2001; **32**: 1458–71.

Osborn A. Vascular malformations. In: *Diagnostic Cerebral Angiography*, 2nd edn. Philadelphia, PA: Lippincott Williams & Wilkins; 1999: 277–312.

The Arteriovenous Malformation Study Group. Arteriovenous malformations of the brain in adults. *N Engl J Med* 1999; **340**: 1812–18.

The ARUBA Study (http://clinicaltrials.gov/ct/show/NCT00389181) The goal of this randomized controlled trial is to determine if the long-term outcomes of patients who receive medical management for symptoms (e.g., headache, seizures) associated with an unruptured brain AVM are superior to those who receive medical management and invasive treatment to eradicate the AVM. Assessment of incident hemorrhage risk and the identification of risk factors for hemorrhage from AVM are other components of this important trial.

Resources for patients

The Aneurysm and AVM Foundation (www.aneurysmfoundation.org/resources.html)

Chapter 4

Other Vascular Malformations

Introduction

This chapter reviews the smaller vascular malformations: cavernous malformations (CMs), developmental venous anomalies (DVAs), and capillary telangiectasias. These lesions are less likely to cause symptoms and major morbidity than arteriovenous malformations (AVMs).

Cavernous malformations

Cavernous malformations (CMs), also known as cavernous angiomas or cavernomas, are benign hamartomas—discrete, walled-off tissue of lobulated sinusoidal spaces lined by a single layer of endothelium and separated by collagenous stroma (**4.1**).[1] CMs are devoid of mature vascular wall elements, such as smooth muscle and elastin. Within the lesion itself, there is no normal brain parenchyma. They may also include a wide range of materials, including cholesterol crystals, calcium, bone, hyalinized tissue, thrombus, and blood-filled cysts (see **case study 1**).

Approximately 80% of CMs are supratentorial (**4.2**). The pons is the most common posterior fossa site (**4.3**). Multiple lesions suggest a hereditary etiology as >75% of familial cases harbor multiple CMs (**4.4, 4.5**).[1]

Epidemiology and natural history

The prevalence of CMs has been estimated at 0.1–0.7% of the general population.[2,3] Natural history data are challenging to obtain, because hemorrhages may often be subclinical, due to the typically small lesion size. Neurologic symptoms such as seizures may or may not be associated with radiologically documented hemorrhage (see **case study 1**).

The diverse clinical and radiological features associated with CM as well as varying reporting standards of CM hemorrhage prompted a recent systematic review.[4] A consensus statement defined CM hemorrhage as a combination of acute or subacute onset symptoms accompanied by evidence of recent extra- or intralesional hemorrhage, most often radiological.

Estimates of symptomatic CM hemorrhage range from 0.25 to 1%/person-year in sporadic cases versus up to 6.5%/person-year for familial lesions.[5,6] The age at presentation is usually 20–40 years. The prospective annual rate of hemorrhage for those without previous hemorrhage is 0.6% versus 4.5% for those with previous hemorrhage.[5]

Lesion behavior for CMs varies widely, and neurological disability depends largely upon location and repeated hemorrhage of individual lesions. Although CMs may be quiescent for years, repeated hemorrhage into eloquent tissue, such as the pons or basal ganglia, can cause severe morbidity and even mortality. A pseudotumoral growth of cavernous matrix due to re-hemorrhaging can be detected on magnetic resonance imaging (MRI).[1] Cavernomas are frequently associated with DVAs (**4.2, 4.3; case study 2**). One study of 57 patients with CM found that those with associated DVA had a higher likelihood of incident hemorrhage than those without DVA.[7] Patients with familial CMs have been demonstrated to develop *de novo* lesions.

Clinical presentation

Symptoms relate to lesion location. The most common cause of neurologic symptoms is hemorrhage into surrounding tissue, and related mass effect, causing seizures and/or headache. Brainstem lesions, due to the dense neuroanatomy, are frequently symptomatic (**4.3, 4.4, 4.6, 4.8**). In some patients, cavernomas develop in eloquent tissue and produce symptoms at an early age of life, regardless of whether or not they hemorrhage (**4.4**).

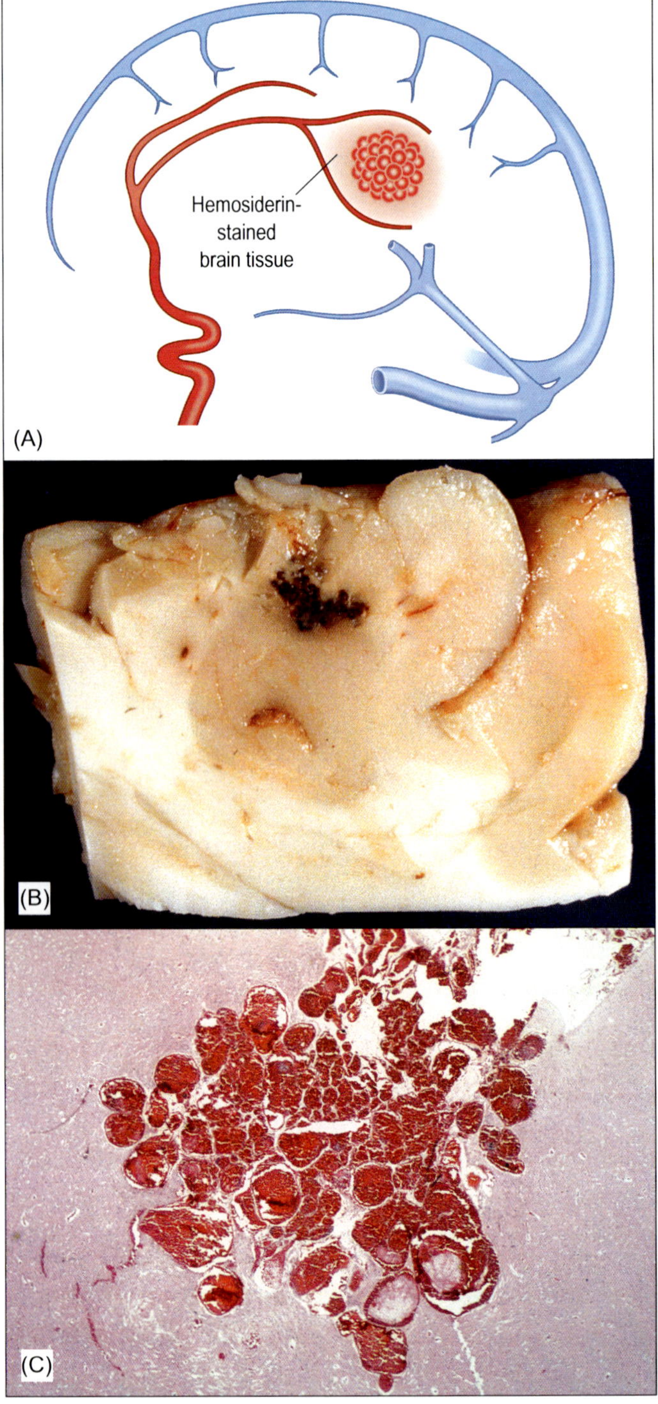

4.1 Cavernoma. An illustration demonstrates the concept of recurrent microhemorrhages, surrounded by a rim of hemosiderin-stained brain tissue (A). (Adapted from Osborn[1]). Gross pathology of a superficial, cortical CM. This lesion does not appear to have a significant capsule that would indicate prior hemorrhage (B). Micropathology shows a collection of simple blood-filled thin-walled endothelial, vascular spaces, without any normal intervening brain parenchyma (H&E, 100×) (C).

Neuroimaging

Cavernomas are considered 'angiographically occult' or 'cryptic' vascular malformations. Unless a CM is associated with a DVA, it should not be detected by conventional angiography. In contrast with AVMs, CMs are usually slow flow lesions, with no large venous outflow vessels or arterialized veins. Gradient-echo (GE) MRI sequences have vastly improved the sensitivity with which CM is detected, particularly in comparison with non-contrast computed tomography (CT) scans (**4.7**).[8] The GE-MRI frequently registers a lesion that appears larger than on other sequences, a so-called 'blooming artifact' (blackness of a lesion) caused by chronic blood products that are strongly paramagnetic, such as hemosiderin (e.g., **4.2**B, **4.3**A, **4.5**C, **4.6**B, **4.7**B, **4.8**A). This artifact occurs, because the GE-MR sequence is especially sensitive to small changes in the magnetic field.

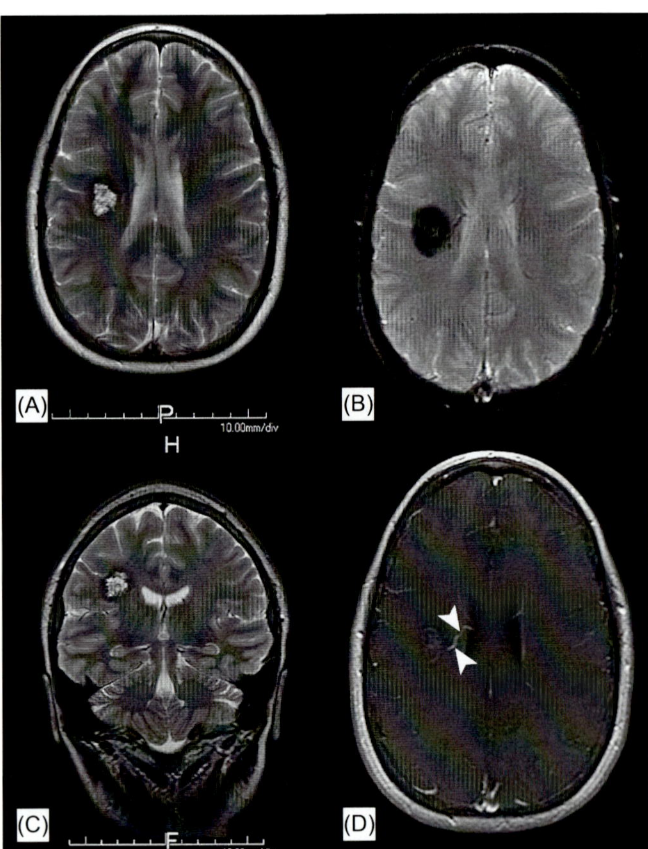

4.2 Large hemispheric CM. MRI sequences: T2-weighted, transaxial (A) and GE (B) sequences; coronal T1WI (C); and T1 with gadolinium (D) show a large CM based in the hemispheric white matter and an associated periventricular DVA (arrowheads). The lesion caused complex partial seizures, but would be high risk for neurosurgical resection, given its proximity to white matter tracts from primary sensory and motor cortex.

Brain MRI studies are also recommended for the screening of family members for occult CM when an inherited form of this disorder is suspected. Magnetic resonance imaging may underestimate the presence of an associated DVA when compared with conventional angiography.[7]

Management and outcomes

As CMs are typically small, benign vascular malformations, with limited symptoms associated with mass effect, neurosurgical resection is only considered in order to prevent morbidity and mortality associated with recurrent hemorrhages. Some CMs cause seizures and/or significant morbidity from repeated hemorrhage into eloquent tissue. Though peripheral lesions can be 'shelled out' by the neurosurgeon, there is some risk when these lesions abut or involve primary motor, sensory, or language areas (**4.2**, **4.8**). Deeper lesions, particularly in the brainstem, unless abutting the ventricular surface, will carry a high surgical morbidity and are often monitored conservatively over time, with clinical and radiographic follow-up evaluations (**4.3**, **4.4**, **4.6**, **4.8**). Newer image-guided modalities improve the localization of CM in deep and eloquent brain areas, facilitating microneurosurgical resection and reducing morbidity.[9] CMs are not directly supplied by large arteries; therefore, they cannot be accessed or treated by endovascular approaches.

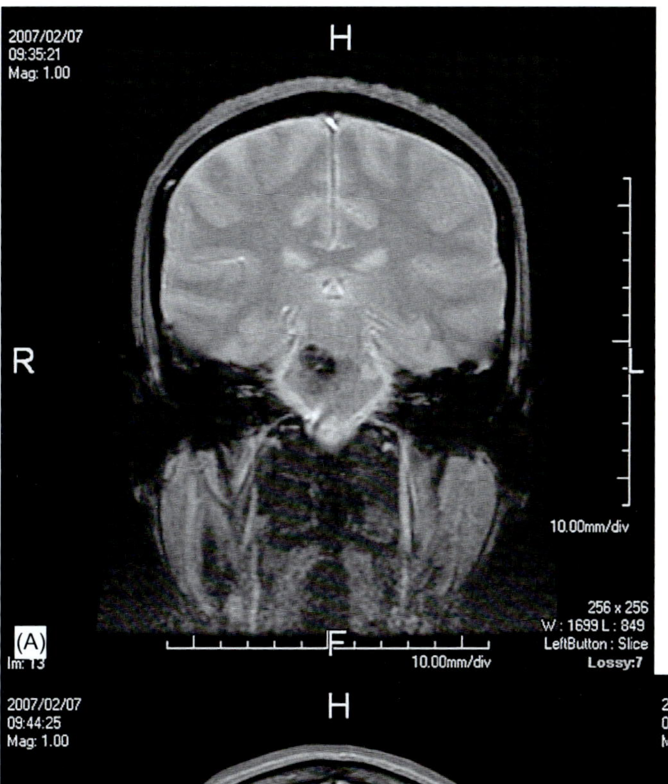

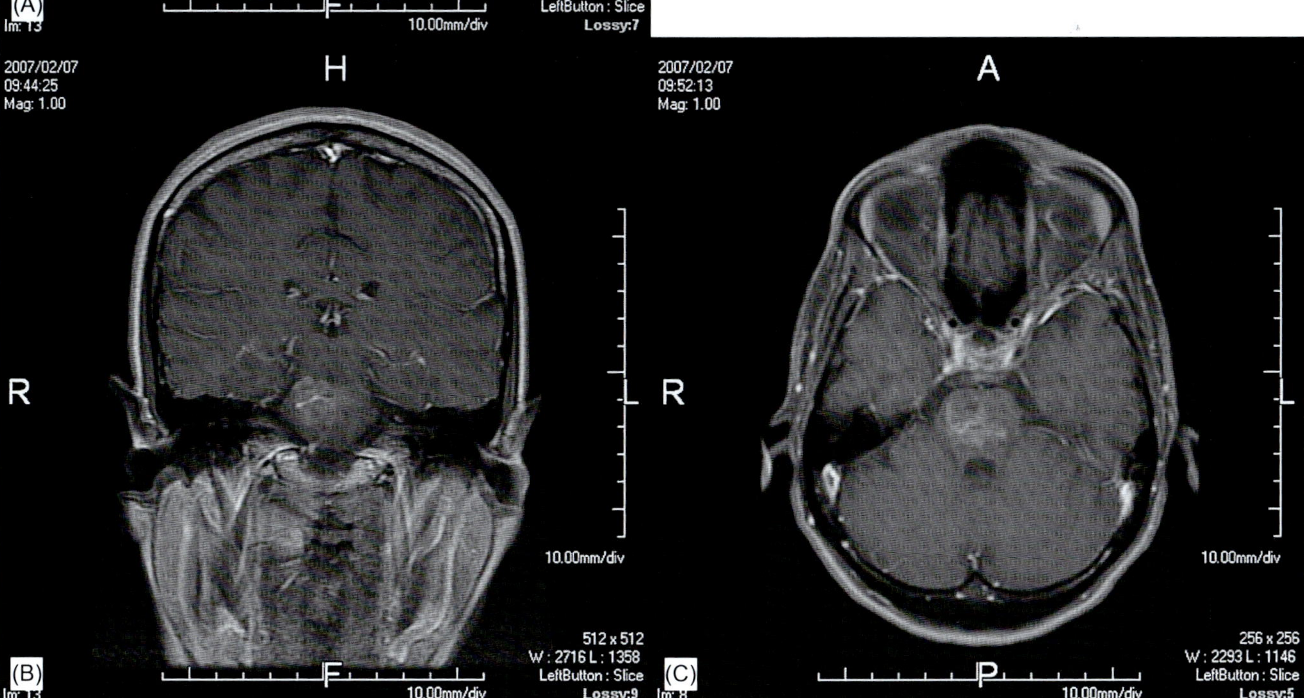

4.3 Pontine CM. A coronal GE-MRI (A); and coronal (B) and transaxial (C) T1WI with contrast sequences show a right pontomedullary lesion. A DVA appears as a contrast-enhancing component situated within the lesion (B,C). This brainstem lesion caused only mild right facial paresis.

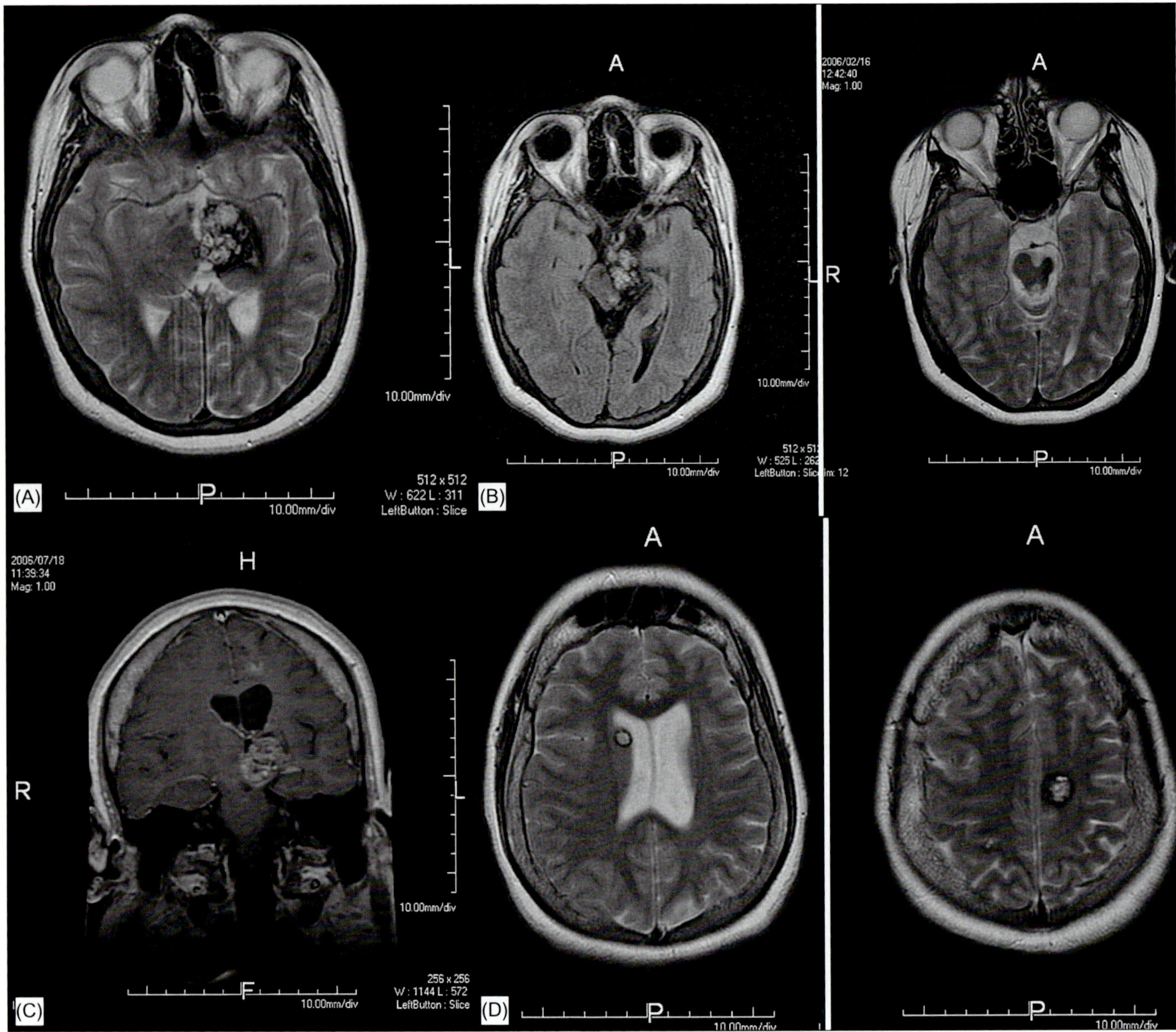

4.4 Multiple CMs. This 40-year-old patient was born with severe right-sided sensorimotor deficits, but MRI was not yet available to ascertain the diagnosis. Instead, the lesion was surmised based on the patient's clinical presentation and a normal conventional angiogram. The primary cause of perinatal morbidity is a large CM based in the left thalamus and midbrain, shown on transaxial T2WI (A) and FLAIR (fluid attenuated inversion recovery) (B, left), and a coronal contrast-enhanced T1WI (C) MRI. The lesion caused significant atrophy of the left cerebral peduncle (B, right; T2WI). Two hemispheric lesions on T2WI (D), adjacent to the right lateral ventricle (left) and in the left frontoparietal white matter (right), were asymptomatic.

Another approach to CM treatment is radiosurgery, particularly in patients with recurrent hemorrhages and whose lesions would carry an unacceptable risk for open neurosurgery. This modality may not help prevent recurrent hemorrhage from CM (or the benefit may be delayed roughly 2 years), but may control epilepsy.[10] In one study of gamma knife surgery, 26 of 49 patients (53%) were seizure-free following radiotherapy, with a highly significant decrease in seizures in 20%. The remaining 26% had little or no improvement.[11]

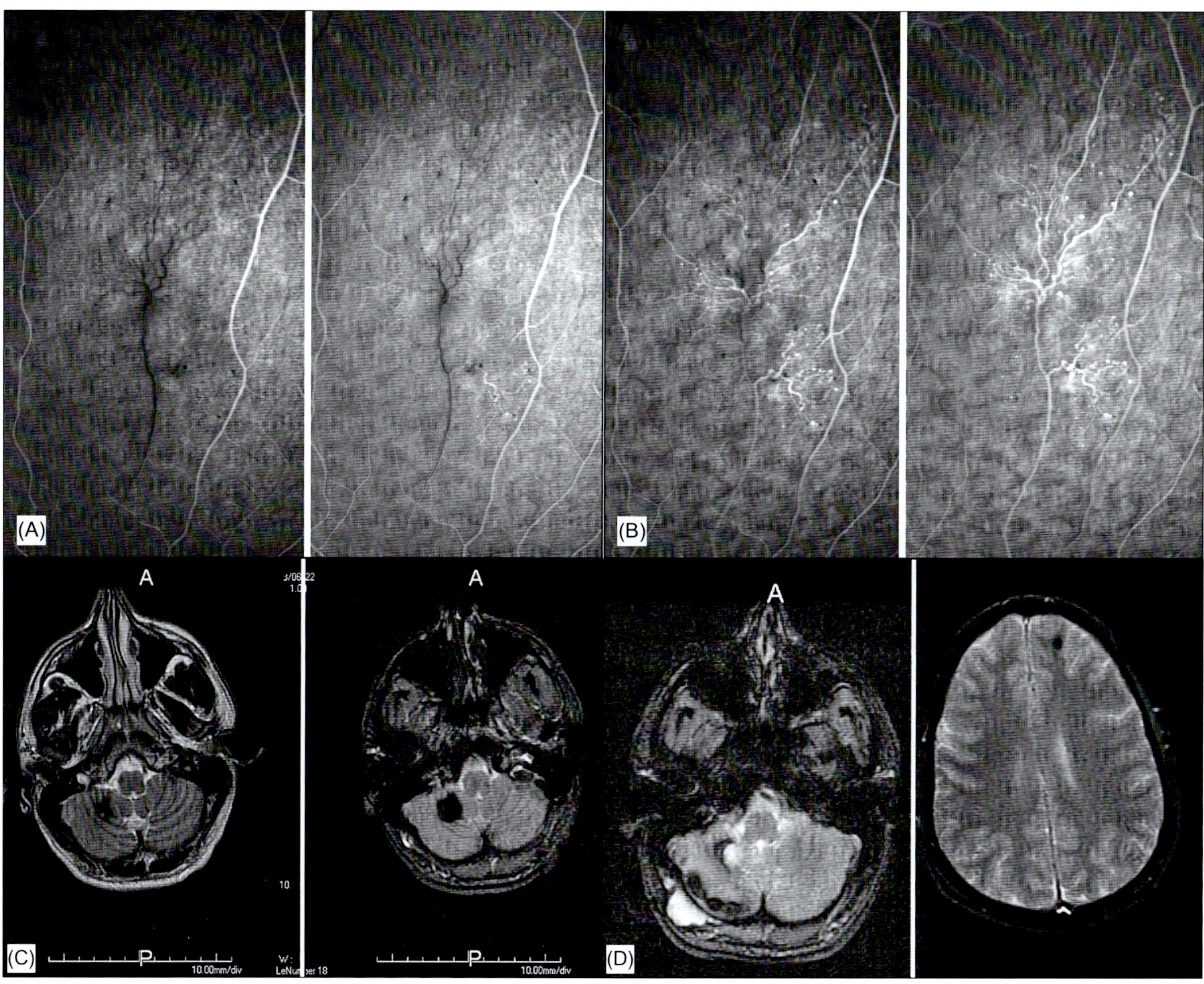

4.5 Cerebral and ocular CMs. A 27-year-old man was incidentally found to have a cavernous hemangioma in the peripheral retina of the right eye. Fluorescein angiography (A,B) shows progressive late filling of the distal most telangiectatic vessels, which demonstrate some local microaneurysms and leakage of dye. The brain was subsequently imaged. The transaxial MR sequences (C), T2WI (left) and GE (right), show a CM in the right cerebellar hemisphere, 2 cm wide, that was resected. A postoperative GE-MRI (D) shows the former lesion site (left) and a 5 mm left frontal CM (right).

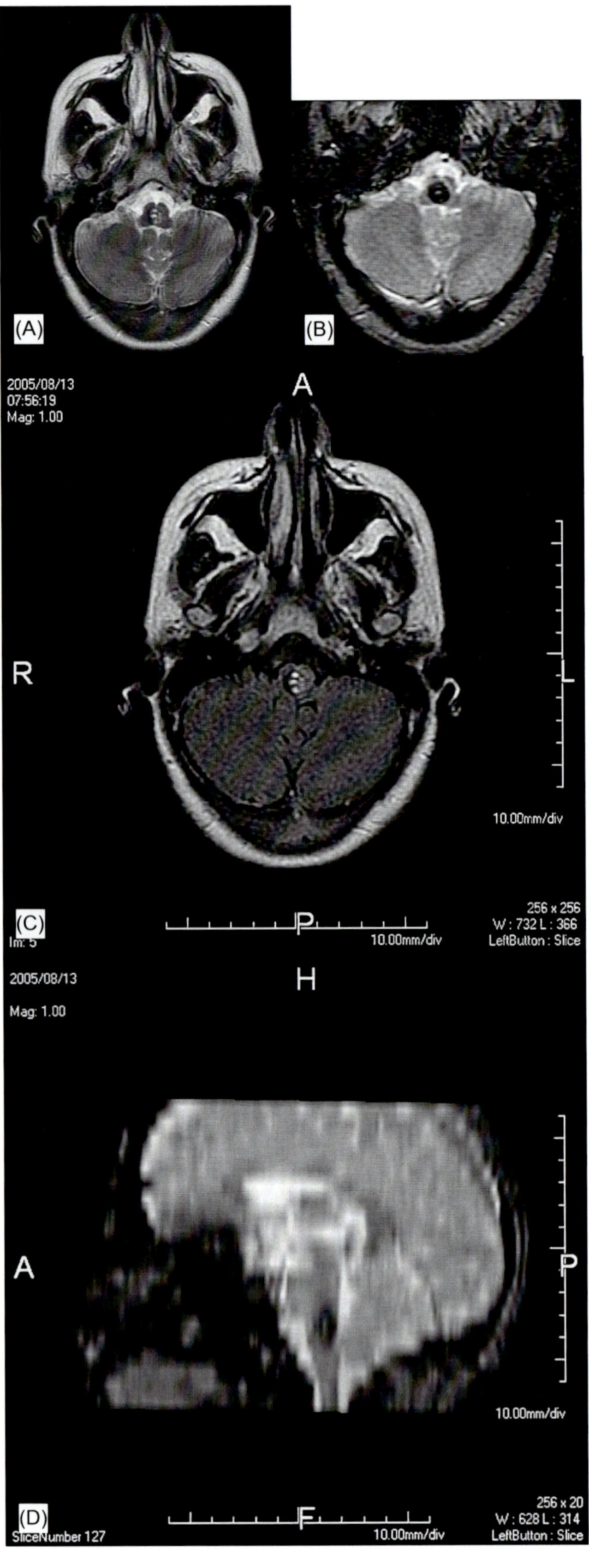

Developmental venous anomalies

Formerly known as venous angiomas, a DVA represents the dilation of a single or cluster of medullary (white matter) veins, particularly in the periventricular regions, converging into an enlarged transcortical or subependymal draining vein (**4.8**).[1] Frequently, these multiple, small branches drain into a single large vein in a 'caput medusae' pattern (**4.9–4.11**).[1] A DVA is composed entirely of thickened, hyalinized veins containing minimal smooth muscle and elastic tissue. Interspersed brain parenchyma is normal.[12] The pattern of venous development in DVA formation is likely a normal congenital variant. One hypothesis is that a DVA represents a developmental arrest, in that the primitive larger venous channels of embryonic life do not fully coalesce, even though normal arterial development is already complete.[1]

Of the four types of vascular malformations, DVA are the most common, accounting for up to 60% of all cerebral vascular malformations at autopsy.[1] Their prevalence may be as high as 3% in the general population.[13] The most common sites are frontal lobe (55.6%) and cerebellum (27%).[14] Lesions in the cerebral hemispheres are usually situated adjacent to the lateral ventricles.

Natural history and clinical presentation

Typically, DVAs are incidental, solitary lesions that do not cause neurologic symptoms.[13-15] The major exception is the frequent association of DVA with CMs that can hemorrhage into adjacent brain tissue (**4.2**, **4.4**; **case study 2**).[13] They may also rarely contribute to the development of seizures, neurologic deficits, and chronic but benign headaches.[13-15] However, DVAs do not change intracranial pressure or cause traction on superficial veins that would be anticipated to precipitate headache. Mechanisms other than hemorrhage for causing symptoms include mechanical (i.e., hydrocephalus or neurovascular compression of cranial nerves) and flow-related (i.e., increased when a DVA is associated with a AV shunt or venous congestion).[16] Two studies document a very low risk of hemorrhage, at 0.15% and 0.34% per year.[13,14]

4.6 Medullary CM. A 45-year-old patient presented with a self-limited episode of hemisensory loss, dysphagia, dizziness, and gait difficulty. The MRI study shows a lesion in the right rostral medulla, approximately 4 mm wide, on transaxial T2WI (A), GE (B), and FLAIR (C) sequences, and a reconstructed sagittal view (D).

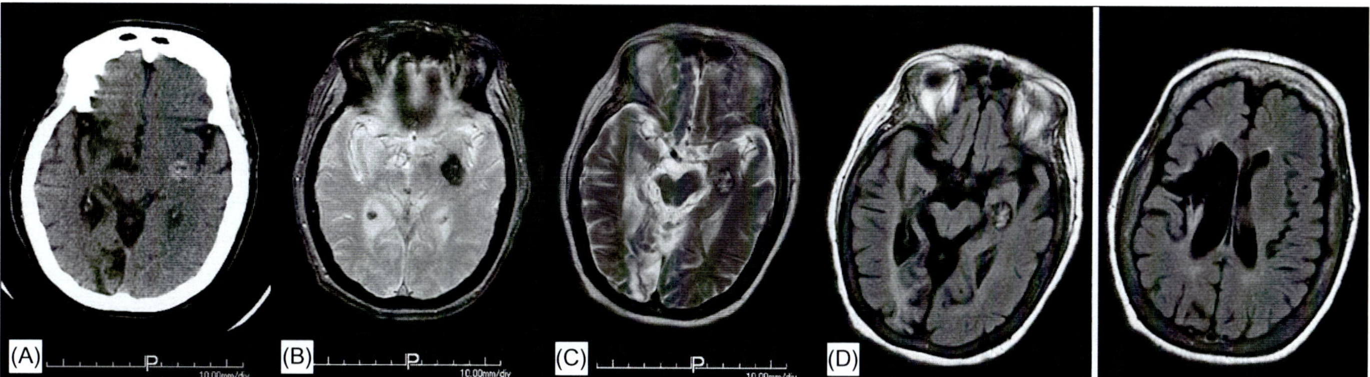

4.7 Cavernoma on CT versus MRI. A non-contrast head CT scan shows a heterogeneous hyperdense lesion in the left medial temporal lobe (A); this hyperdensity could be due to calcification or microhemorrhage. Transaxial GE (B), T2WI (C), and FLAIR (D, left) sequences demonstrate that this lesion has the typical 'popcorn' appearance of a CM. Unrelated to the CM, a chronic, right MCA stroke (D), is also evident, with *ex vacuo* enlargement of the adjacent lateral ventricle (right) and Wallerian degeneration, evidenced by atrophy of the right cerebral peduncle (left).

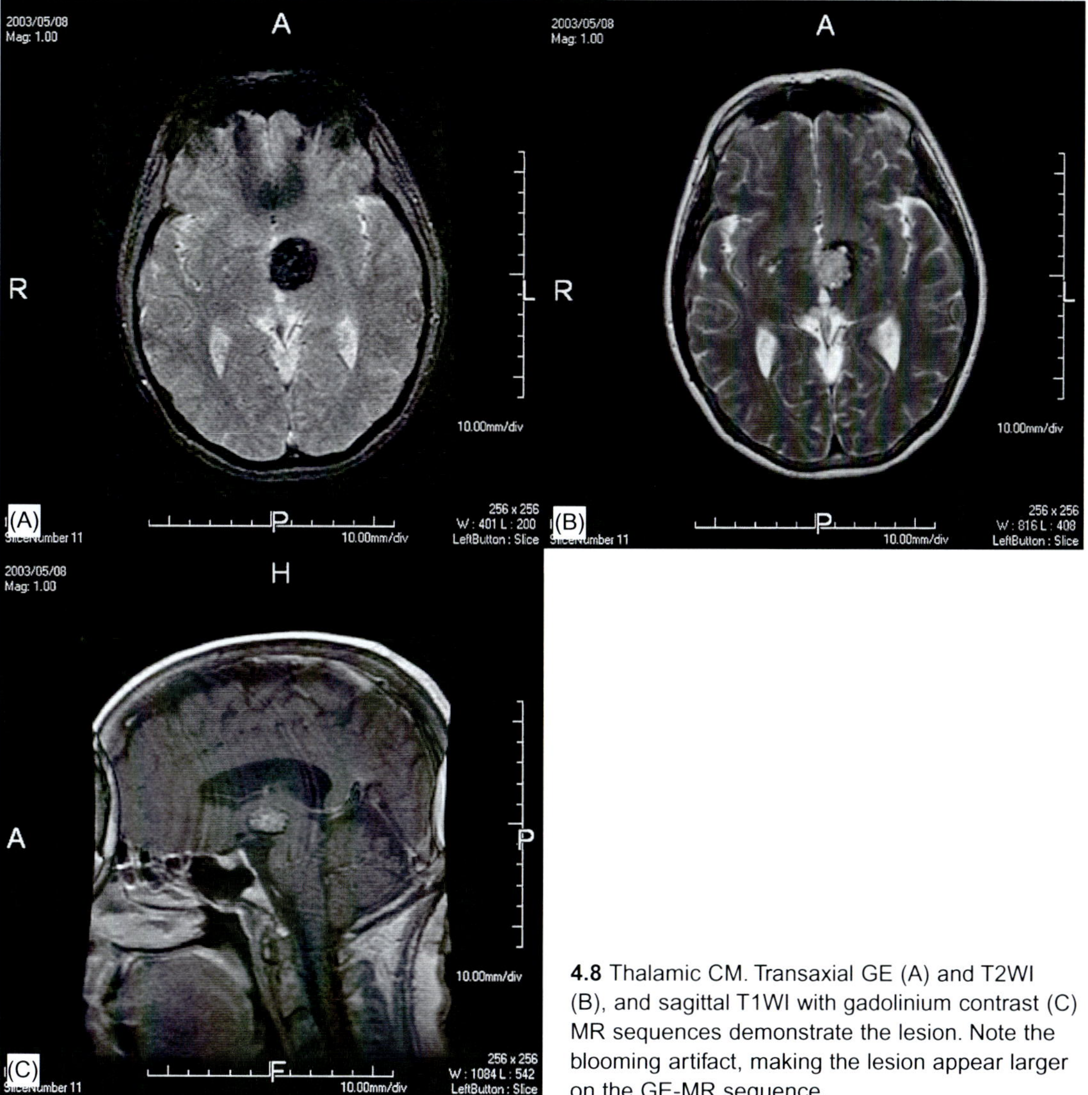

4.8 Thalamic CM. Transaxial GE (A) and T2WI (B), and sagittal T1WI with gadolinium contrast (C) MR sequences demonstrate the lesion. Note the blooming artifact, making the lesion appear larger on the GE-MR sequence.

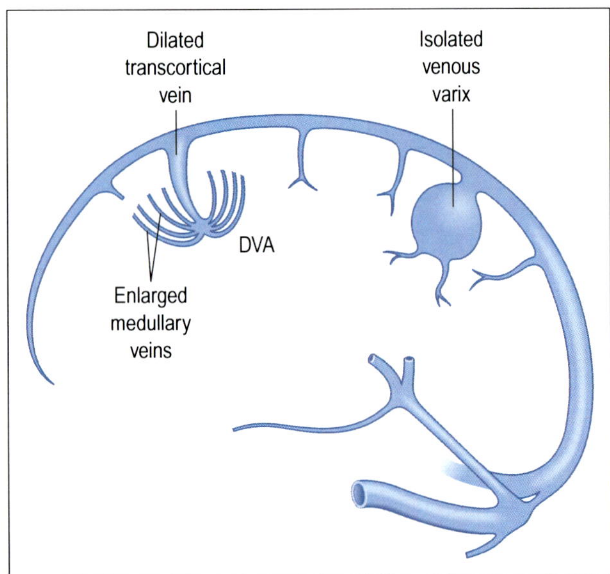

4.9 Venous malformations. This illustration shows two types of venous malformations. A DVA or venous angioma, is an umbrella-shaped collection of enlarged medullary veins that drain a dilated transcortical vein. An isolated venous varix, a dilatation of cerebral veins that more often is associated with a vein of Galen malformation (**4.14**) or other high-flow vascular shunts, is also depicted (adapted from Osborn[1]).

Neuroimaging

The caput medusae pattern of DVAs is evident in the late venous phase of angiography (**4.10**; **case study 3**), though circulation time and arterial phases of this study are normal.[14] On MRI, the lesion typically is contrast enhancing (**4.11, 4.12**; **case studies 2 and 3**).

Management

The low morbidity and hemorrhage rates of DVAs dictate conservative management.[13,14] Because they drain normal intervening parenchyma, DVAs should usually not be removed surgically.[16] The primary risk of surgery is venous infarction with local edema and/or hemorrhage into normal brain tissue.[13] Neurosurgical intervention may rarely be indicated for refractory seizures or acute hemorrhage, but in most of these cases, an associated CM is the target for resection (**case study 2**). Small branches of the caput medusae may be sacrificed if necessary, but most of the venous anatomy should be preserved.[13] There is no evidence that antithrombotic agents pose greater hemorrhage risk for patients with DVA. There is no recommended restriction from normal activities or pregnancy due to the presence of a DVA.

Atypical developmental venous anomalies

Occasionally, DVAs may assume diverse and large patterns that contribute to a markedly abnormal early development of the venous system (see **case study 3**). A rare but important cause of perinatal morbidity is the vein of Galen malformation (VGM) (**4.13**). Usually, a vein of Galen malformation presents in the newborn or infants with high-output congestive heart failure, due to extensive shunting of blood to this malformation and away from the body (**4.14**). Associated symptoms of the vein of Galen malformation may be tachycardia, respiratory distress, cyanosis, and cranial bruit, while complications include obstructive hydrocephalus, venous thrombosis, and hemorrhage; atrophy of adjacent structures due to compression, steal phenomena, or frank ischemia; and periventricular leukomalacia.

Capillary telangiectasias

Capillary telangiectasias, also called capillary malformations, are small nests of dilated capillaries interspersed with normal brain tissue, usually <2.0 cm in diameter.[1,17,18] Their walls resemble normal capillaries, without smooth muscle or elastic fibers (**4.15**). They are the second most common developmental anomaly after DVA, with an estimated prevalence at autopsy of 0.4%.[18] They may be found anywhere in the central nervous system, though the pons is the most common site. The cerebellum, diencephalic regions, and spinal cord are also frequently involved.[18]

It is believed that capillary telangiectasias are virtually always asymptomatic. Hemorrhages are usually subclinical, incidental findings on MRI. Before the advent of MRI, they were solely identified at autopsy, as they are too small to confidently be identified by CT imaging. On GE-MRI sequences, capillary telangiectasias may manifest as areas of signal loss. These lesions also have homogeneous contrast enhancement, but lack the hemosiderin rim of CMs.[18,19] With the exception of telangiectasias associated with DVA, these lesions are not identified by conventional cerebral angiography, as they are too small and isolated from the major cerebral vasculature.

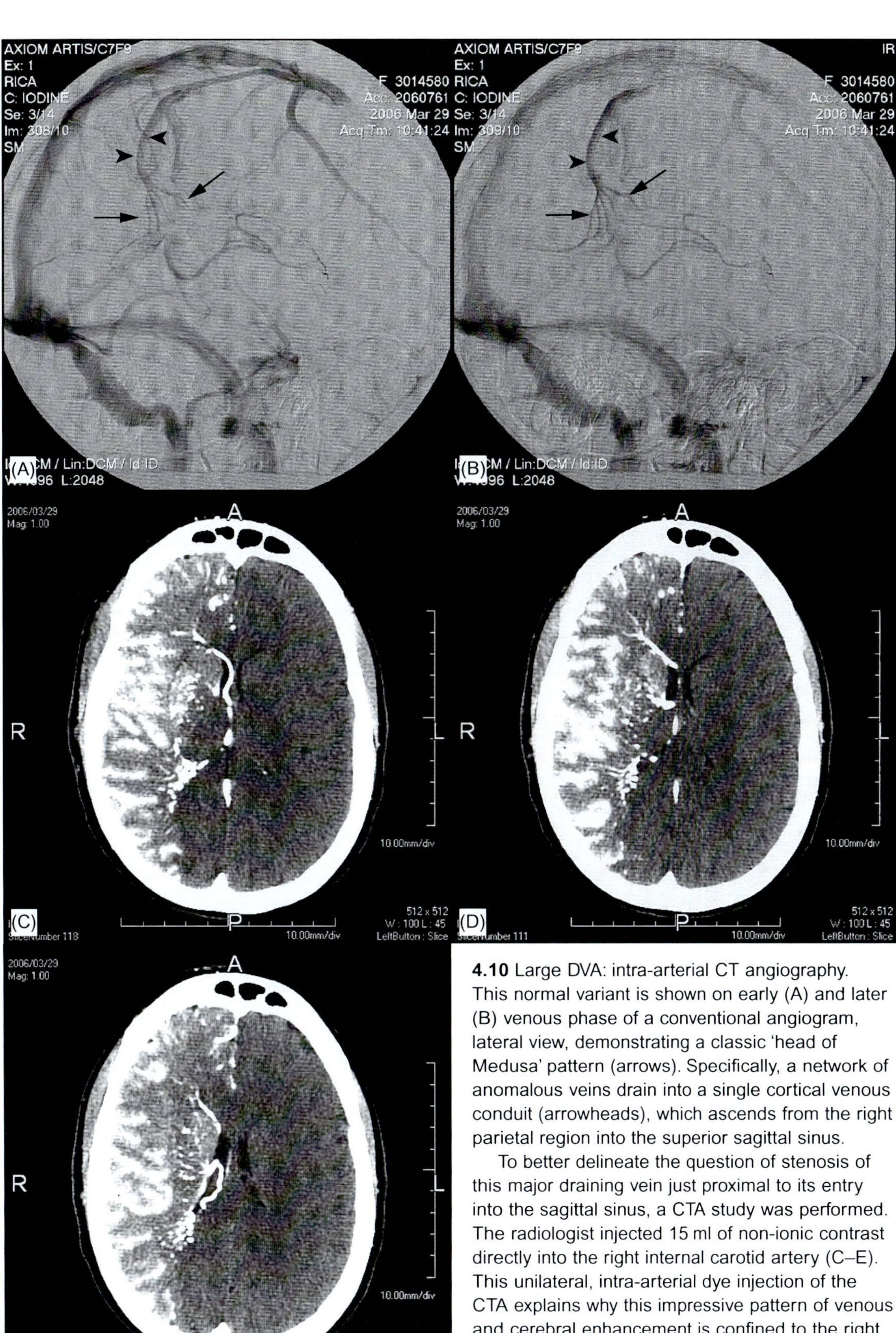

4.10 Large DVA: intra-arterial CT angiography. This normal variant is shown on early (A) and later (B) venous phase of a conventional angiogram, lateral view, demonstrating a classic 'head of Medusa' pattern (arrows). Specifically, a network of anomalous veins drain into a single cortical venous conduit (arrowheads), which ascends from the right parietal region into the superior sagittal sinus.

To better delineate the question of stenosis of this major draining vein just proximal to its entry into the sagittal sinus, a CTA study was performed. The radiologist injected 15 ml of non-ionic contrast directly into the right internal carotid artery (C–E). This unilateral, intra-arterial dye injection of the CTA explains why this impressive pattern of venous and cerebral enhancement is confined to the right hemisphere (radiologic study processed by Gary Spiegel, MD).

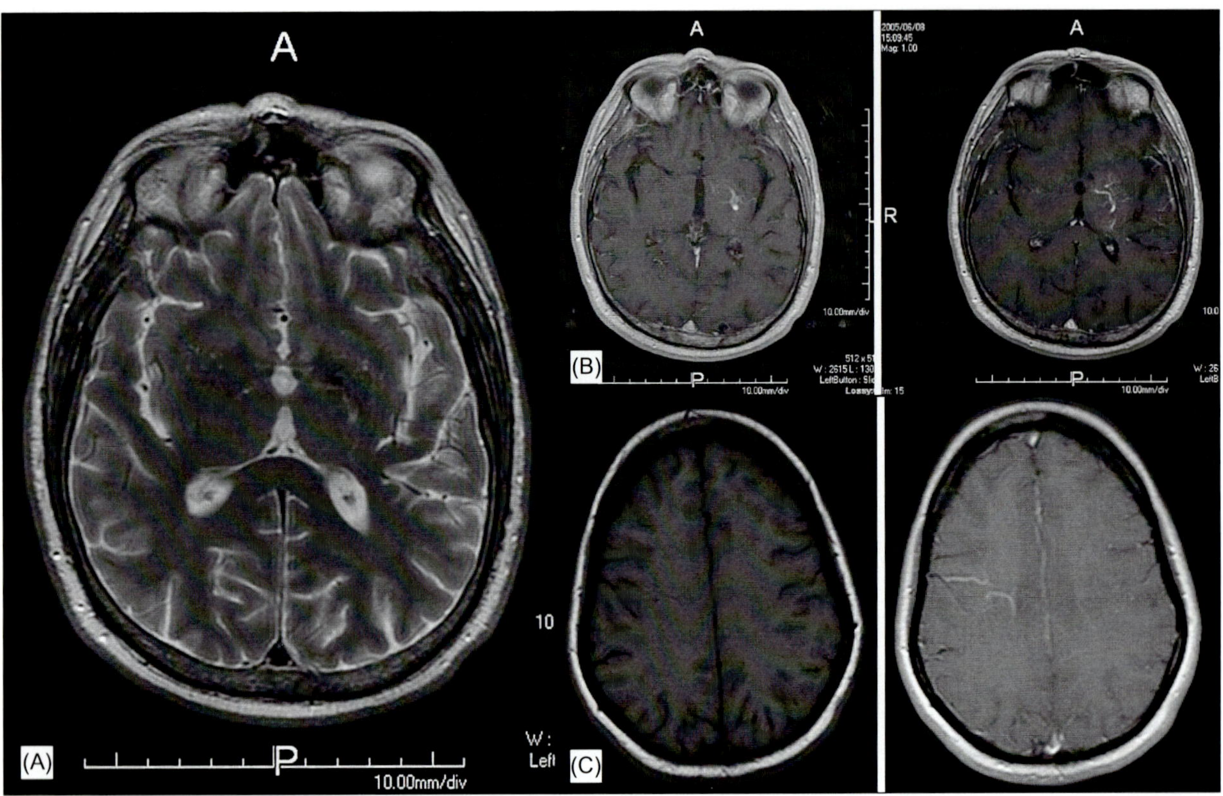

4.11 Contrast-enhanced MRI of DVAs. Two typical DVAs are shown on MRI sequences, without and with gadolinium. The first is shown on a T2WI sequence (A), followed by two adjacent slices of the T1WI with gadolinium (B). The second is shown as a T1WI without (C, left) and with gadolinium (C, right). Often, contrast administration is essential to detecting a DVA.

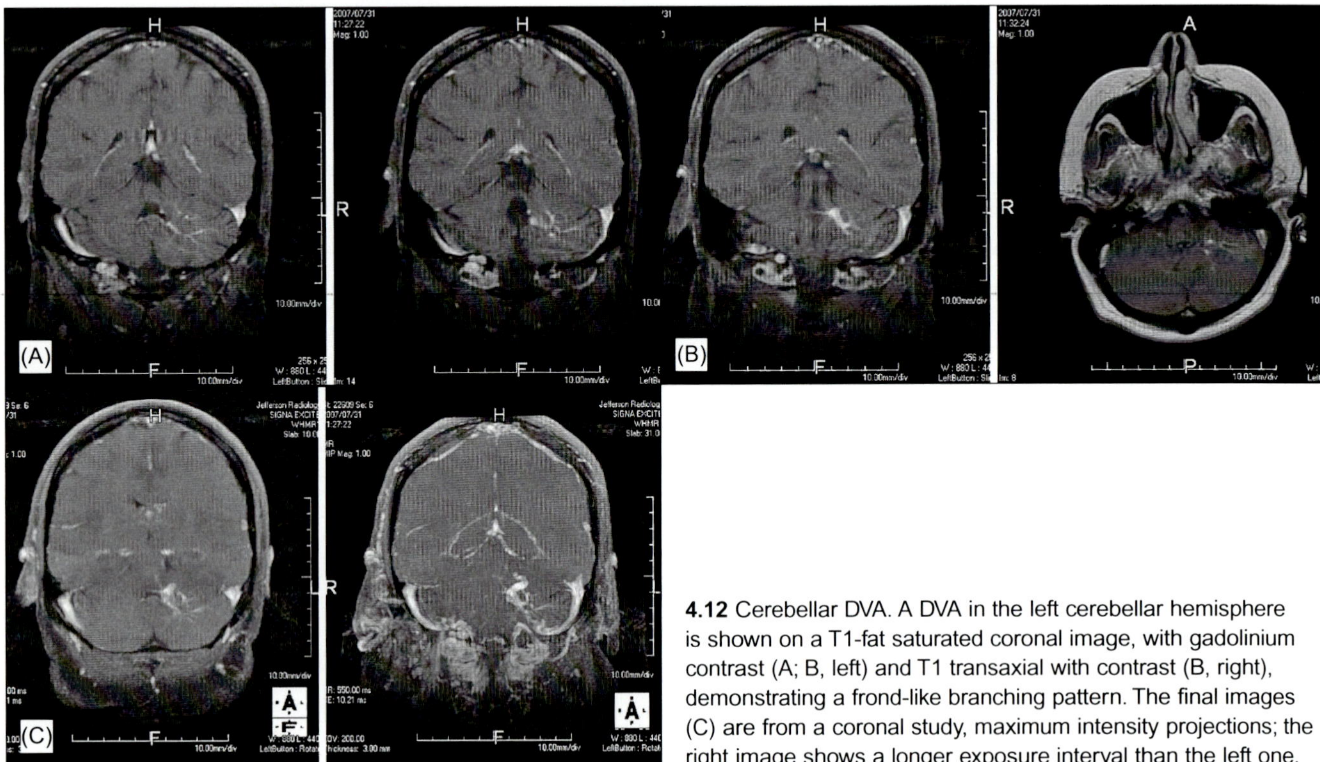

4.12 Cerebellar DVA. A DVA in the left cerebellar hemisphere is shown on a T1-fat saturated coronal image, with gadolinium contrast (A; B, left) and T1 transaxial with contrast (B, right), demonstrating a frond-like branching pattern. The final images (C) are from a coronal study, maximum intensity projections; the right image shows a longer exposure interval than the left one.

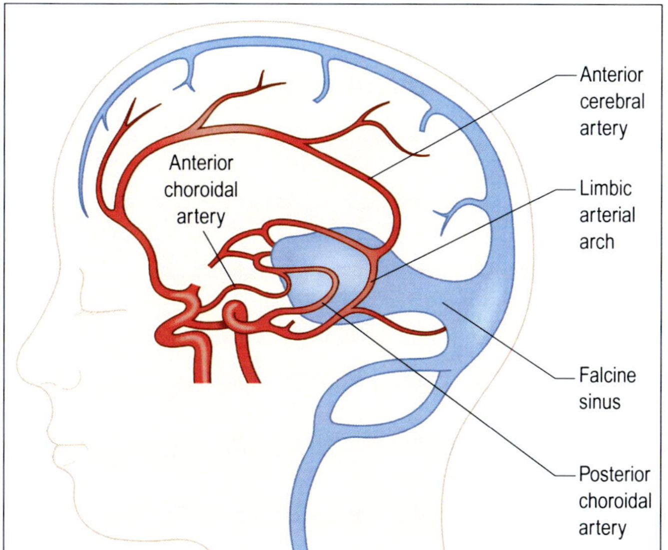

4.13 Vein of Galen malformation anatomy. The pathophysiology of this lesion involves a massively enlarged galenic (neonatal) venous system from a thalamic AVM or choroidal AV fistula, due to the persistence of an embryonic vascular channel, the median prosencephalic vein. Enlarged choroidal and pericallosal (anterior cerebral artery) branches drain, via direct, mural-type fistulae, into a primitive accessory sinus, the falcine sinus. (adapted with permission from Osborn[1]).

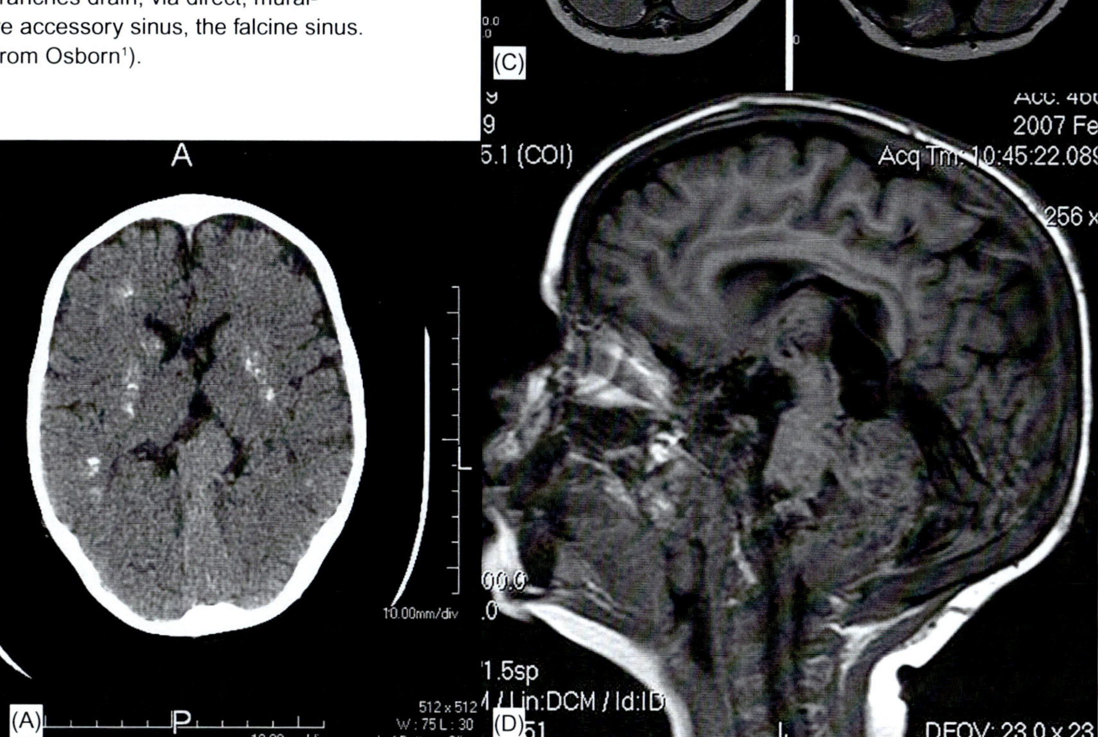

4.14 Vein of Galen malformation. This newborn's non-contrast head CT scan (A) shows bilateral calcifications (hyperdensities) in the hemispheric white matter and external capsules, bilaterally. This dystrophic calcification in a neonate may be attributed to subacute venous ischemia. The lesion is appreciated on transaxial (B) and coronal (C) T2-weighted MR sequences, as well as a sagittal T1-weighted image (D). In addition to the massive midline venous structure, the coronal study (C, right) suggests an AVM in the region of the left thalamus (arrows).

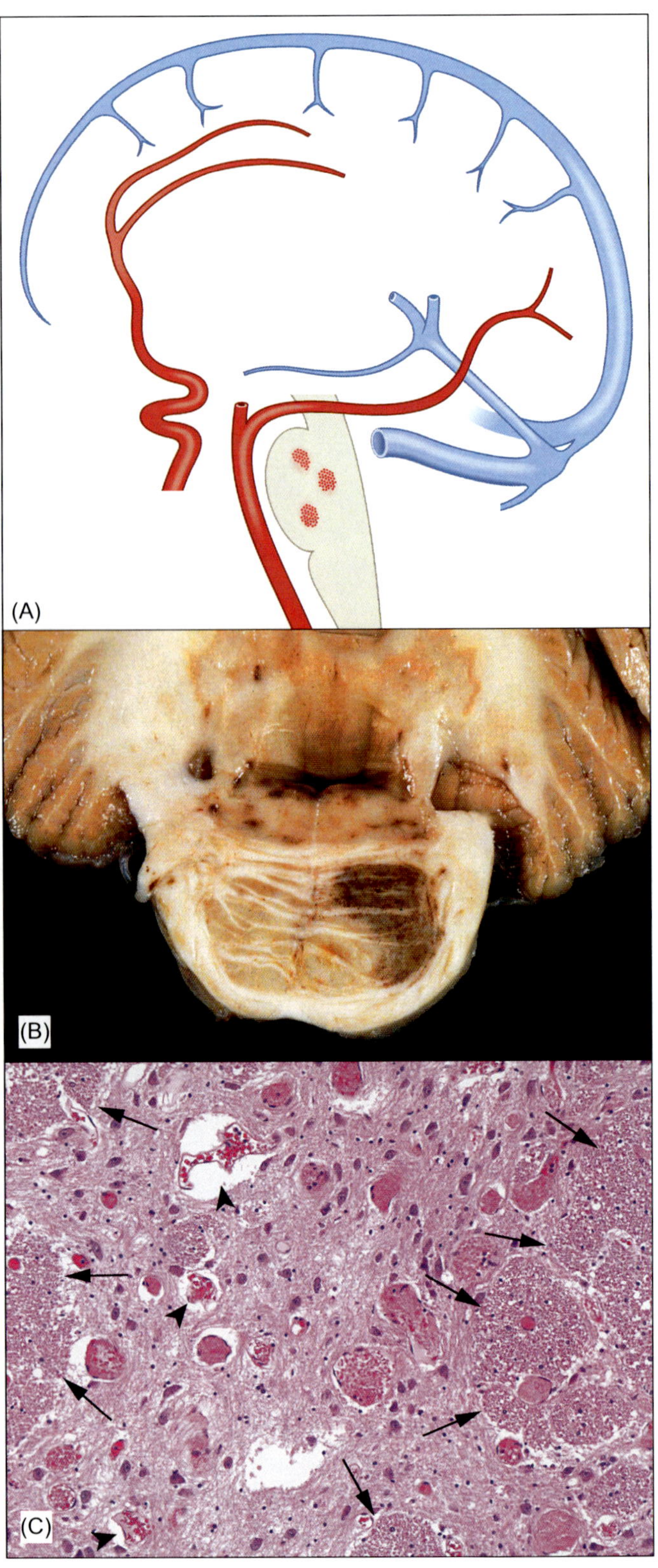

4.15 Capillary telangiectasia. Illustration of capillary telangiectasias, punctate lesions often found in the pons (A) (illustration adapted from Osborn[1]). Gross pathology of a red-brown lesion in the lateral pons (B). On micropathology (H&E stain, 100×) (C), the lesion consists solely of dilated capillaries with normal walls (arrowheads), surrounded here by normal intervening brain tissue. This capillary telangiectasia involves the more medial motor tracts (fibrillary pattern) of the pons situated in the central two-thirds of the image, and the sensory tracts (bundled pattern; arrows) along both lateral margins.

Case studies

Case study 1. Temporal lobe cavernoma, resected

A 40-year-old right-handed woman presented with complex partial seizures. During one episode of loss of consciousness that occurred while she was driving (preceded by facial and hand posturing), her husband had to take over steering the motor vehicle in order to avert an accident.

The cause of her seizures was a 1 cm×2 cm CM in the right superior mesiotemporal lobe, with adjacent ventricular enlargement. This lesion is shown pre-operatively on MR sequences (**CS 1.1**): transaxial T2-weighted image (T1WI) (A), with gadolinium (B), GE-MRI (C), before (left) and following surgery (right). The surgical approach is evident as a lateral area of encephalomalacia (arrowheads).

Micropathology of this lesion (**CS 1.2**) is shown as hematoxylin and eosin (H&E) stain (100×) (**CS 1.2**A,C); H&E (40×) (**CS 1.2**B) and elastin stain (100×) (**CS 1.2**D). The following features are demonstrated: (1) calcification (purple staining, arrows) (**CS 1.2**A); (2) hemosiderin (light brown, arrowhead) (**CS 1.2**B); (3) fibrillary gliosis (arrows) (**CS 1.2**C); and (4) variable, irregular wall thickness, with minimal well-formed internal elastic lamina, demonstrated by the lack of dark staining within the arterial walls (arrowheads) (**CS 1.2**D). Some of these features (i.e., calcification, gliosis, arterial wall fragmentation) are more typical of AVM than of CM.

Comments

This patient wished to pursue elective neurosurgery because of intolerance to several anticonvulsant medications. The surgery to the non-dominant medial temporal lobe held a reasonably low risk. Although this patient's epilepsy resolved following removal of the lesion, she had a residual left quadrantanopia due to damage to the optic radiations of Meyer's loop during surgery.

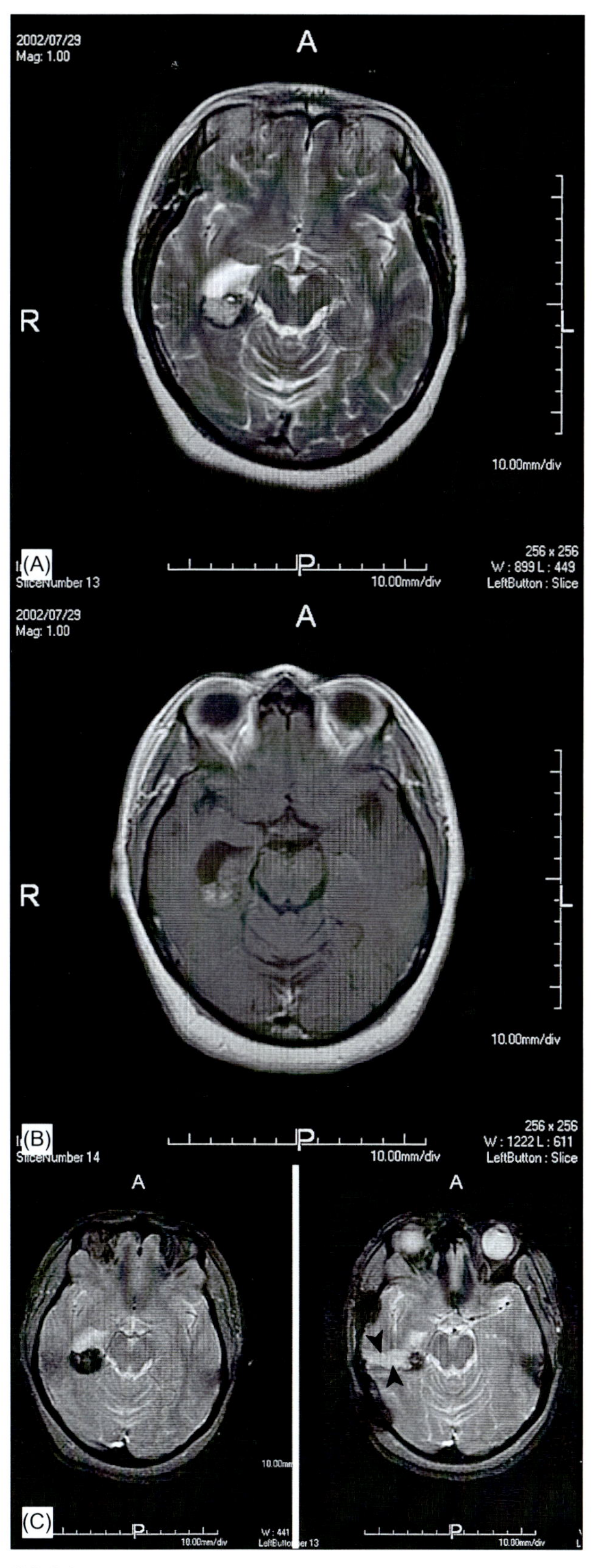
2002/07/29
Mag: 1.00
A
R
L
10.00mm/div
(A)
P
256 x 256
W : 899 L : 449
SliceNumber 13
LeftButton : Slice
2002/07/29
Mag: 1.00
A
R
L
10.00mm/div
(B)
P
256 x 256
W : 1222 L : 611
SliceNumber 14
LeftButton : Slice
A
A
(C)
P
P
10.00mm/div

CS 1.1

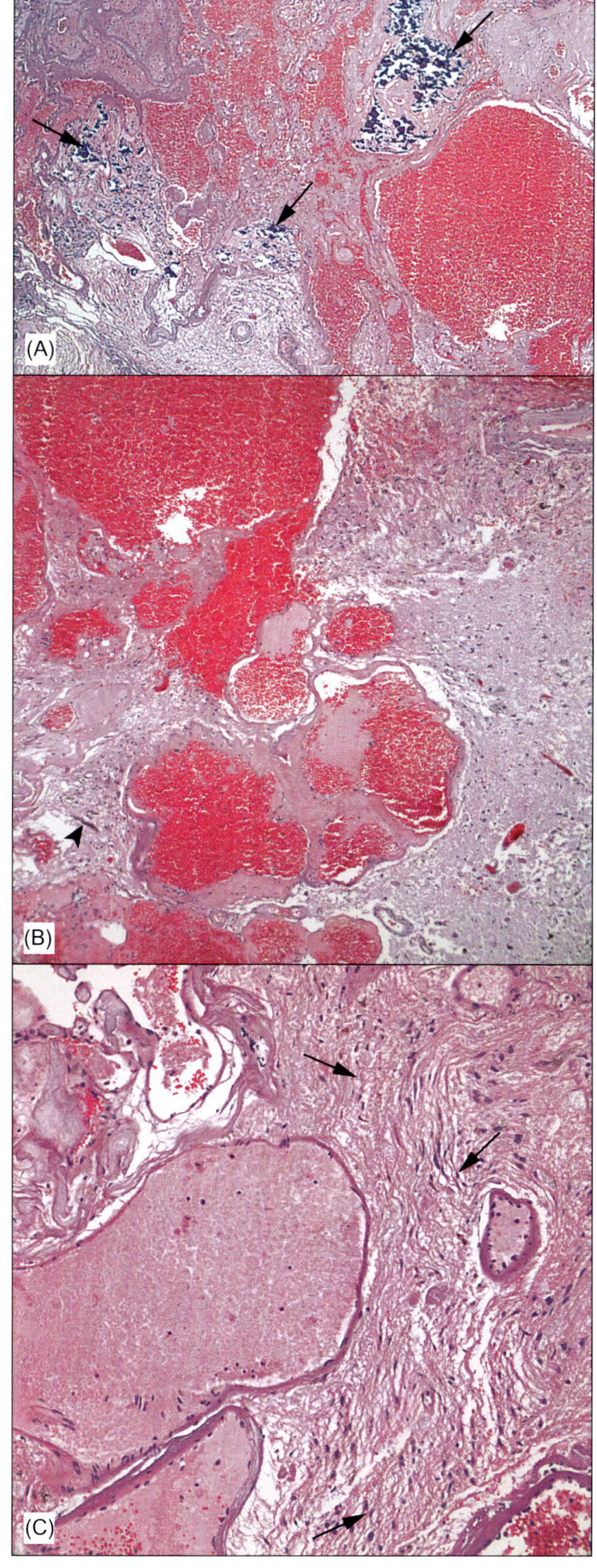
(A)
(B)
(C)

CS 1.2

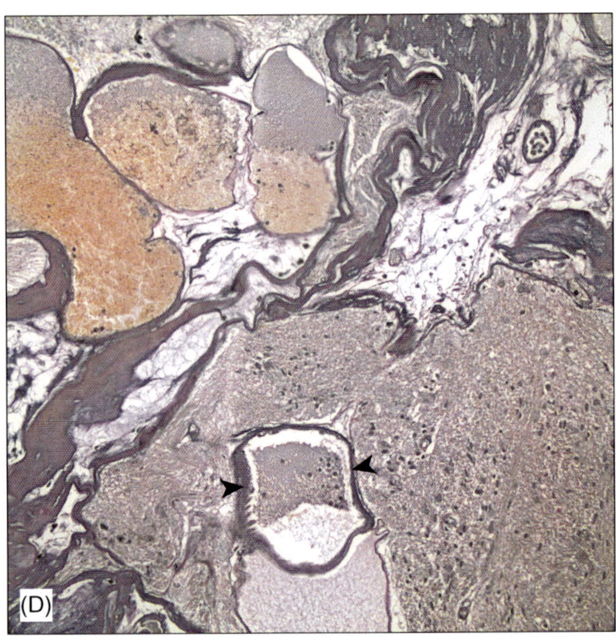

CS 1.2 (*continued*)

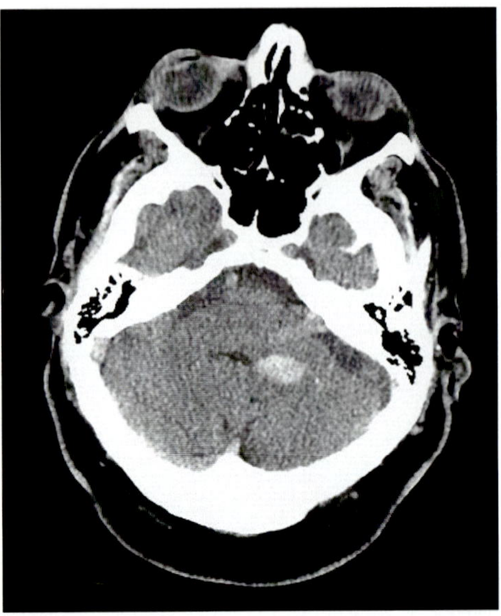

CS 2.1

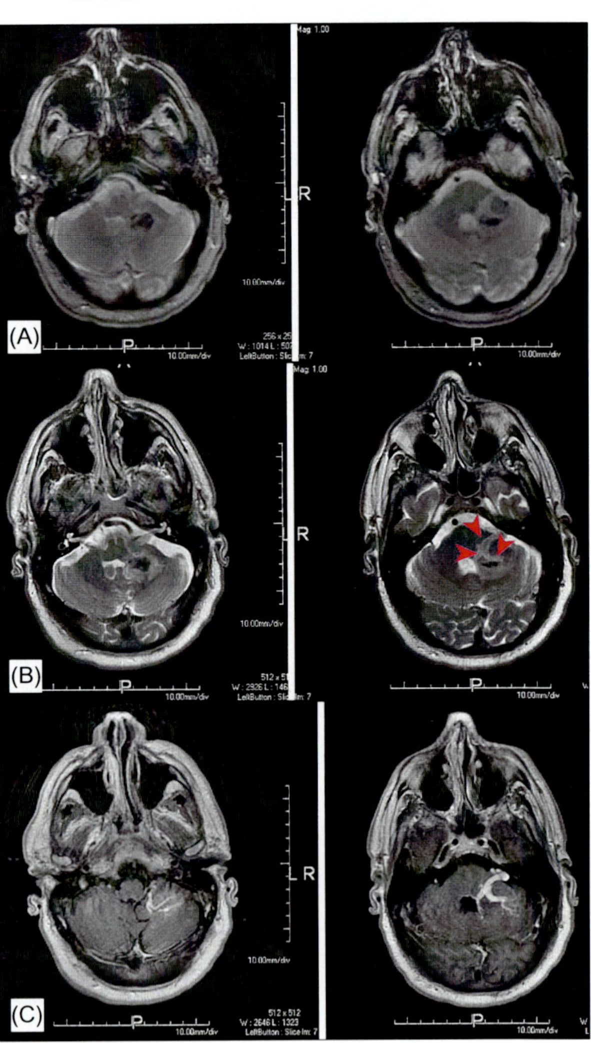

CS 2.2

Case study 2. Resection of cerebellar cavernoma, sparing associated DVA

A 51-year-old patient presented initially with vertigo, dysarthria, and gait ataxia. Admission CT scan showed an acute hemorrhage adjacent to the fourth ventricle (**CS 2.1**). The initial MRI scan (**CS 2.2**) shows an area of hemorrhage on GE sequence (**CS 2.2**A) and T2WI without contrast (**CS 2.2**B), raising the question of an adjacent vascular structure (B, right; arrowheads). This finding is readily discerned as a large DVA on the T1WI with gadolinium study (**CS 2.2**C). The lack of other findings (i.e., for AVM) on conventional angiography (not shown) suggested that the source of hemorrhage was a CM.

The patient presented on a second occasion 6 weeks later, with vertical diplopia, dizziness, nausea, and vomiting; these new symptoms raised the clinical concern for a recurrent local hemorrhage. The lesion was then electively resected via an occipital craniotomy. Note on the postoperative scans (**CS 2.3**) that the adjacent DVA has been carefully spared: CT scan (**CS 2.3**A, left) and MRI studies, GE sequence (**CS 2.3**A, right), and the T1 with gadolinium (**CS 2.3**B).

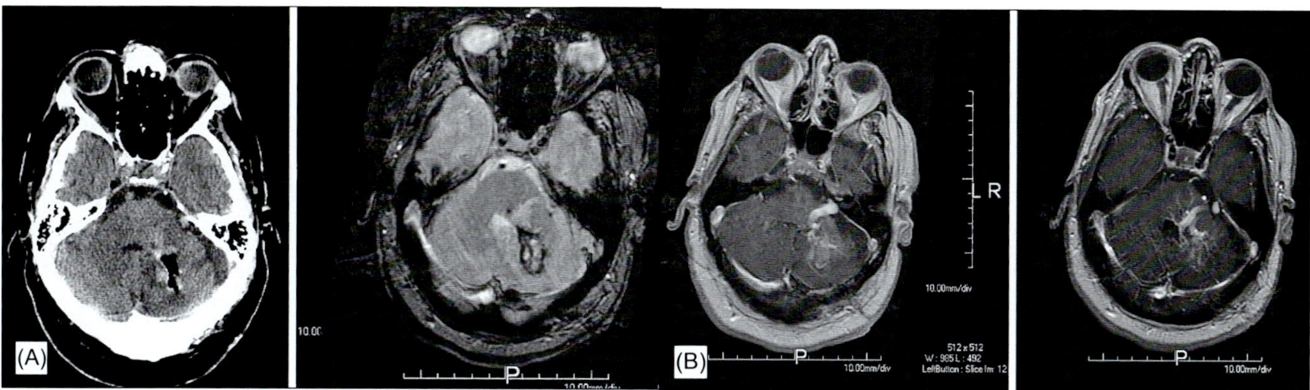

CS 2.3

Comments

The concern prompting neurosurgical resection of the CM was recurrent symptoms likely due to rebleeding of a lesion abutting the brainstem. The critical management consideration was to avoid injury to the large DVA during microsurgery, as this venous structure was an important component of the deep venous system. This patient made an excellent recovery, with only mild residual gait imbalance.

Case study 3. Persistent falcine sinus, with straight sinus aplasia

A congenital, massive DVA was identified during the diagnostic work-up of a healthy 35-year-old woman for chronic headaches. On non-invasive neuroimaging (**CS 3.1**), the lesion is appreciated along the midline in a sagittal (**CS 3.1**A) T2WI with gadolinium MRI sequence. The lesion appears similarly on transaxial T2WI with gadolinium MRI (**CS 3.1**B) and a CT scan with contrast (**CS 3.1**C).

The venous structure is best appreciated on conventional angiography (**CS 3.2**). In the absence of a straight sinus, there is instead a large persistent (embryonic) anomalous, falcine venous channel ascending superiorly from the level of the vein of Galen and draining into the superior sagittal sinus. An extensive 'caput medusae' pattern of radiating branches is appreciated in the lateral views (**CS 3.2**A). The relative components of venous drainage in the right and left hemispheres are appreciated on coronal (anteroposterior) views (**CS 3.2**B), venous phases of right (left image) and left (right image) ICA injections. Note the large, superficial cortical vein (arrowheads) (**CS 3.2**B, right) that originates

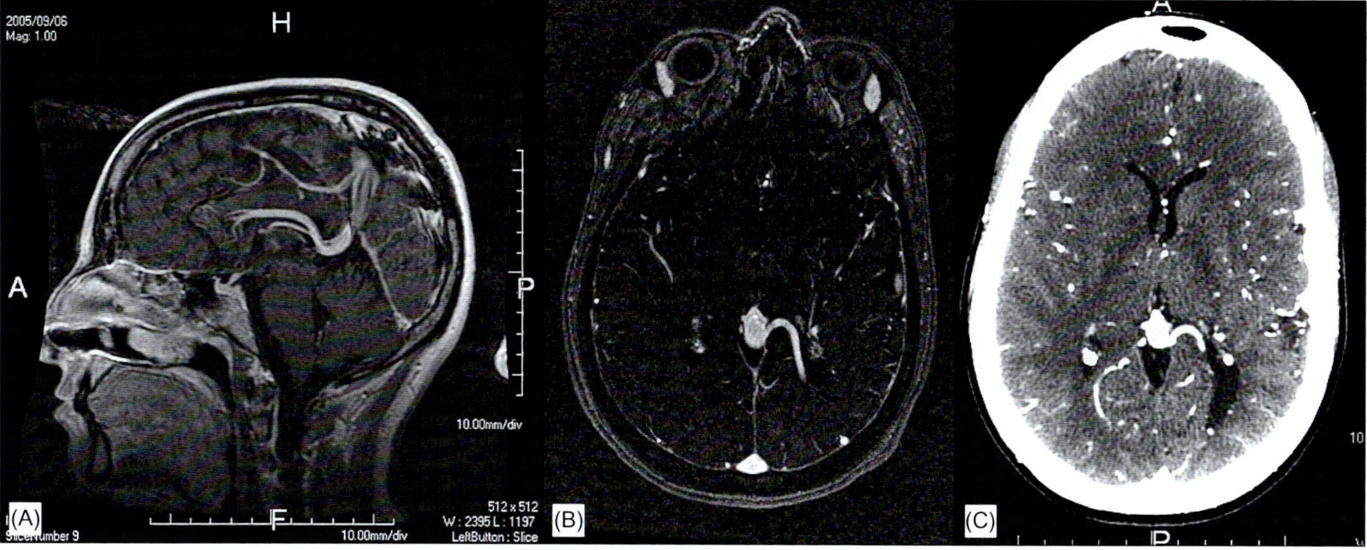

CS 3.1

at the anterior cranial fossa and courses over the lateral cerebral convexity to drain into the sagittal sinus. This lesion is also prominent on lateral views (**CS 3.2**A), particularly a late arterial phase (**CS 3.2**C).

Comments

Compare the radiating anatomy of the large venules comprising this DVA with that of the more typical DVA shown in **4.10**. These lesions probably represent arrested development at different locations within the embryonic venous system. The large, unique DVA in this case study could conceivably contribute to headache symptoms by causing venous hypertension. Acetazolamide, an agent that reduces intracranial pressure by decreasing cerebrospinal fluid production, was administered as a potential headache treatment for this patient. The lesion was fortunately not associated with a cavernoma or other vascular malformation, as this DVA is too complex to engineer any interventional treatment.

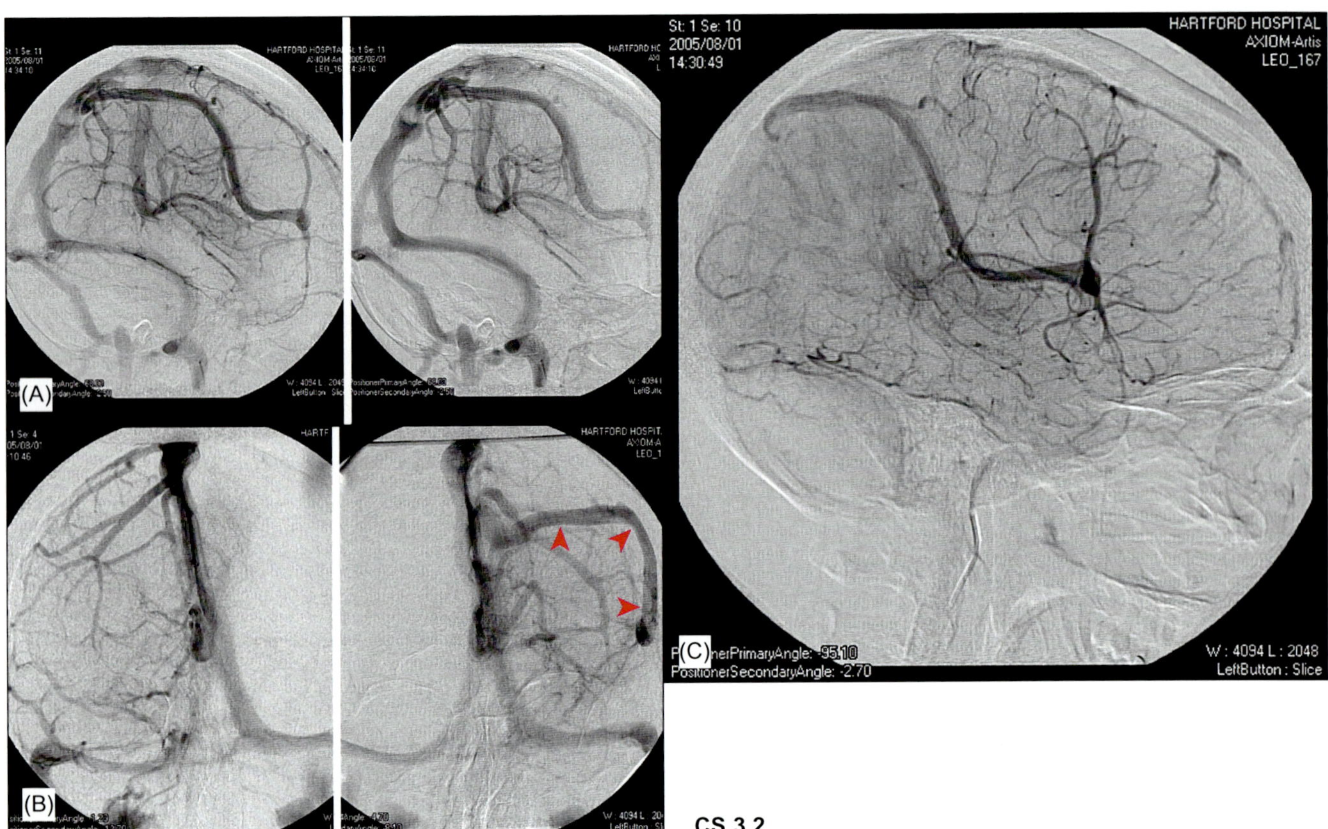

CS 3.2

References

1. Osborn A. Vascular malformations. In: *Diagnostic Cerebral Angiography*, 2nd edn. Philadelphia, PA: Lippincott Williams & Wilkins; 1999: 277–312.
2. Retta S, Avolio M, Francalanci F, *et al.* Identification of Krit1B: a novel alternative splicing isoform of cerebral cavernous malformation gene-1. *Gene* 2004; **325**: 63–78.
3. Zabramski J, Wascher T, Spetzler R, *et al.* The natural history of familial cavernous malformations: results of an ongoing study. *J Neurosurg* 1994; **80**: 422–32.
4. Al-Shahi Salman R, Berg MJ, Morrison L, Awad IA. Hemorrhage from cavernous malformation of the brain: definition and reporting standards. *Stroke* 2008; **39**: 3222–30.
5. Kondziolka D, Lunsford L, Kestle J. The natural history of cerebral cavernous malformations. *J Neurosurg* 1995; **83**: 820–4.
6. Kupersmith M, Kalish H, Epstein F, *et al.* Natural history of brainstem cavernous malformation. *Neurosurgery* 2001; **48**: 47–53.
7. Kamezawa T, Hamada J, Niiro M, Kai Y, Ishimaru K, Kuratsu J. Clinical implications of associated venous

drainage in patients with cavernous malformation. *J Neurosurg* 2005; **102**: 24–8.

8. Lehnhardt F, von Smekal U, Ruckriem B, *et al.* Value of gradient-echo magnetic resonance imaging in the diagnosis of familial cerebral cavernous malformation. *Arch Neurol* 2005; **62**: 653–8.
9. Conrad M, Schonauer C, Morel C, Pelissou-Guyotat I, Deruty R. Computer-assisted resection of supratentorial cavernous malformation. *Minim Invasive Neurosurg* 2002; **45**: 87–90.
10. Hasegawa T, McIerney J, Kondziolka D, Lee J, Flickinger J, Lunsford L. Long-term results after stereotactic radiosurgery for patients with cavernous malformations. *Neurosurgery* 2002; **50**: 1190–7.
11. Regis J, Bartolomei F, Kida Y, *et al.* Radiosurgery for epilepsy associated with cavernous malformation: retrospective study in 49 patients. *Neurosurgery* 2000; **47**: 1091–7.
12. Osborn A. Intracranial vascular malformations. In: *Diagnostic Neuroradiology*. St Louis, MO: Mosby; 1994: 284–329.
13. McLaughlin M, Kondziolka D, Flickinger J, *et al.* The prospective natural history of cerebral venous malformations. *Neurosurgery* 1998; **43**: 195–201.
14. Naff NJ, Wemmer J, Hoenig-Rigamonti K, Rigamonti DR. A longitudinal study of patients with venous malformations: documentation of a negligible hemorrhage risk and benign natural history. *Neurology* 1998; **50**: 1709–14.
15. Hon JML, Bhattacharya JJ, Counsell CE, *et al.* The presentation and clinical course of intracranial developmental venous anomalies in adults: a systematic review and prospective, population-based study. *Stroke* 2009; **40**: 1980–5.
16. Pereira VM, Geibprasert S, Krings T, *et al.* Pathomechanisms of symptomatic developmental venous anomalies. *Stroke* 2008; **39**: 3201–15.
17. Robinson J, Jr, Awad I, Masaryk T, Estes M. Pathological heterogeneity of angiographically occult vascular malformations of the brain. *Neurosurgery* 1993; **33**: 547–55.
18. Lee R, Becher M, Benson M, Rigamonti D. Brain capillary telangiectasia: MR imaging appearance and clinicohistopathologic findings. *Radiology* 1997; **205**: 797–805.
19. Scaglione C, Salvi F, Riguzzi P, Tassinari C. Symptomatic unruptured capillary telangiectasia of the brainstem: report of three cases and review of the literature. *J Neurol Neurosurg Psychiatry* 2001; **71**: 390–3.

Further reading

Al-Shahi Salman R, Berg MJ, Morrison L, Awad IA. Hemorrhage from cavernous malformation of the brain: definition and reporting standards. *Stroke* 2008; **39**: 3222–30.

Chaloupka J, Huddle D. Classification of vascular malformations of the central nervous system. *Neuroimaging Clin North Am* 1998; **8**: 295–321.

Hon JML, Bhattacharya JJ, Counsell CE, *et al.* The presentation and clinical course of intracranial developmental venous anomalies in adults: a systematic review and prospective, population-based study. *Stroke* 2009; **40**: 1980–5.

Osborn A. Vascular malformations. In: *Diagnostic Cerebral Angiography*, 2nd edn. Philadelphia, PA: Lippincott Williams & Wilkins; 1999: 277–312.

Resources for patients

Cavernous Malformations (www.angiomaalliance.org)

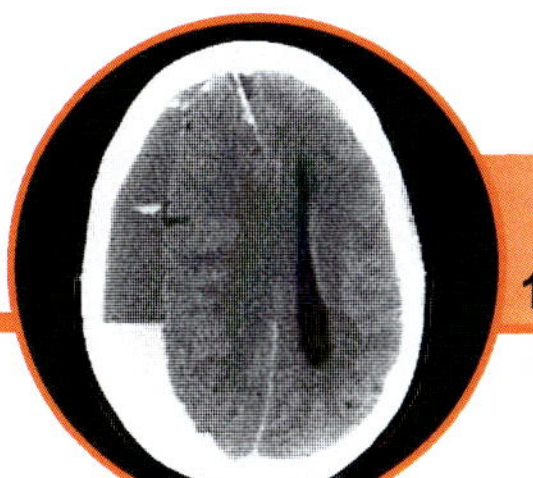

Chapter 5

'Extreme' Neurovascular Disorders

Introduction

Some neurovascular disorders do not readily fit into the categories outlined in the previous chapters. Other cases reflect atypical or extreme examples of conditions discussed in those chapters. Often, 'extreme' neurovascular disorders imply serious, life-threatening pathology, but not always. In contrast to the focus on acute and common initial presentations in the two volumes of this book up to this point, this final chapter focuses on neurovascular pathology that may be rare (e.g., intravascular lymphomatosis, cerebral autosomal dominant arteriopathy with subcortical infarcts and leukoencephalopathy (CADASIL)), chronic (e.g., calcification), and even reversible (e.g., the posterior leukoencephalopathy syndrome).

Neurovascular disorders also occur in locations of the central nervous system other than the brain, in particular, the eye and the spinal cord. A few examples of retinal stroke were shown within volume 1 on ischemic stroke, and a brief introduction to spinal cord syndromes is included here.

The topics included in this chapter are listed in *Table 5.1*, and are presented in a survey, case-based format.

Table 5.1 Topics covered: extreme neurovascular disorders

- Dural AV shunts
- The reversible posterior leukoencephalopathy syndrome
- Subdural hematoma
- Intravascular lymphomatosis
- Phakomatoses
- Cerebral autosomal dominant arteriopathy with subcortical infarcts and leukoencephalopathy (CADASIL)
- Calcifications and other hyperdensities
- Intracranial dolichoectasia
- Radiation arteriopathy
- Sickle cell disease
- Spinal cord infarction and vascular malformations

Dural AV shunts (5.1–5.4)

In contrast to most pial AVMs (Chapter 3), dural-based lesions lack a nidus. Rather, numerous abnormal direct communications – called shunts, or fistulae – exist between dural arteries and dural or cortical (intracranial) veins. The shunt is situated within the dural wall of a venous sinus, rather than within the sinus itself (**5.1**A).[1–3] Typically situated in or around the skull base and posterior fossa, the most common arterial feeders are meningeal branches of the external carotid artery (ECA) and the occipital artery. The most common venous sinuses involved are the transverse–sigmoid sinus junction (**5.1**B, **5.2**) and the cavernous sinus (CS) (**5.3**).[1,2]

The presentation of dural-based arteriovenous lesions may be quite subtle. Symptoms may include headache and auditory phenomena, such as pulsatile tinnitus (and an associated bruit over the skull on examination) when the transverse or sigmoid sinuses are involved. Other phenomena such as proptosis, chemosis, ophthalmoplegia, other cranial neuropathies, and retro-orbital pain, suggest involvement of the cavernous sinus.[1,2] The classification scheme of dural arteriovenous shunts is complex.[1,3] Clinical outcomes depend on the venous drainage patterns, with venous ectasias carrying a worse prognosis.[1,3] The treatment approach is typically endovascular embolization, sometimes with adjunct vascular neurosurgery.

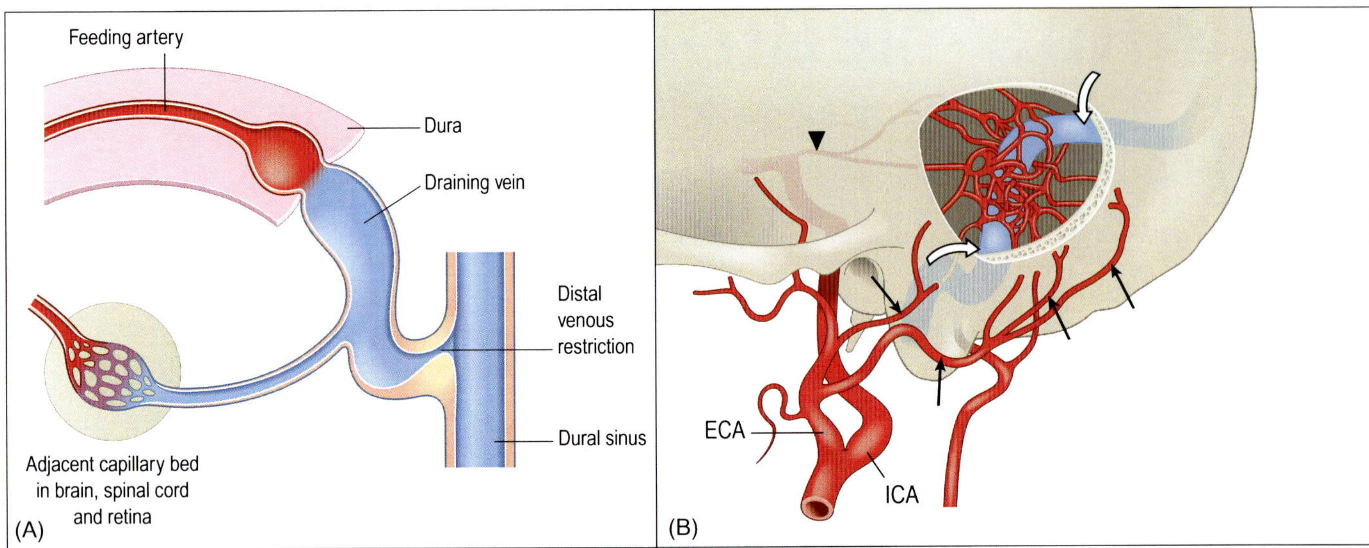

5.1 Dural AV shunt. Distal venous restriction, resulting in venous hypertension, is believed to play a major role in the development of dural AV shunts (A) (figure adapted from Bederson[1]).

A window in the skull base (B) depicts a dural AV shunt at the transverse–sigmoid sinus junction supplied by numerous branches of the external carotid artery (ECA; arrows), as well as the meningohypophyseal trunk (arrowhead), a branch of the internal carotid artery (ICA). A collection of microfistulae exists within the dural wall of the sinus, and drain in an anterograde direction through a patent transverse-sigmoid sinus (curved white arrows).

A dural AV shunt may recruit arterial feeders from adjacent (i.e., meningeal and/or adjacent scalp–pial tissue) sources (figure adapted from Osborn[2]).

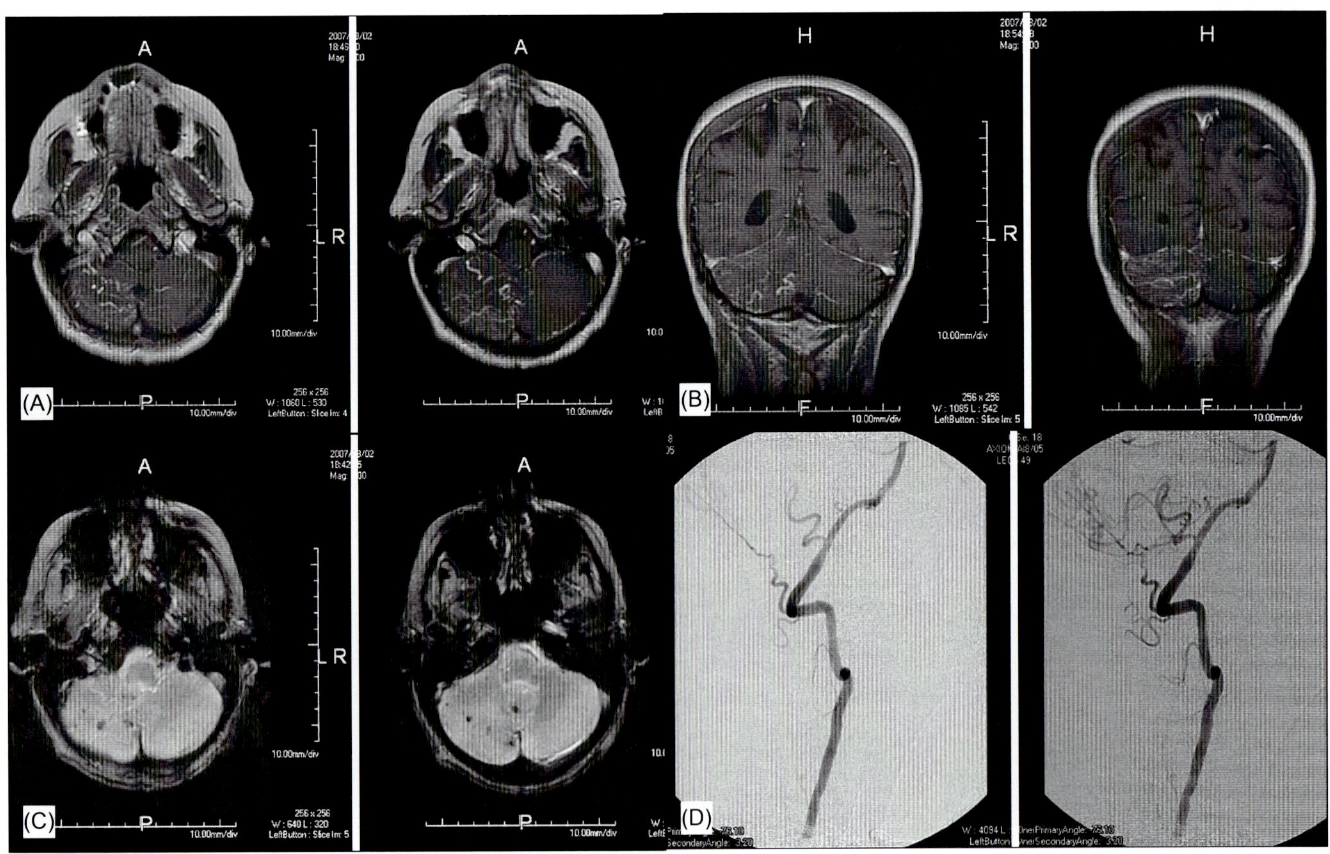

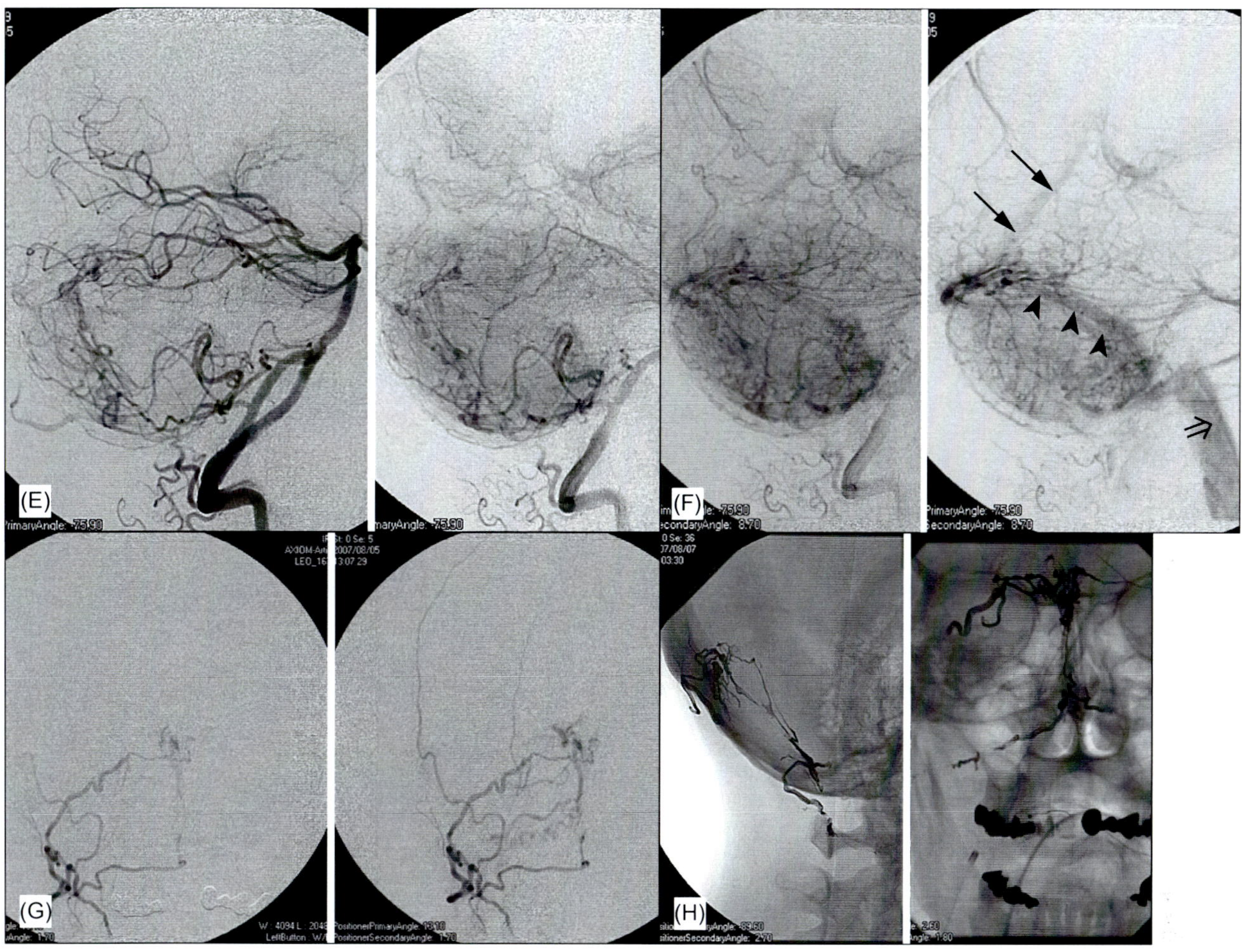

5.2 Multifocal cerebellar dural AV fistulae. An 81-year-old woman presented to another hospital with diplopia and gait ataxia. Her MRI scan prompted a transfer to the regional Stroke Center for further work-up. This T1-weighted MRI scan with gadolinium showed enlarged, tortuous vessels on transaxial (A) and coronal (B) images. Multiple punctate areas of magnetic susceptibility are scattered throughout the right cerebellar hemisphere on the GE-MR sequence (C), likely due to venous infarcts with associated microhemorrhages. A FLAIR (fluid attenuated inversion recovery) sequence (not shown) demonstrated edema, from venous congestion, throughout the right cerebellar hemisphere.

On conventional angiography, AV shunts exist at the level of the inferior aspect of the torcula, supplied by several extracranial arteries: the posterior meningeal branches arising from each of the vertebral arteries (VAs), the right occipital artery, and both middle meningeal arteries. The fistulae communicated directly to veins in the right cerebellar hemisphere that were engorged and showed poor drainage, causing edema and punctuate hemorrhages. Parts of this angiographic study are reproduced here.

First, a series of an injection into the left VA, is shown on lateral, subtracted views, both cervical (D) and intracranial (E,F). The last image (F) demonstrates the relative location of the straight (arrows) and sigmoid (arrowhead) sinuses, and the internal jugular vein (large arrow) (F). Lateral views of the cerebellum demonstrate increased arterial flow (E) and early venous filling (F). Second, an injection into the right occipital artery (G), a branch of the ECA (anteroposterior (AP) projection), on early (left) and mid-arterial (right) phase, also demonstrates early venous filling consistent with fistulization.

During the first of several embolization procedures, the posterior meningeal branch of the left VA was occluded with n-butyl cyanoacrylate, unsubtracted views (H), lateral (left) and AP (right). The cast of radio-opaque substance is situated extracranially, outside the skull (left); note the position of the embolic material relative to the orbits, nasal turbines, and dental fillings (right).

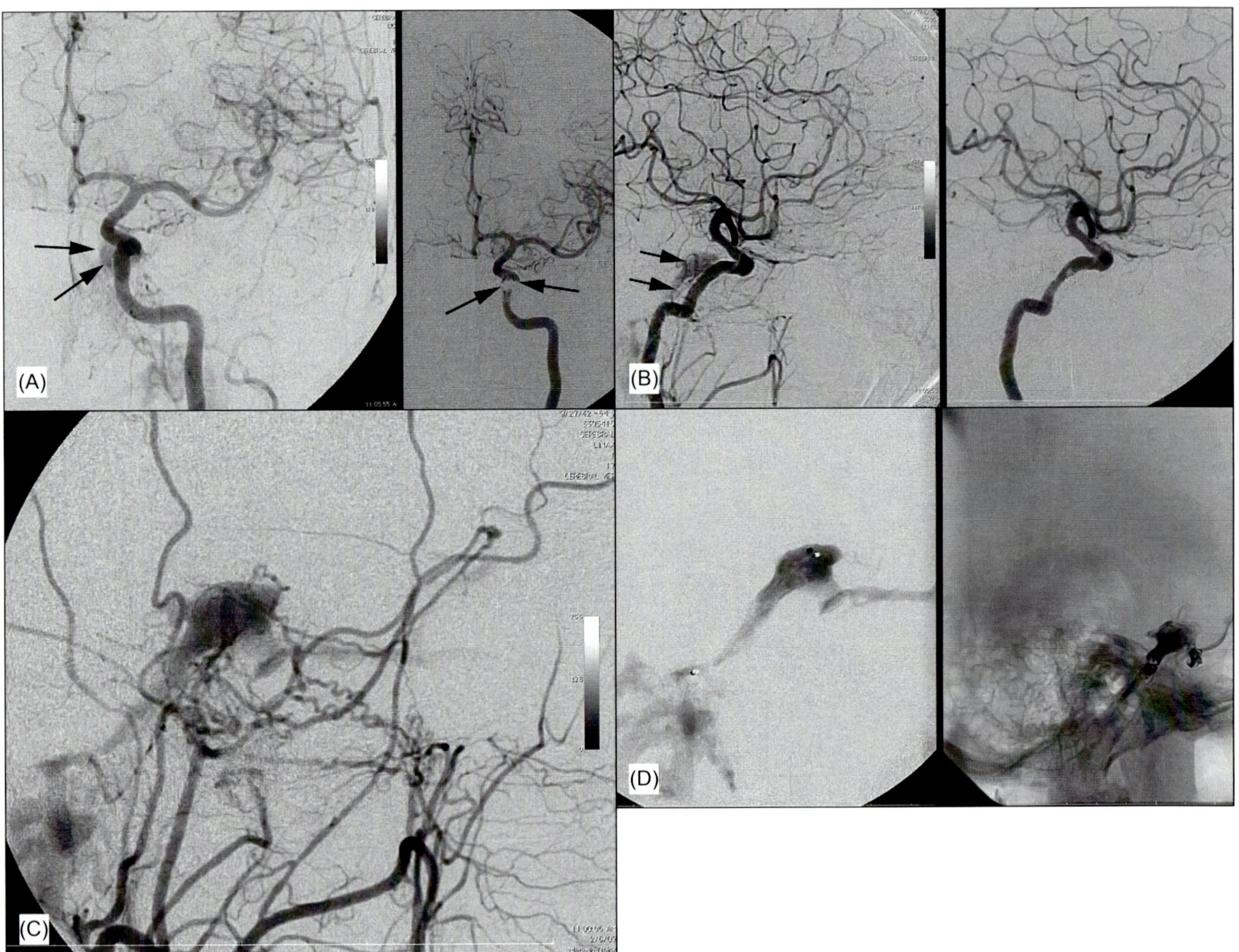

5.3 Cavernous sinus AV fistula. A 75-year-old woman presented with bilateral conjunctival injection, periorbital edema, and horizontal diplopia, and was referred to the Neurovascular Clinic by an ophthalmologist. A CT angiography study (not shown) initially documented early opacification and enlargement of the superior division of the left ophthalmic vein along with the left cavernous sinus and retroclinical plexus, concerning for a dural AV lesion.

Conventional angiography, a selected study of the left ICA, showed a component fistulous supply to the cavernous sinus. The first two images, an AP (A) and lateral (B) projections, show some abnormal blush (arrows) adjacent to the ICA (on the left images) that resolved following embolization (the right images). The point of fistulization was the posterior compartment of the left cavernous sinus, draining primarily into the inferior petrosal sinus and the left orbital venous system. Selective studies of the left ECA, including a lateral view of an injection into the internal maxillary branches (C), suggest multiple abnormal fistulous communications to the posterior aspect of the left cavernous sinus. The arterial supply to this dural AV fistula (AVF) arose from various ECA branches (both ascending pharyngeal arteries, both middle meningeal arteries, and other branches of the left internal maxillary artery), as well cavernous branches of both ICAs.

Endovascular occlusion of this AVF was carried out by initial coil embolization of the communication between the left posterior cavernous sinus and the orbital venous system, followed by coil occlusion of the medial channel of the left inferior petrosal sinus with the cavernous sinus. Finally, liquid embolization of the cavernous sinus was then carried out using Onyx®, with complete occlusion of the AVF. Another comparison of pre- and post-treatment angiography is shown in the final image, a lateral view, ICA injection, of the cavernous sinus (D). First, subtracted, the fistulous pouch (left) is evident, and then, unsubtracted, the cast of embolic material is visualized in this same space (right), just above the skull base.

More than one month post-embolization, the patient had slight residual proptosis and incomplete abduction, consistent with a partial sixth-nerve palsy, of the left eye. The periorbital edema had resolved. No residual fistulization appeared on the follow-up angiography 8 months later.

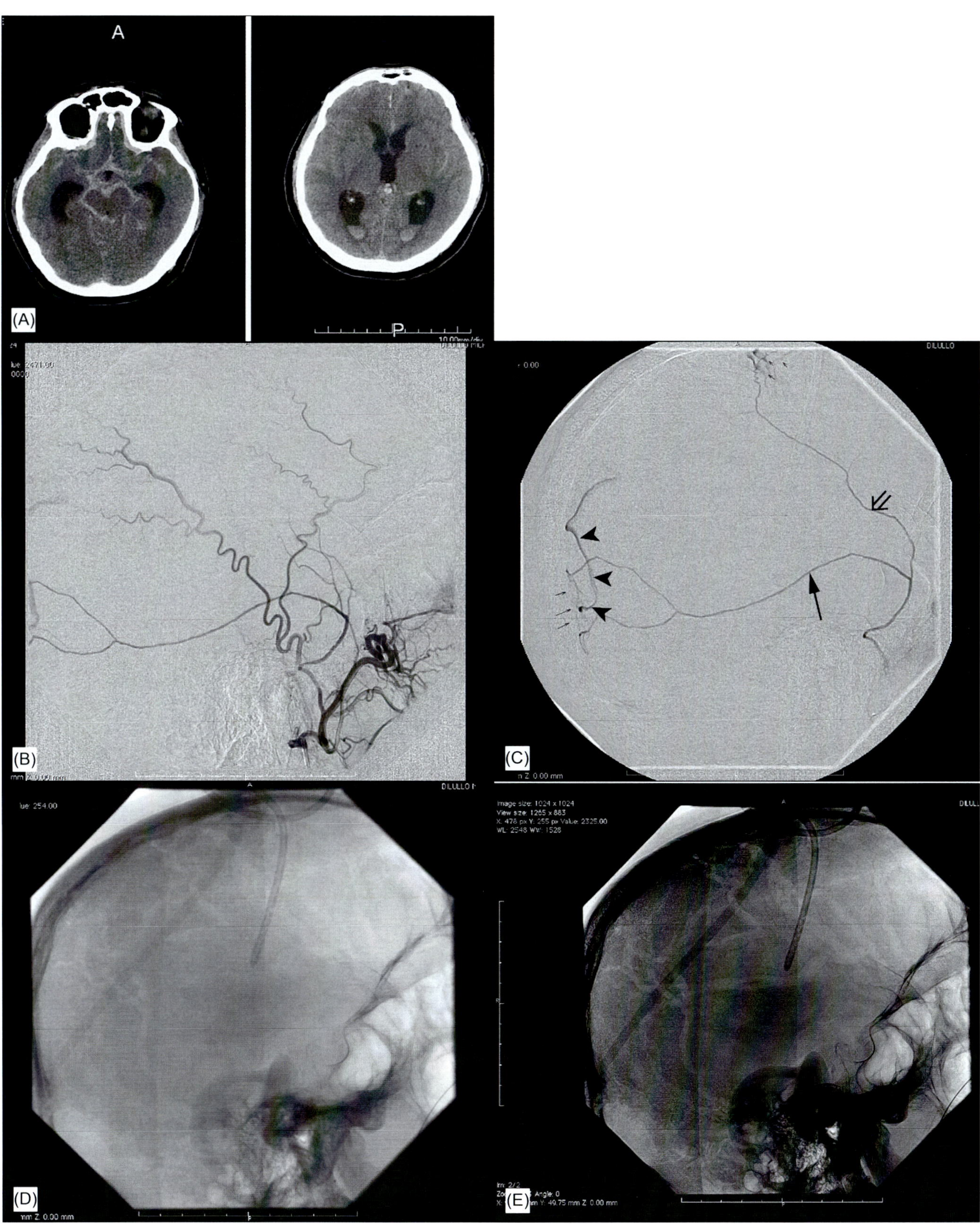

5.4 Dural AV fistulae, with calvarial grooves. (*caption on following page*).

5.4 Dural AV fistulae, with calvarial grooves. This 65-year-old man presented with delirium, associated with this subarachnoid and intraventricular hemorrhage on head CT scan at admission (A). Progressive hydrocephalus prompted placement of an external ventricular drain. The lesion causing this hemorrhage was a multifocal dural AVF.

Conventional angiography: an injection into the internal maxillary artery, a branch of the external artery, is first shown (B). Two foci of fistulization are observed with a more selective injection into the right middle meningeal artery (C), the linear branch of the internal maxillary artery. These two fistulae are marked with small black arrows at the left and at top of the image: (1) a posterior division of the middle meningeal artery (large arrow) that localized to the occiput just above the torcula, with early filling of a cortical vein (arrowheads) that drains into the sagittal sinus; and (2) an anterior division of the middle meningeal artery coursing to the convexity (open arrow), with rapid filling of a cortical vein (not well visualized here).

An extraordinary radiographic observation, shown on the unsubtracted skull X-ray (D) and again, maximizing the black–white contrast (E), are a plethora of widened vascular grooves over the calvarium (although the venous structures that likely caused these vascular grooves did not opacify during any portion of the exam). It is possible that, given their lack of apparent blood flow, these bony grooves were venous channels that thrombosed some time in the distant past.

The cerebral venous system and dural sinuses were otherwise intact, with normal antegrade flow. The two sites of fistulization (C) were later embolized with liquid embolic material, n-butyl cyanoacrylate (not shown). The patient made a complete cognitive recovery.

The reversible posterior leukoencephalopathy syndrome (5.5–5.8)

In this syndrome, vasogenic edema develops in the white and gray matter, most commonly in the posterior parieto-occipital region. The causes are diverse and may reflect acute hyperperfusion and/or a toxic compromise of the blood–brain barrier. The most common causes include hypertensive encephalopathy, eclampsia, and immunosuppressive drugs.[4]

Subdural hematoma (5.9–5.12)

Subdural hematomas (SDHs) may mimic other neurovascular disorders, causing acute and recurrent neurologic symptoms either by mass effect or by causing seizures. They also may evolve over a long time interval, with recurrent hemorrhages in the setting of coagulopathies, such as alcohol abuse, and head trauma.

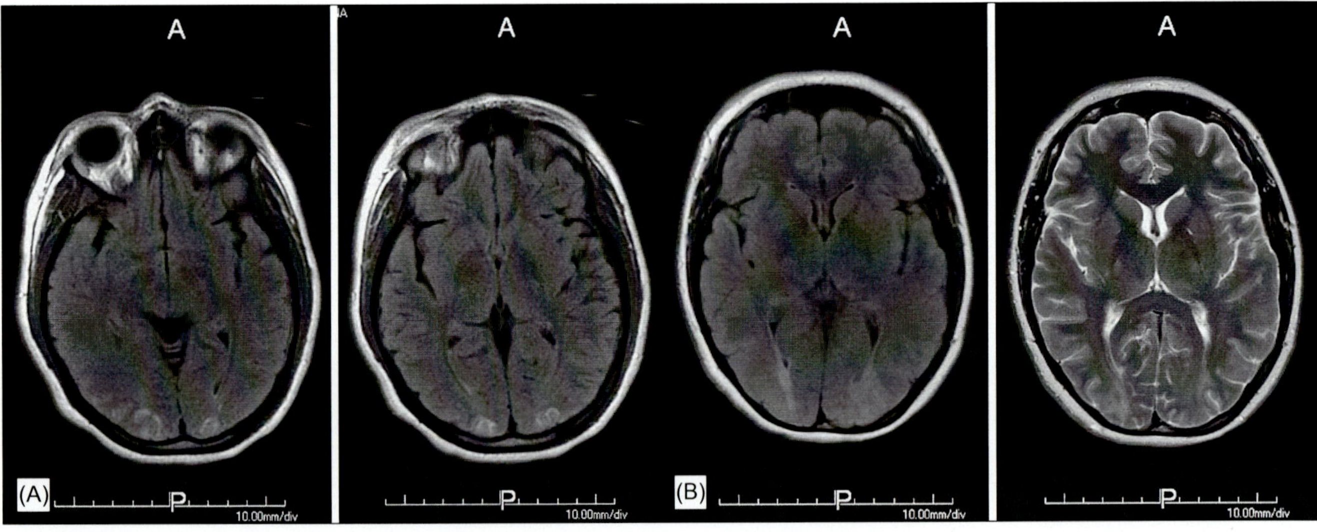

5.5 Mild disease, post-partum. Two cases (A,B) of mild eclampsia and peripartum headache and visual loss are shown. The posterior edema registers most readily on FLAIR sequence (A; B, left), but to a lesser extent on T2-weighted images (WI) (B, right), also. Both patients' symptoms spontaneously resolved, with careful titration of blood pressure.

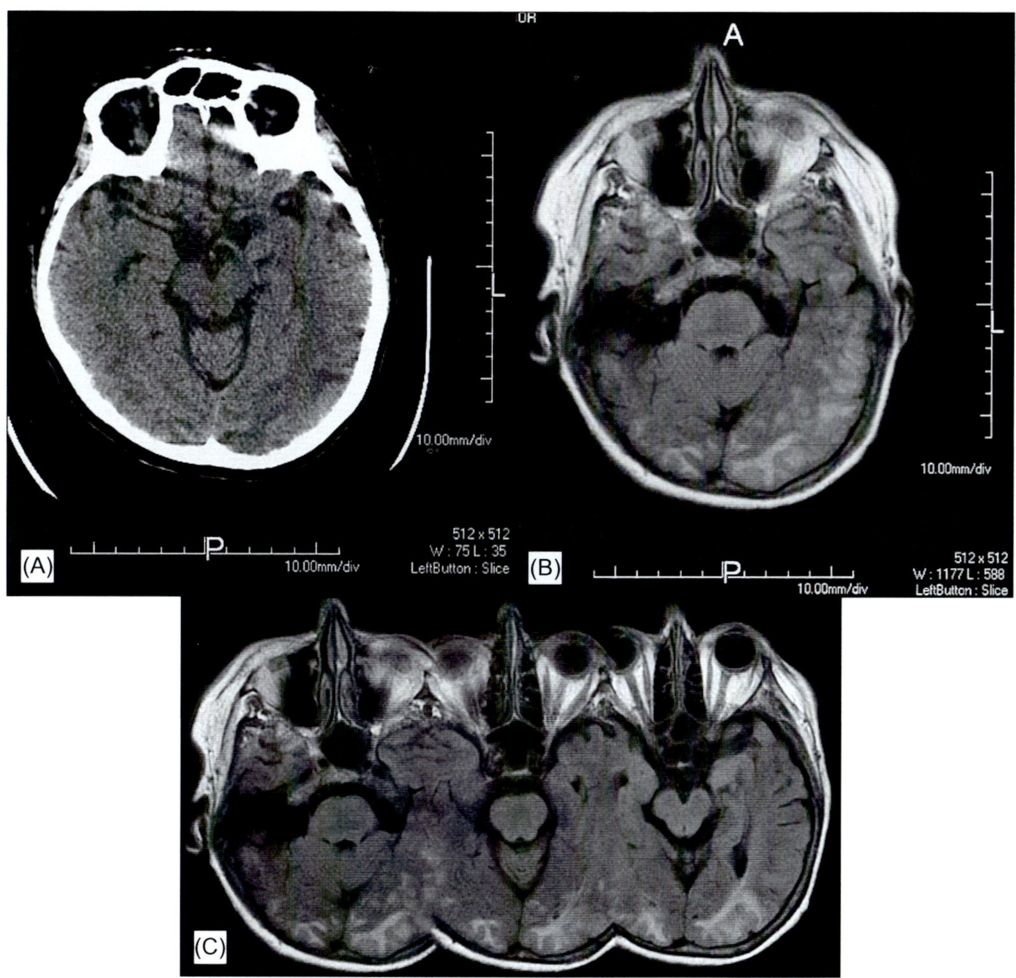

5.6 Moderate disease. This patient presented with delirium and visual hallucinations, associated with recent exposure to chemotherapy. Neuroimaging shows initial CT scan (A) and extensive temporo-occipital changes on the FLAIR MR sequence (B). The final image (C) is a composite of three adjacent transaxial slices juxtaposed to demonstrate the tracking of vasogenic edema along the white matter.

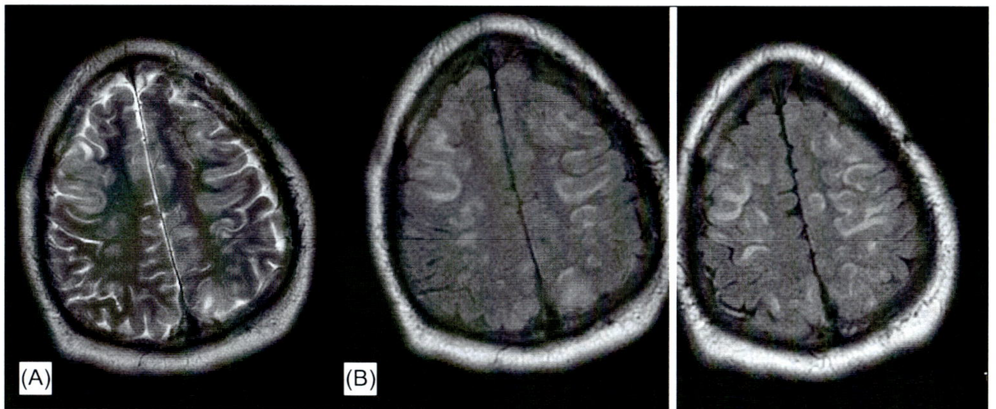

5.7 Extensive frontoparietal involvement from hypertensive encephalopathy. In this patient, MR changes were more prominent in frontoparietal regions than the posterior cerebral hemispheres. The images shown are T2WI (A) and FLAIR (B) sequences. The lesions predominate within the cortical gyri.

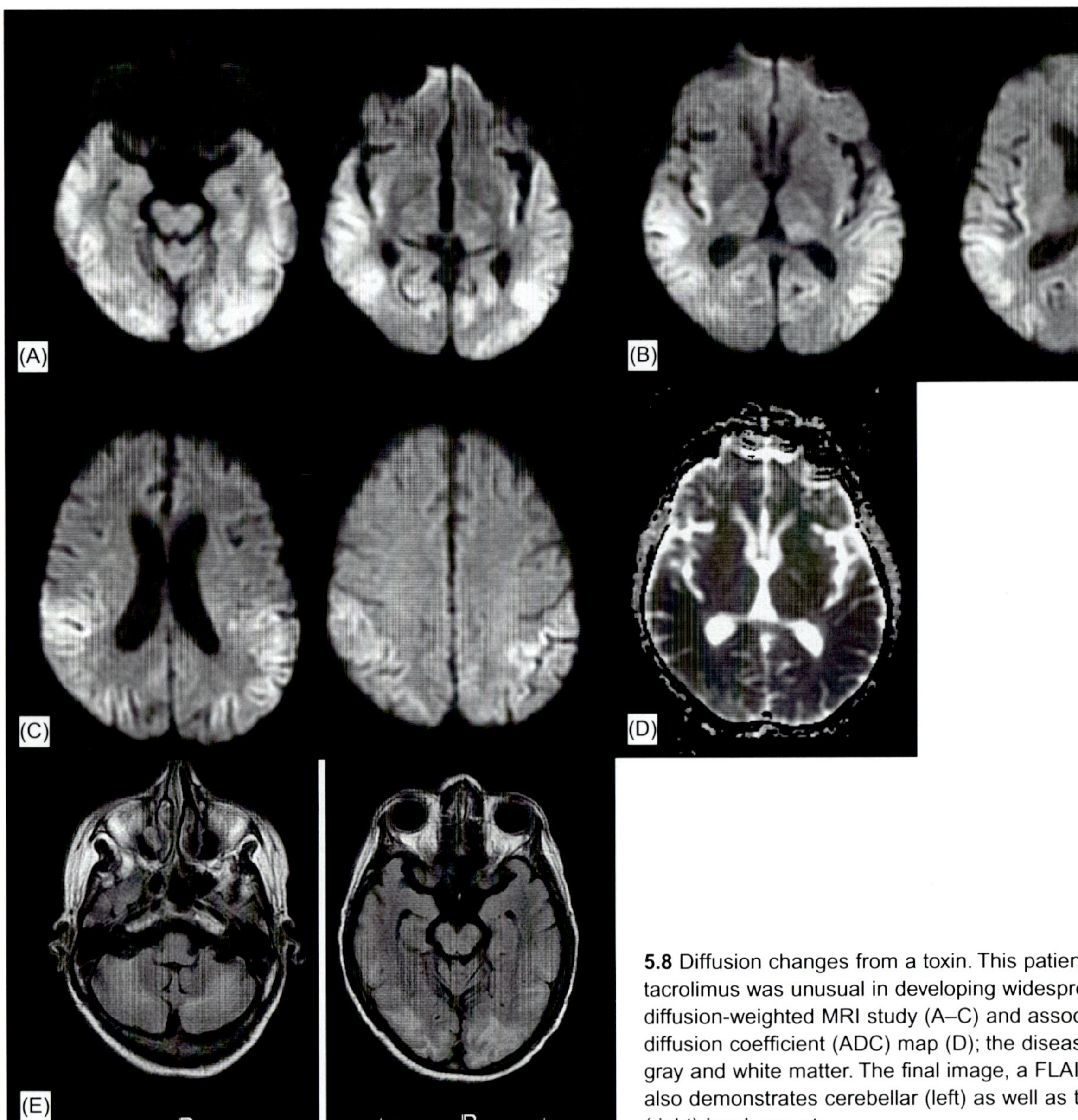

5.8 Diffusion changes from a toxin. This patient with toxicity from tacrolimus was unusual in developing widespread lesions on a diffusion-weighted MRI study (A–C) and associated apparent diffusion coefficient (ADC) map (D); the disease involves both gray and white matter. The final image, a FLAIR sequence (E) also demonstrates cerebellar (left) as well as temporo-occipital (right) involvement.

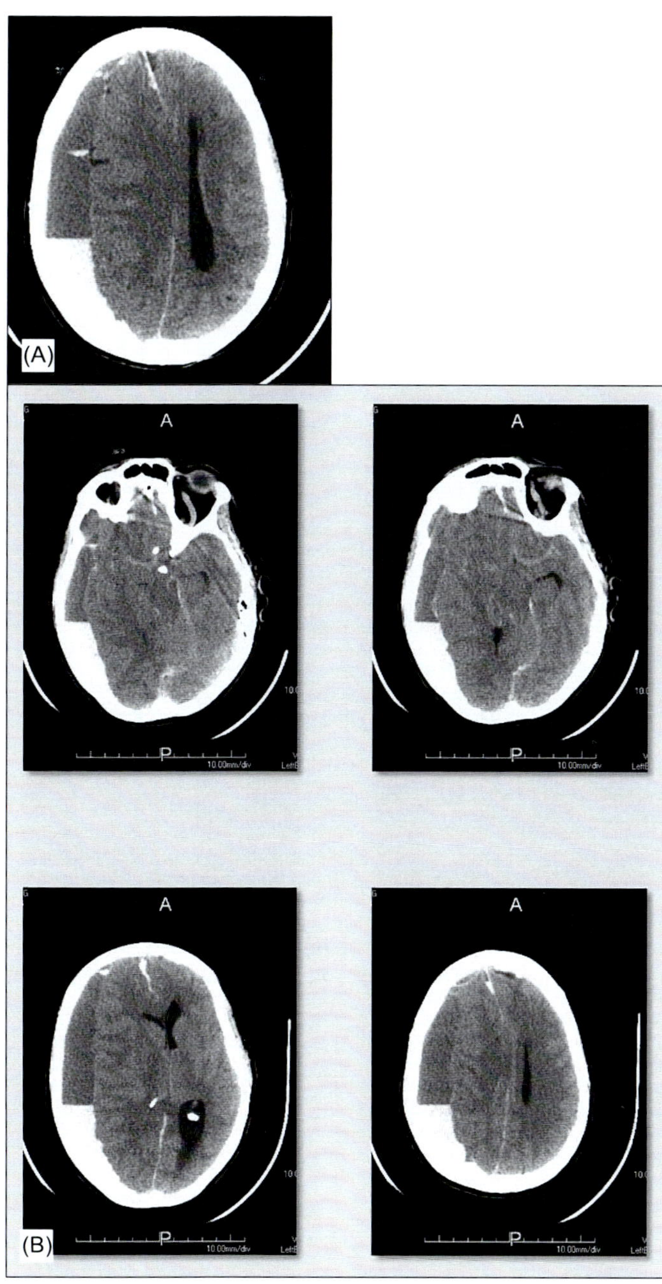

5.9 Acute-on-chronic subdural hematoma (SDH). An acute, posterior hyperdense hematoma adds to the mass effect of the more anterior lesion, to efface the entire right lateral ventricle (A). A composite image (B) shows the severe mass effect in the posterior fossa, with absence of the basal cisterns. Elevated intracranial pressure is also evidenced by the absence of sulcal markings throughout the hemispheres.

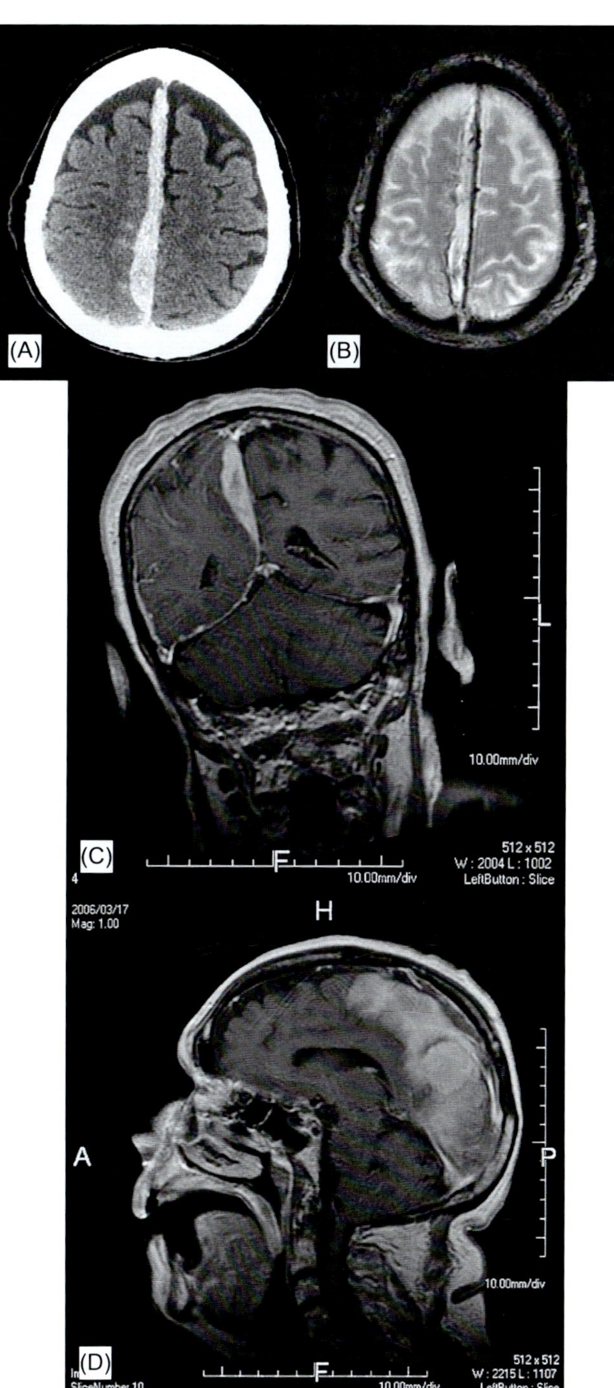

5.10 Falcine SDH. A large SDH along the falx is seen on transaxial non-contrast CT scan (A) and GE-MRI sequence (B). The coronal (C) and sagittal (D) T1-weighted MRIs with gadolinium provide documentation of the extent of this lesion, which did not require neurosurgical drainage.

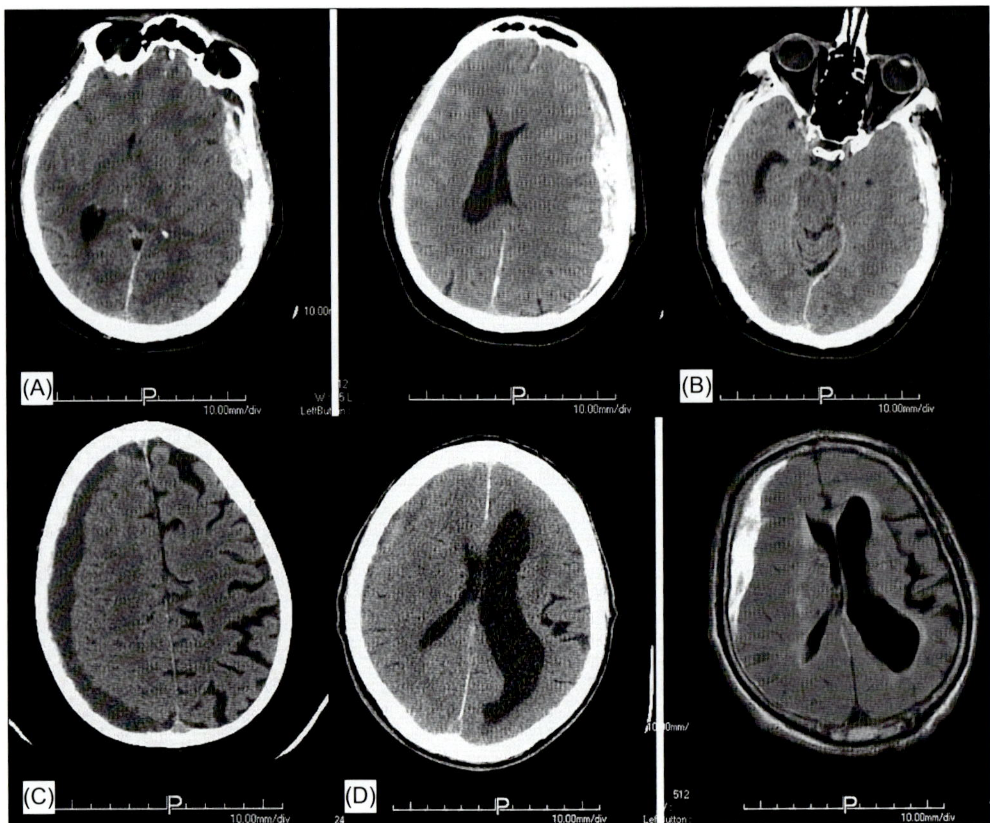

5.11 Acute versus chronic hemispheric SDH. The first lesion (A,B) is a large acute left hemispheric SDH on initial CT scan. Owing to diminished sensorium, a sign of impending herniation, the patient underwent emergent neurosurgical drainage, and made a complete recovery. Note the mass effect along the midline (A) and compressing the midbrain (B).

The next two SDHs are two chronic right hemispheric lesions: first, a CT scan (C), and second, another lesion (D) on CT (left) and FLAIR MRI (right). Note the continued mass effect, evidenced by effacement of the adjacent gyri and reduced size of the lateral ventricle, but the relative lack of midline shift.

Intravascular lymphomatosis (5.13)

Intravascular lymphomatosis is a rare neoplastic disease characterized by the intraluminal proliferation of malignant cells of B-cell lineage. Typically, small arteries become occluded, causing ischemic infarction, most often in the central nervous system and skin.

The diagnosis, also known as intravascular lymphoma or malignant angioendotheliomatosis, is a favorite of clinicopathologic conferences, as the disorder is a master of mimicry, both in its diverse clinical presentation and its neuroimaging findings.[5] The presenting symptoms include a progressive or relapsing-remitting multifocal neurologic syndrome (comparable with multiple sclerosis) but with recurrent infarctions in different vascular territories; a progressive or acute myelopathy; cognitive impairment (dementia, delirium); or peripheral neuropathy and mononeuritis multiplex.

On neuroimaging, intravascular lymphomatosis may most resemble central nervous system vasculitis, with strokes involving both cortical gray matter and subcortical white matter. However, vasculitis more often has more peripherally located lesions as well as meningeal involvement. In addition, patients with intravascular lymphomatosis will not respond to the aggressive immunosuppressive treatment that may help those with vasculitis improve. No established treatment for this neoplasia exists, largely because the disease is too rare to systematically study.

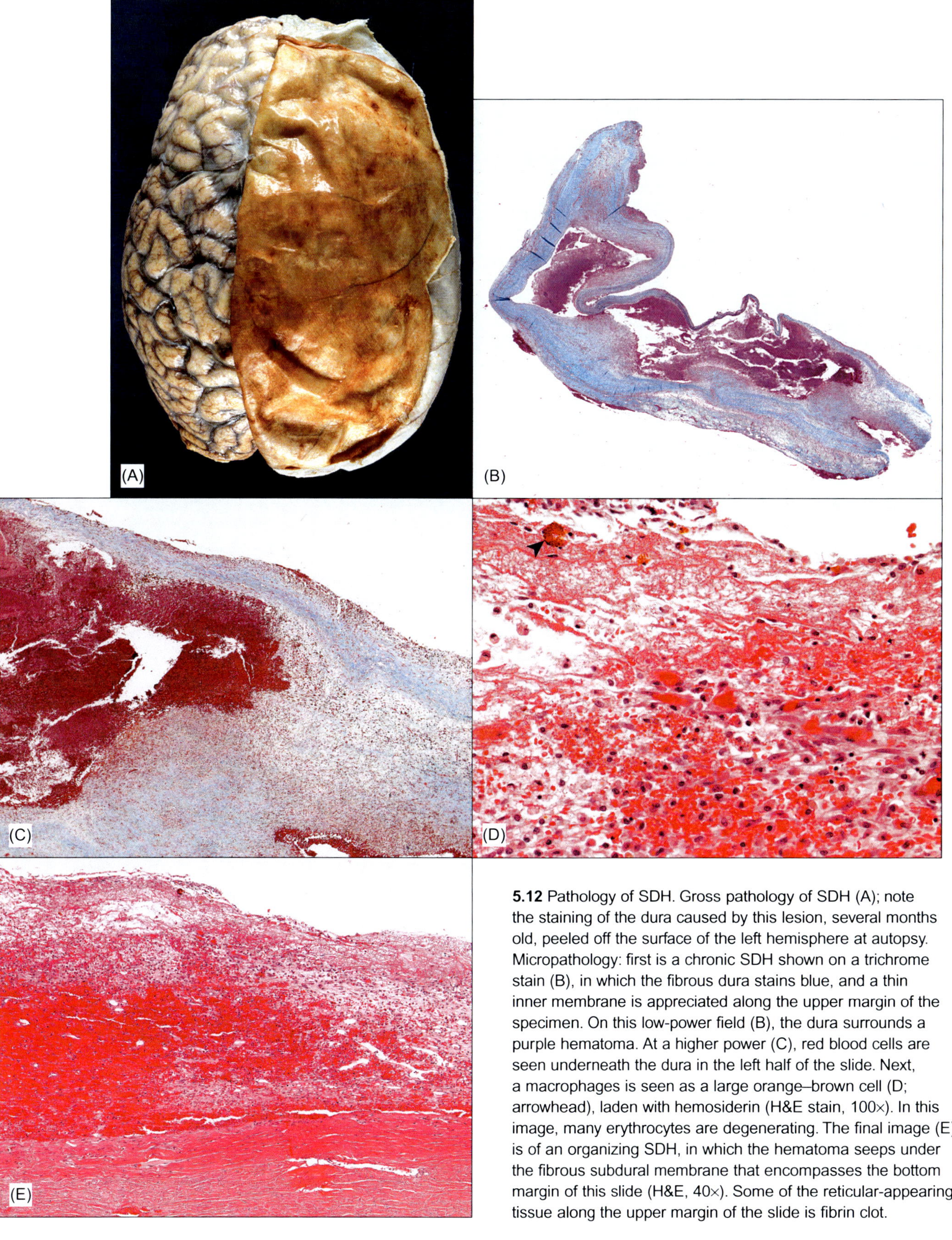

5.12 Pathology of SDH. Gross pathology of SDH (A); note the staining of the dura caused by this lesion, several months old, peeled off the surface of the left hemisphere at autopsy. Micropathology: first is a chronic SDH shown on a trichrome stain (B), in which the fibrous dura stains blue, and a thin inner membrane is appreciated along the upper margin of the specimen. On this low-power field (B), the dura surrounds a purple hematoma. At a higher power (C), red blood cells are seen underneath the dura in the left half of the slide. Next, a macrophages is seen as a large orange–brown cell (D; arrowhead), laden with hemosiderin (H&E stain, 100×). In this image, many erythrocytes are degenerating. The final image (E) is of an organizing SDH, in which the hematoma seeps under the fibrous subdural membrane that encompasses the bottom margin of this slide (H&E, 40×). Some of the reticular-appearing tissue along the upper margin of the slide is fibrin clot.

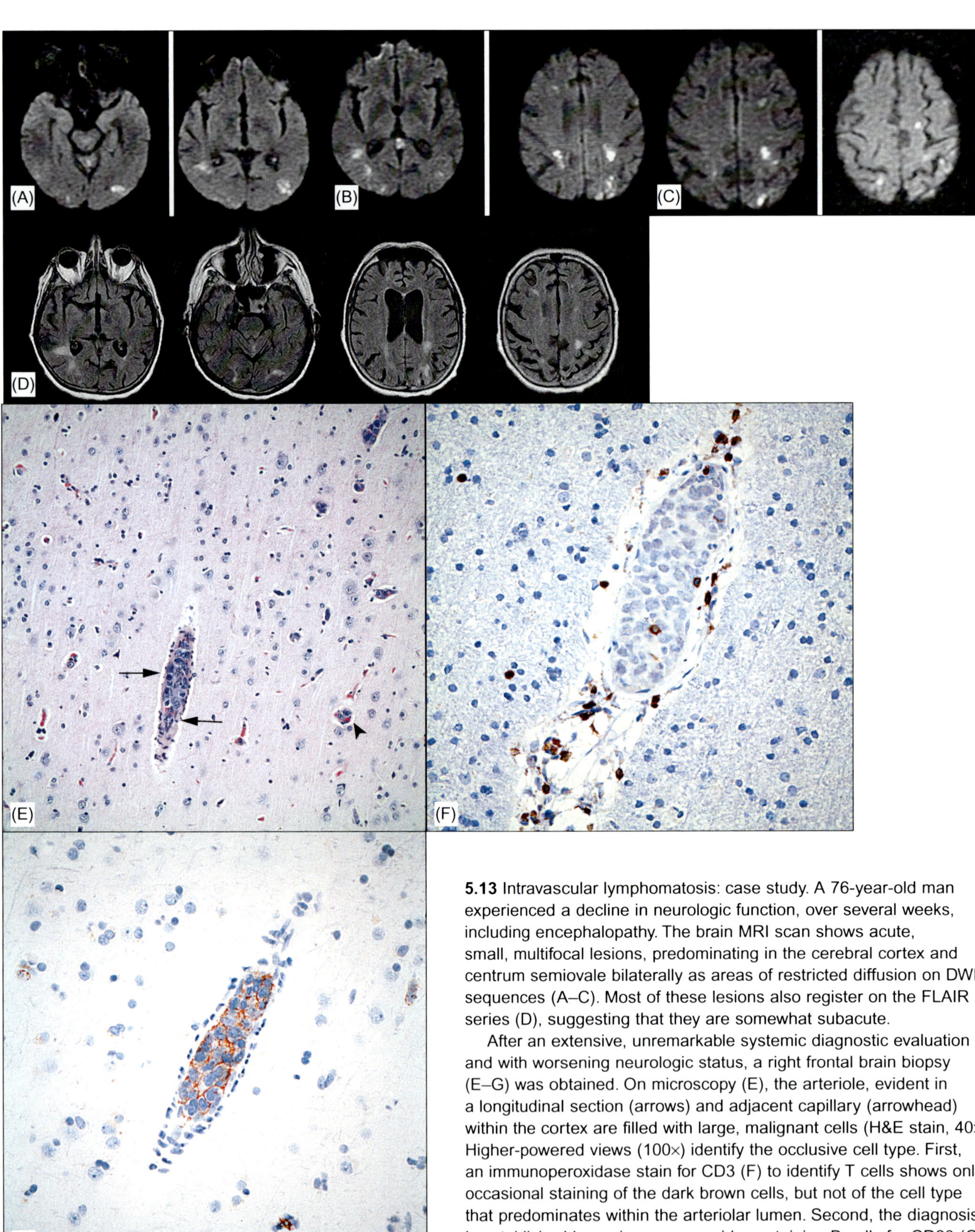

5.13 Intravascular lymphomatosis: case study. A 76-year-old man experienced a decline in neurologic function, over several weeks, including encephalopathy. The brain MRI scan shows acute, small, multifocal lesions, predominating in the cerebral cortex and centrum semiovale bilaterally as areas of restricted diffusion on DWI sequences (A–C). Most of these lesions also register on the FLAIR series (D), suggesting that they are somewhat subacute.

After an extensive, unremarkable systemic diagnostic evaluation and with worsening neurologic status, a right frontal brain biopsy (E–G) was obtained. On microscopy (E), the arteriole, evident in a longitudinal section (arrows) and adjacent capillary (arrowhead) within the cortex are filled with large, malignant cells (H&E stain, 40×). Higher-powered views (100×) identify the occlusive cell type. First, an immunoperoxidase stain for CD3 (F) to identify T cells shows only occasional staining of the dark brown cells, but not of the cell type that predominates within the arteriolar lumen. Second, the diagnosis is established by an immunoperoxidase staining B cells for CD20 (G); the lumen is filled with these large, blue-staining B cells.

Phakomatoses (5.14, 5.15)

The phakomatoses are a diverse group of disorders involving skin and the central nervous system, several with a defined genetic basis. A subset of the phakomatoses are notorious for neurovascular involvement, in particular the Sturge–Weber syndrome and Von Hippel–Lindau (VHL) disease, shown here.[6,7] Others are listed in *Table 5.2*.

CADASIL (5.16)

CADASIL (cerebral autosomal dominant arteriopathy with subcortical infarcts and leukoencephalopathy) is a syndrome characterized by ischemic stroke in the young, as well as migraine and progressive cognitive impairment. White matter lesions in the temporal lobe and external capsule are an early sign of CADASIL,[9] though severe white matter disease eventually develops, including involvement of the U-fibers underlying the cortex. Mutations to the *notch-3* gene on chromosome 19, responsible for a large transmembrane protein, cause this syndrome.

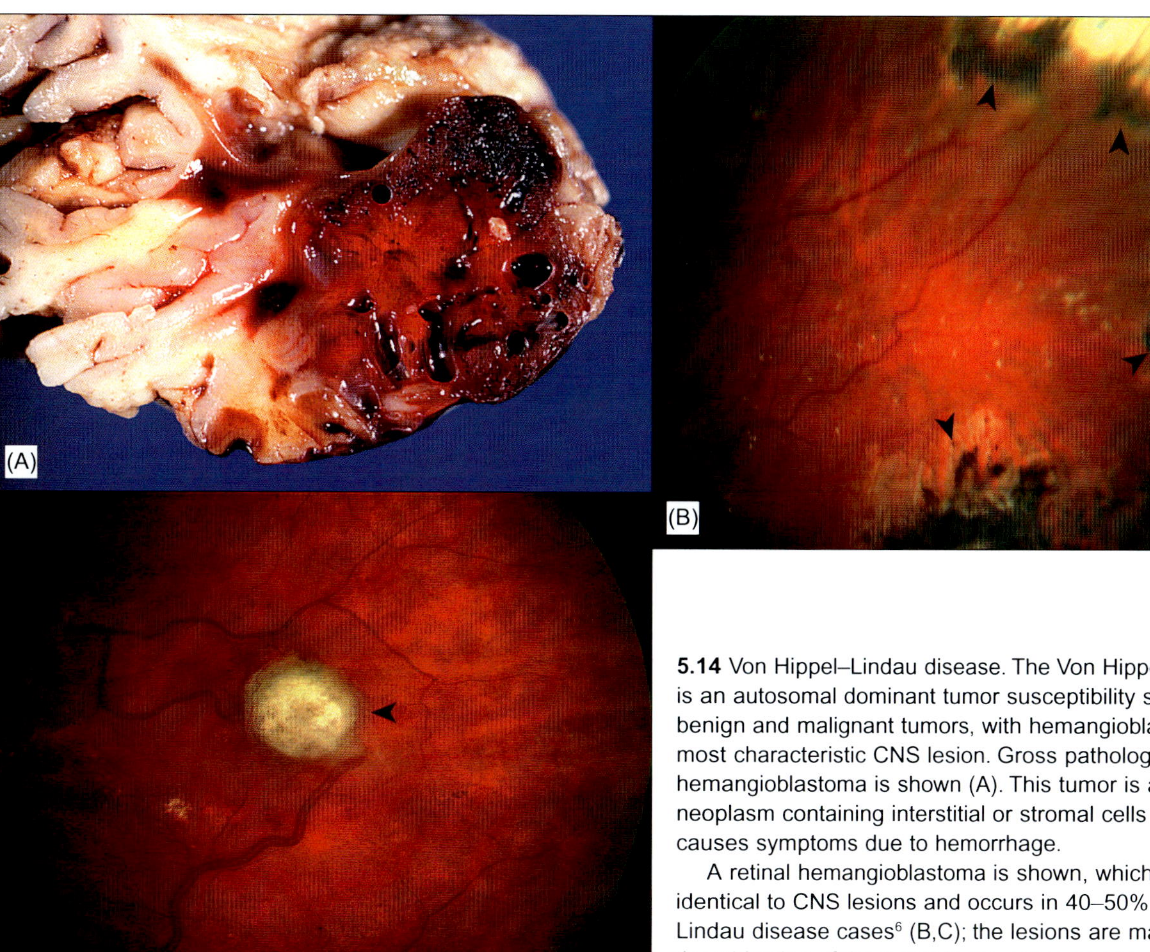

5.14 Von Hippel–Lindau disease. The Von Hippel–Lindau disease is an autosomal dominant tumor susceptibility syndrome of benign and malignant tumors, with hemangioblastoma being the most characteristic CNS lesion. Gross pathology of a cerebellar hemangioblastoma is shown (A). This tumor is a capillary-rich neoplasm containing interstitial or stromal cells that uncommonly causes symptoms due to hemorrhage.

A retinal hemangioblastoma is shown, which is histologically identical to CNS lesions and occurs in 40–50% of Von Hippel–Lindau disease cases[6] (B,C); the lesions are marked (arrowheads); the whitening of the tumor in the second image (C) is due to previous laser therapy (funduscopic images courtesy of Paul Gaudio, MD).

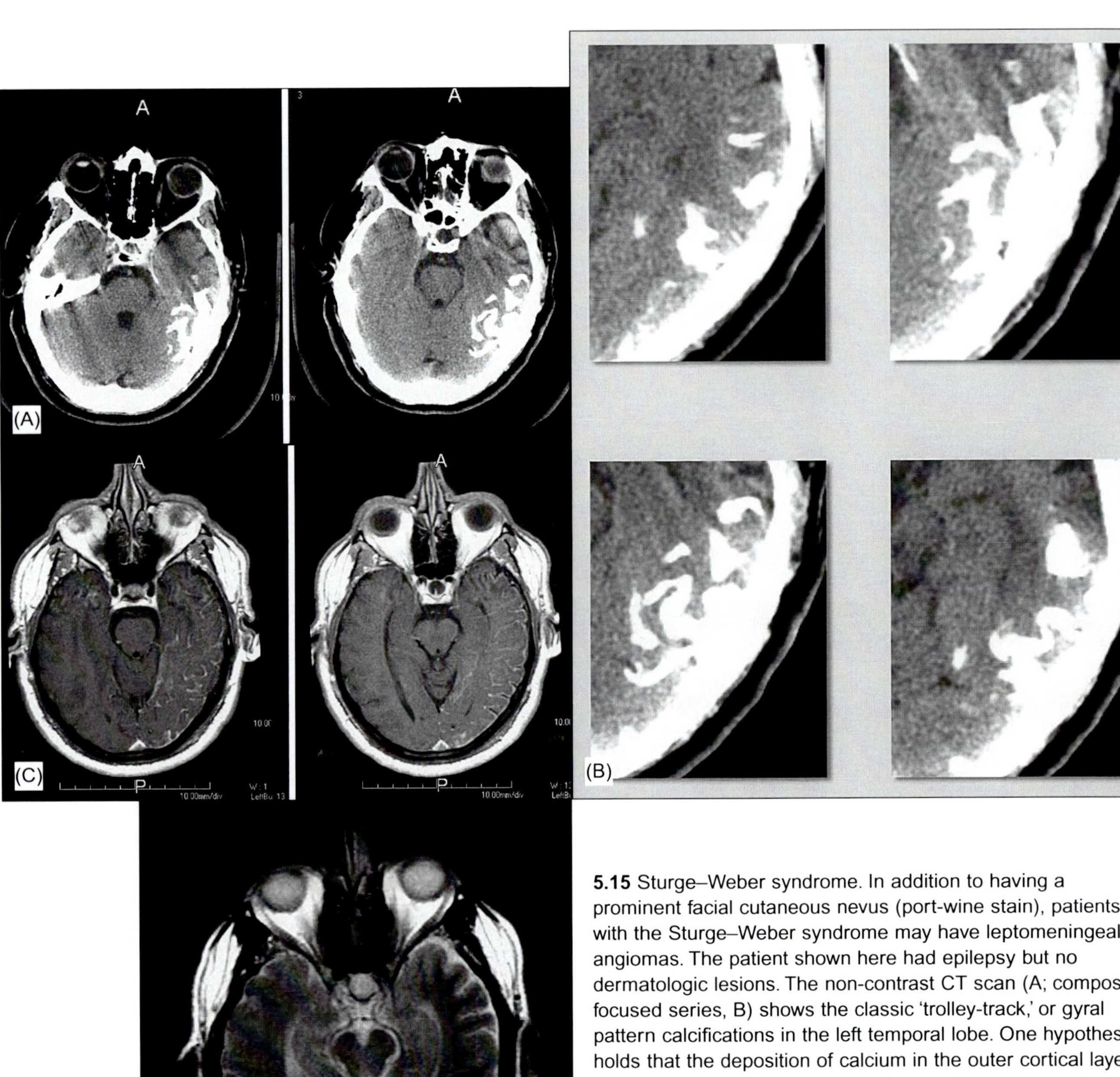

5.15 Sturge–Weber syndrome. In addition to having a prominent facial cutaneous nevus (port-wine stain), patients with the Sturge–Weber syndrome may have leptomeningeal angiomas. The patient shown here had epilepsy but no dermatologic lesions. The non-contrast CT scan (A; composite, focused series, B) shows the classic 'trolley-track,' or gyral pattern calcifications in the left temporal lobe. One hypothesis holds that the deposition of calcium in the outer cortical layers is due to chronic venous stasis with anoxic damage to the nearby cortex.[7]

The MRI study, T1WI with gadolinium (C) and non-contrast T2WI (D) sequences, shows gadolinium enhancement and decreased signal intensity throughout this temporo-occipital region. The leptomeninges are thickened by increased vascularity, and the angiomatous vessels (primarily thin-walled veins) in this patient appear to enter the superficial brain parenchyma and possibly the ipsilateral choroid plexus, and may obliterate the subarachnoid space.[7]

Table 5.2 Neurovascular disorders involving skin and connective tissue[6-8]

Disorder	Stroke type	Stroke mechanism
Behçet's disease	AIS, Venous infarction	Small vessel disease, Hypercoagulability
Ehlers–Danlos syndrome	AIS, SAH	Cervical artery dissection Intracranial aneurysms Carotid-cavernous fistulae
Epidermal nevus syndrome	AIS	Large vessel intracranial dysplasia
Fabry disease	AIS, ICH	Glycolipid accumulation in small- and medium-sized arteries
Hereditary—hemorrhagic Telangiectasias	AIS ICH	Paradoxical embolism via pulmonary AVF Intracranial AVM, CMs
Marfan syndrome	AIS	Aortic and cervical artery dissection
Neurofibromatosis	AIS, SAH	Moyamoya syndrome; intracranial aneurysms; tumor mass effect
Pseudoxanthoma elasticum	AIS	Small vessel and large vessel disease; cervical artery dissection
Sturge–Weber syndrome	SAH	Leptomeningeal angiomatosis
Von Hippel–Lindau disease	ICH	Cerebellar and retinal hemangioblastomas

AIS, acute ischemic stroke; AVM/F, arteriovenous malformation/fistula; CM, cavernous malformation (angioma); ICH, intracerebral hemorrhage; SAH, subarachnoid hemorrhage.

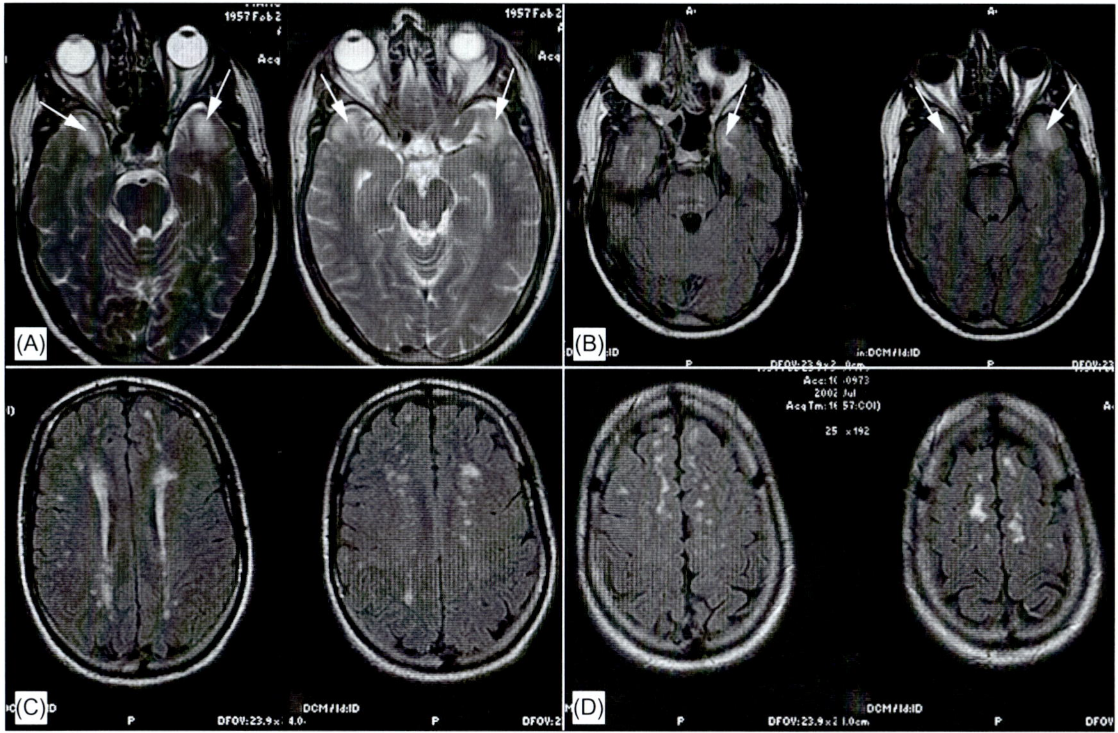

5.16 CADASIL: case study. A healthy 45-year-old man presented with a headache as well as some left body focal symptoms, such as numbness of his hand and lower lip, prompting neuroimaging. The brain MRI sequences (T2WI in A; FLAIR in B–D) showed white matter lesions diffusely, but especially prominent in anterior temporal lobes (arrows). The patient's serum tested positive for a mutation of the *notch-3* gene. There was no known previous family history for CADASIL.

Calcifications and other hyperdensities (5.17–5.21)

Hyperdensities on computed tomography (CT) scan typically signify bone, blood, or calcium but may also indicate metallic foreign materials, such as aneurysm clips and coils, arterial stents or contrast dye. Calcium may become deposited in the intima and media of intracranial and extracranial arteries, and within aneurysmal walls (e.g., **2.9**). The deposition of calcium into vascular walls becomes dysregulated in atherosclerosis, as well as chronic renal disease, diabetes mellitus, and normal aging.[16] Calcification of the intracerebral and extracerebral arteries is a useful marker of atherosclerosis, and a predictor of myocardial infarction and death.[17]

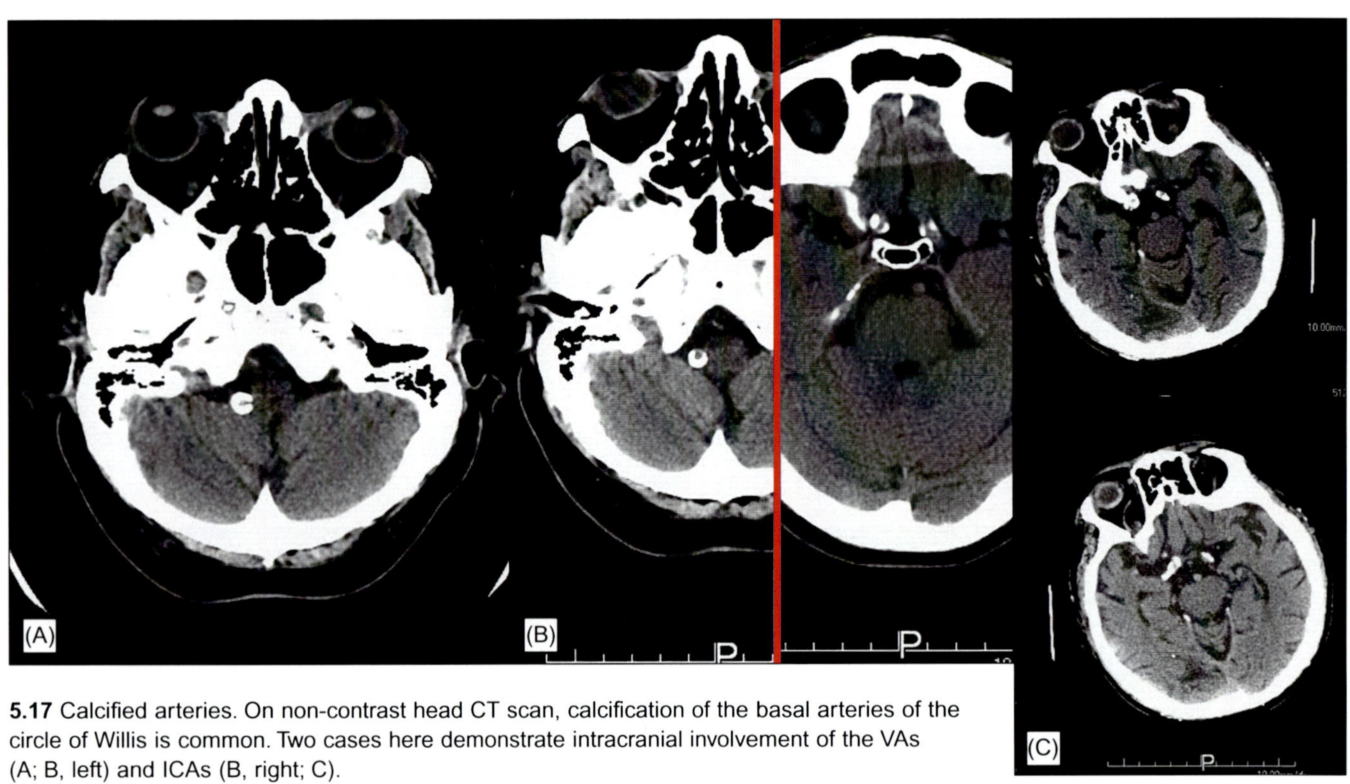

5.17 Calcified arteries. On non-contrast head CT scan, calcification of the basal arteries of the circle of Willis is common. Two cases here demonstrate intracranial involvement of the VAs (A; B, left) and ICAs (B, right; C).

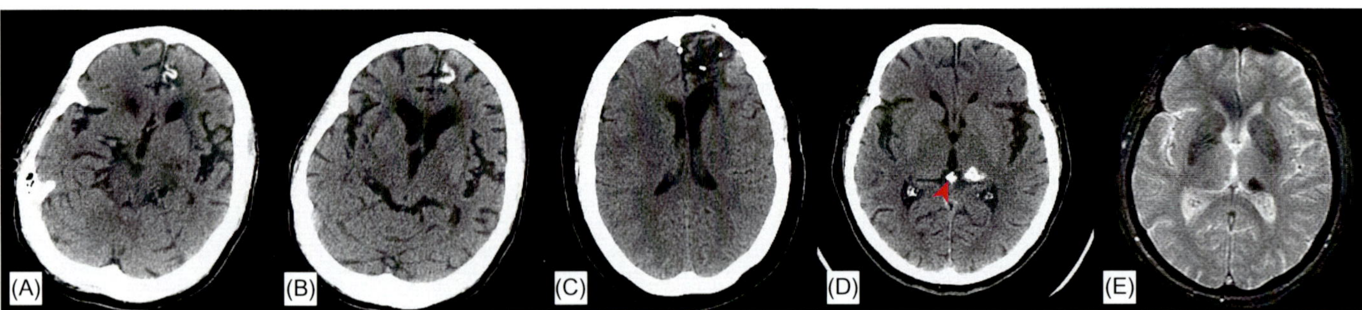

5.18 Calcified stroke. Parenchymal calcification of an old ischemic stroke or hemorrhage is rare.[10] Two examples here demonstrate that calcium may take a gyriform pattern (A,B) or mark an old hypodensity with a multifocal punctuate pattern (C). Finally, calcification of a small, chronic hemorrhage based in the medial thalamus is shown on admission head CT scan (with comparable hyperdensity to the adjacent, midline calcified pineal gland; arrowhead) (D) and on the associated GE-MRI sequence (E).

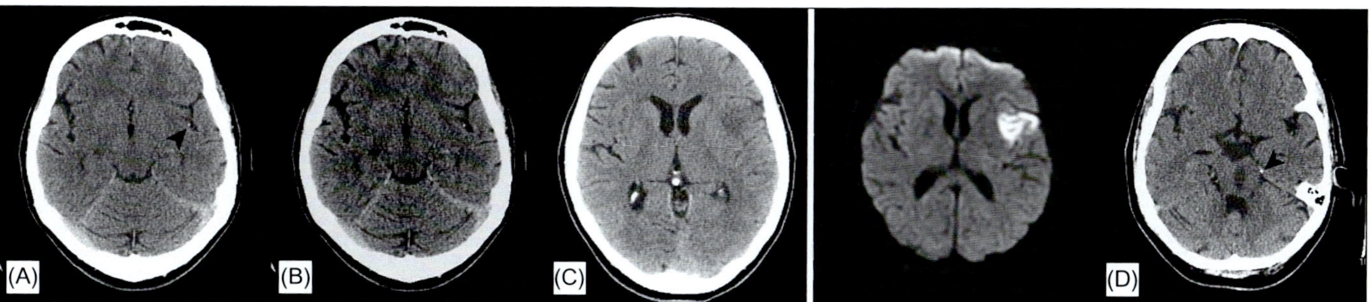

5.19 Hyperdense middle cerebral artery (MCA) dot sign. Acute thrombus, consistent with stagnant blood flow within an artery, is most often seen on non-contrast CT scan as a hyperdense MCA sign, consistent with an M1 and/or M2 thrombosis. It is a predictor of poor outcomes from hemispheric stroke.[11] A more subtle and analogous finding, the MCA 'dot sign', has been validated by catheter angiography as a sensitive and specific indicator of acute thrombosis in M2 or M3 MCA branches.[12]

Here, a left MCA dot sign is shown in the superior Sylvian fissure on the admission non-contrast CT scan of a patient (arrowhead) (A) as well as the same study with a darkening in the level of brightness (B). The acute stroke in the distribution of an anterior M3 branch involves the insular cortex on a more superior transaxial cut of this CT scan (C, left) and the DW-MRI sequence (C, right).

Finally, a possible hyperdense posterior cerebral artery (PCA) dot sign (arrowhead) (D) is shown in a patient with an adjacent, old left paramedian stroke. Alternatively, this hyperdensity could be a focal calcification in this artery's wall.

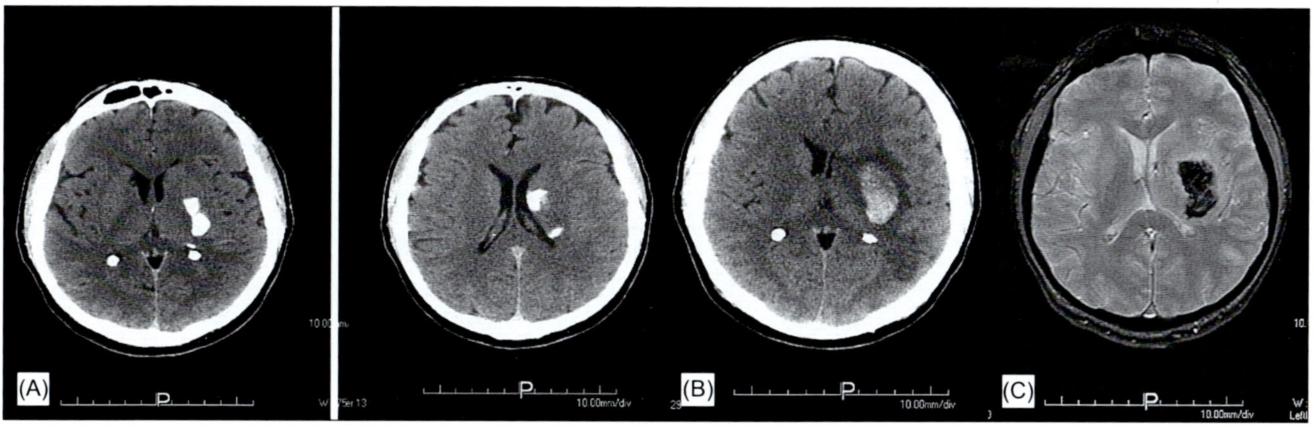

5.20 Contrast extravasation. Contrast extravasation has been defined as a hyperdense lesion with a maximum Hounsfield units >90 on CT that persists on a follow-up CT scan.[13] It has been noted to be a poor prognostic indicator in primary intracerebral hemorrhage,[14,15] as well as a predictor of symptomatic parenchymal hemorrhage following intra-arterial treatment for acute ischemic stroke.[13] The patient shown here was treated with IV and intra-arterial thrombolysis. The initial head CT scan (A) shows contrast extravasation into the periventricular white matter and the putamen. This hyperdensity faded on a follow-up head CT scan 5 days later, in a manner typical of contrast extravasation (B). A GE-MRI sequence 1 day after the initial head CT scan registers the local hemorrhagic transformation (C). Another case of contrast extravasation, during AVM embolization, is shown elsewhere (**3.9**).

Intracranial dolichoectasia (5.22, 5.23)

The development of dolichoectasia (elongation and tortuosity) of the intracranial arteries has a predilection for the posterior circulation.[18,19] Patients may develop stroke due to localized ischemia of the paramedian pontine perforators from the basilar artery (BA), causing lesions in the brainstem and cerebellum, and/or artery-to-artery embolism to the distal territories of the cerebellum, occipital lobe, and thalamus.[18]

Radiation arteriopathy (5.24–5.26)

Radiation exposure causes an arteriopathy in the large cervical arteries comparable with atherosclerosis, though potentially in atypical locations (e.g., within the cervical vertebral artery (VA) and common carotid arteries (CCA) depending upon the local site receiving radiotherapy. The arterial layers most affected appear to be the intima and endothelium, although to some extent, pathologic changes develop in all components of the vascular wall.[20]

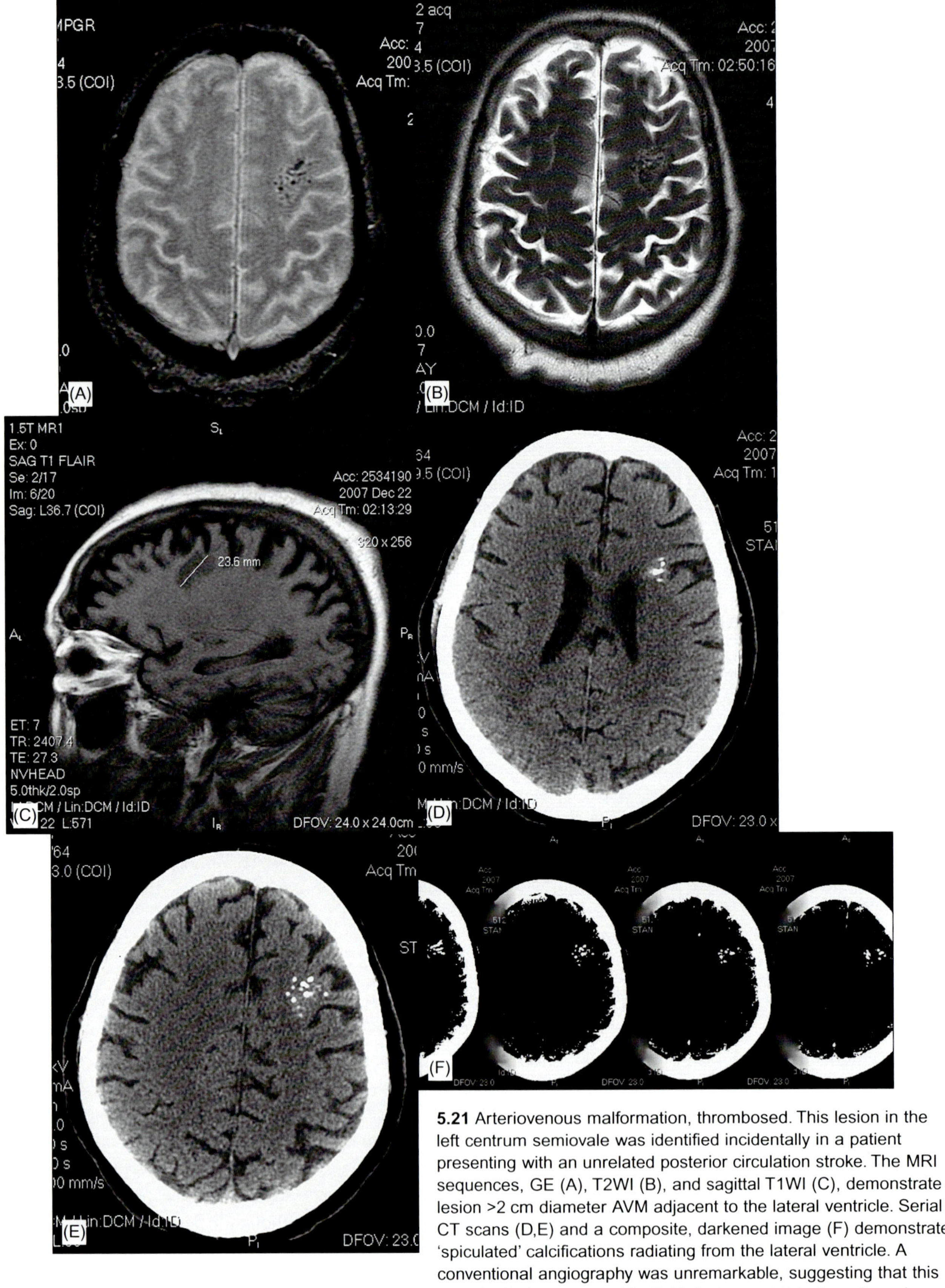

5.21 Arteriovenous malformation, thrombosed. This lesion in the left centrum semiovale was identified incidentally in a patient presenting with an unrelated posterior circulation stroke. The MRI sequences, GE (A), T2WI (B), and sagittal T1WI (C), demonstrate a lesion >2 cm diameter AVM adjacent to the lateral ventricle. Serial CT scans (D,E) and a composite, darkened image (F) demonstrate 'spiculated' calcifications radiating from the lateral ventricle. A conventional angiography was unremarkable, suggesting that this vascular lesion, a probable AVM, had completely thrombosed.

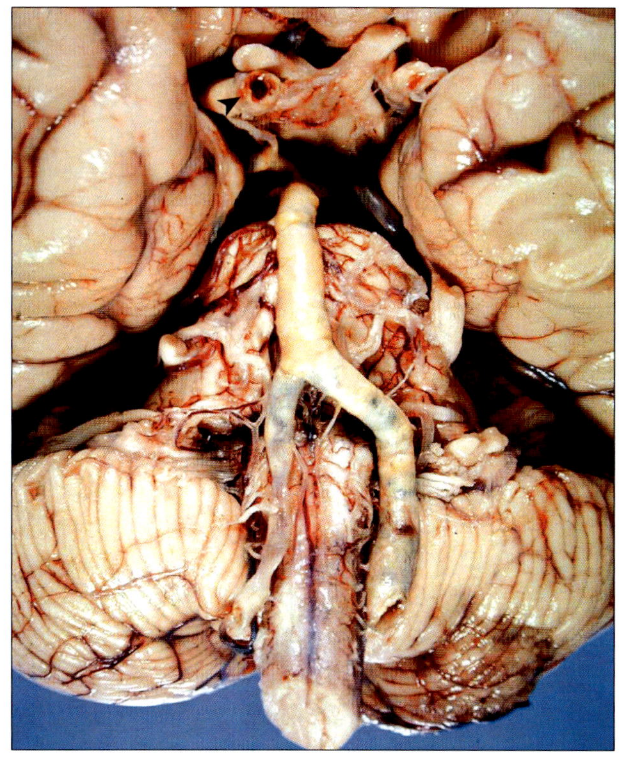

5.22 Vertebrobasilar atherosclerosis. Gross pathology of a markedly enlarged vertebrobasilar system, with plaque diffusely lining the walls of the large arteries. The BA and left VAs appear to have a diameter comparable with the distal right ICA (arrowhead) (pathology courtesy of Louis Caplan, MD).

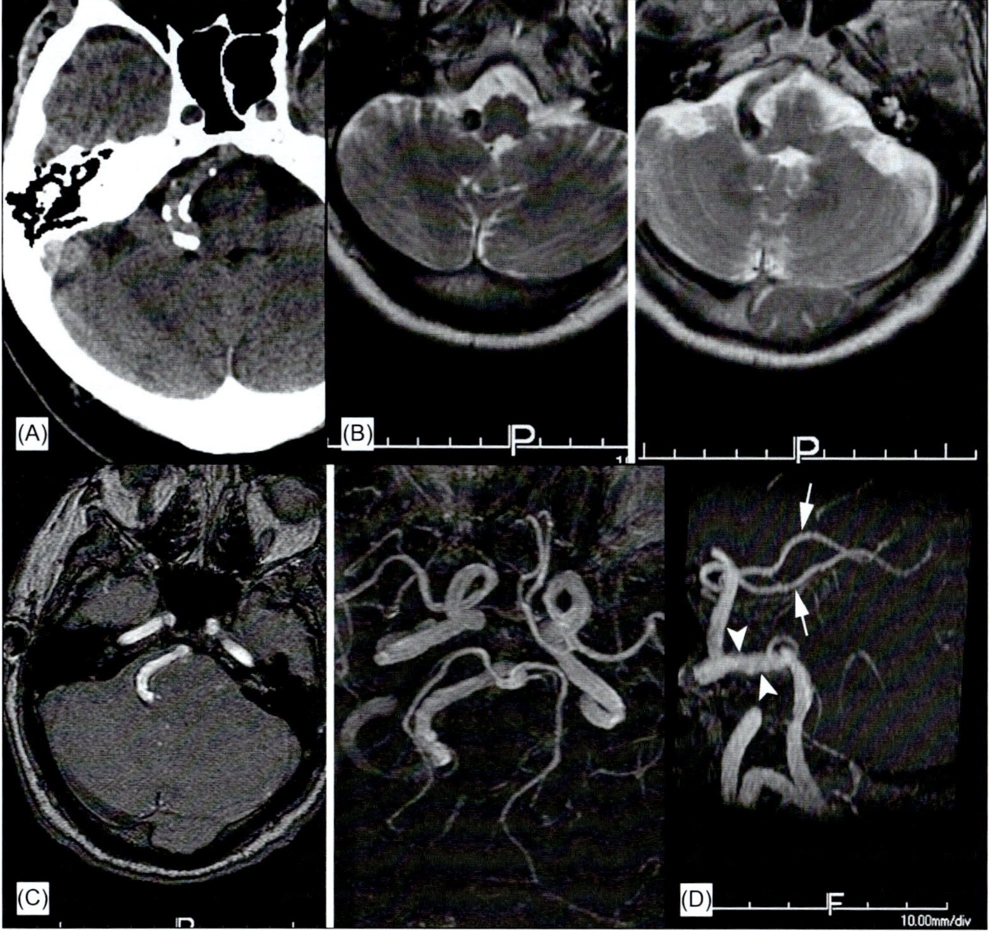

5.23 Vertebrobasilar dolichoectasia. A 70-year-old man presented with a small ventral pontine stroke causing sixth- and seventh-nerve paresis. The admission CT scan (A) shows an enlarged, calcified right VA with some mass effect on the medulla. The T2-weighted MRI study (B) better shows the relationship of the dilated vertebrobasilar complex to the adjacent medulla. Source images from magnetic resonance angiography (MRA) (C, left) and an intracranial MRA study (C, right) demonstrate that the vertebrobasilar system has an enlarged diameter comparable with the ICAs. Finally, a sagittal MRA (D) shows the severe tortuosity, in which the dolichoectatic VA segment courses horizontally (arrowheads), parallel to the PCA (arrows), prior to its continuation as the BA.

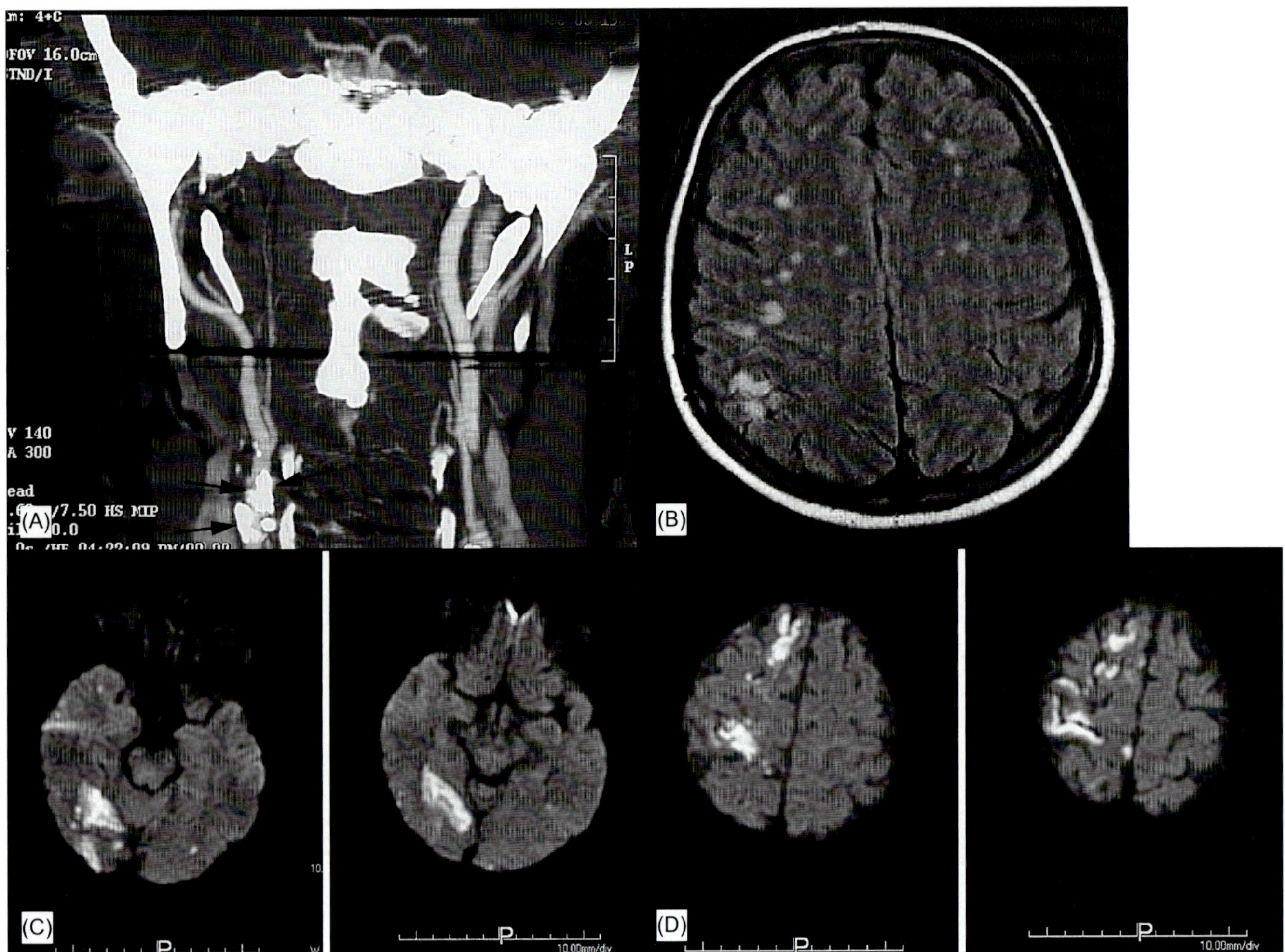

5.24 Carotid bifurcation disease. This patient had severe ICA disease that progressed to occlusion; this cervical CT angiography study (A) shows extensive calcification of the right carotid system (arrows), making it difficult to ascertain flow through the ICA at its origin. There was a history of tobacco use and remote radiation therapy to the breast and axillary region (for breast cancer), and stenosis of the right subclavian artery. The FLAIR study (B) shows a predominance of right- greater than left-sided lesions in the centrum semiovale, a common finding in advanced proximal ICA disease. The patient later presented with a right hemispheric stroke, suggestive of both embolic and border zone lesions. The DW-MRI sequences show acute infarcts within the right PCA territory (there was a right fetal PCA) (C) and the right ACA/MCA border zone (D).

Common treatment sites resulting in radiation arteriopathy responsible for stroke include tumors in the neck (e.g., lymphoma, thyroid carcinoma) or brain (e.g., optic tract glioma, meningioma). Revascularization of cervical arteries that accumulate radiation arteriopathy is typically undertaken as an endovascular procedure. Proximal lesions of the ICA are usually treated with balloon angioplasty and stenting, because radiation arteriopathy makes standard carotid endarterectomy more difficult technically than for typical atherosclerotic disease.

Sickle cell disease (5.27)

This hematologic disorder may cause ischemic stroke, intracerebral hemorrhage, and venous infarction.[21] In time, patients may develop a large vessel intracranial arteriopathy consistent with moyamoya syndrome. Intracranial sickle cell disease should be monitored by transcranial Doppler neurosonology, as plasmapheresis has been demonstrated to be efficacious in primary and secondary stroke prevention.[22,23]

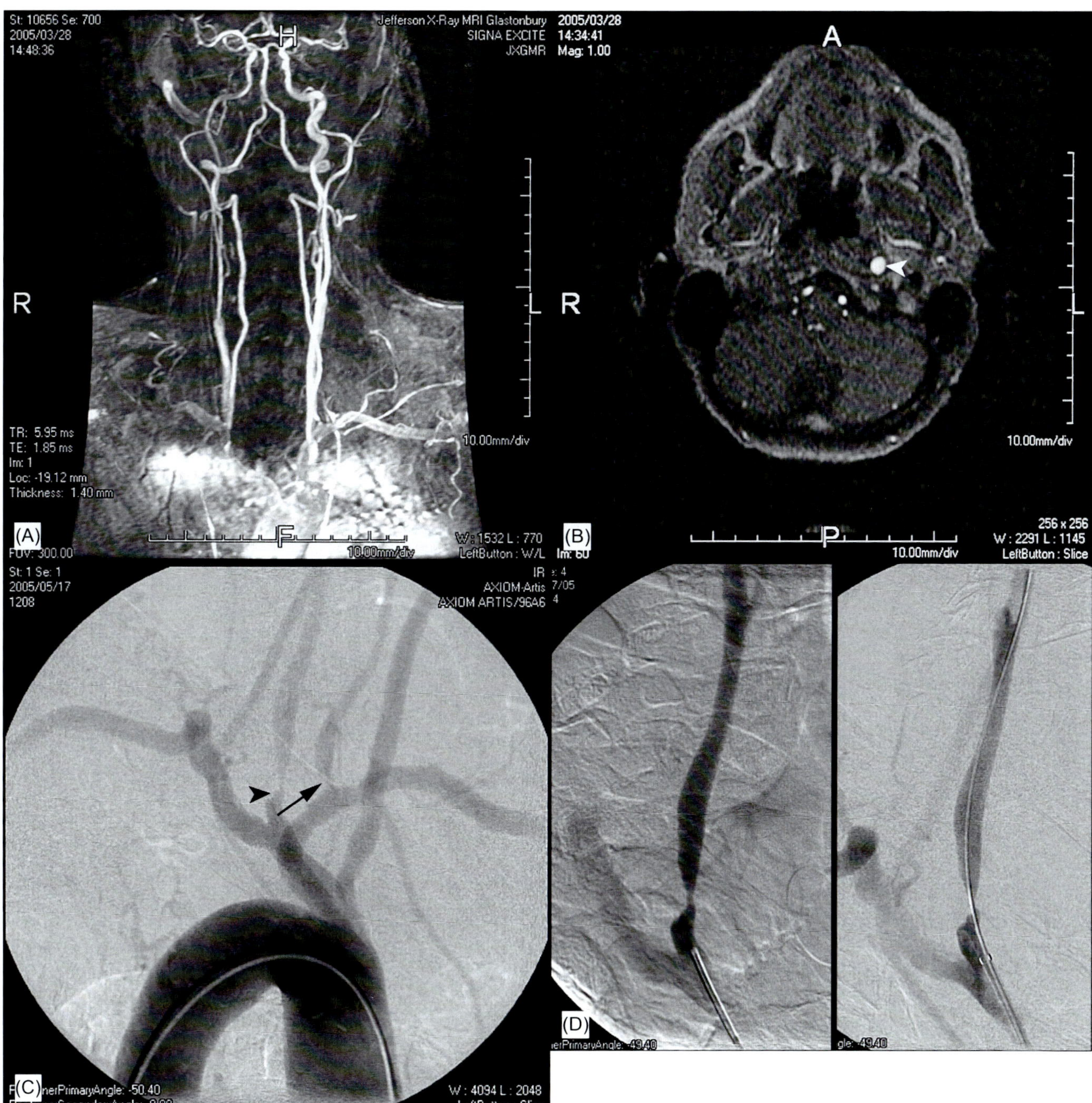

5.25 Common carotid artery (CCA) disease. A 62-year-old man was treated 12 years earlier for non-small cell lung cancer with local radiation therapy and chemotherapy, and his cervical artery disease was identified during an outpatient evaluation for dizziness. The coronal cervical MRA (A) suggests diminished flow from the right mid-CCA through the course of the cervical and intracranial ICA. On a transaxial source image (B), flow is readily appreciated in the left intracranial ICA (arrowhead), but not the right, suggestive of occlusion of the latter. On conventional angiography of the aortic arch (C), all of the major cervical arteries appear to originate from the same single trunk. Stenoses of the proximal left VA (arrow) and right CCA (arrowhead) are visualized. The CCA lesion (D) is isolated (left), and a guidewire is threaded beyond the catheter tip, through the lesion (right), in preparation for angioplasty and stenting of this stenotic segment.

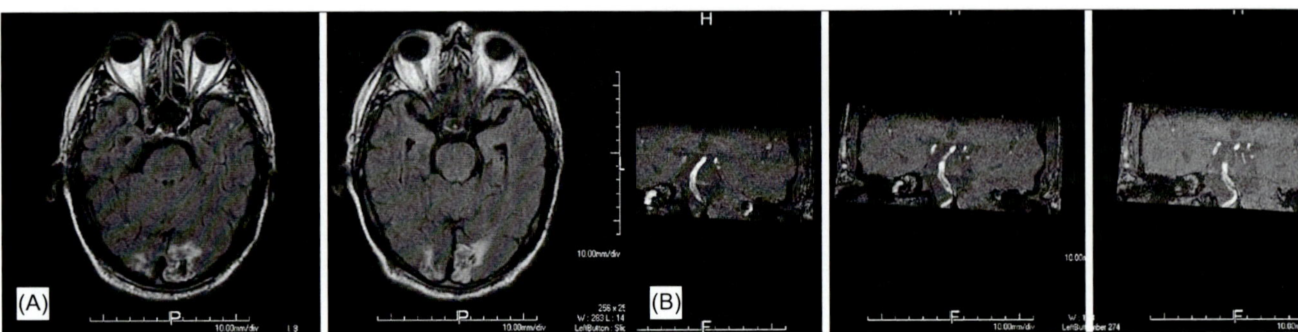

5.26 Basilar artery disease. A 70-year-old man had a left cerebellopontine angle tumor, reportedly a meningioma, treated with surgery and later radiotherapy. He presented 5 years later with right hemifield visual loss, and bilateral PCA territory infarcts, shown here on FLAIR sequence (A). An MRA study (not shown) suggested high-grade proximal BA stenosis, the probable source of this large vessel thromboembolic stroke. Angioplasty of the BA disease was thus undertaken. On a composite view of several adjacent coronal slices from a follow-up MRA study (B), obtained 4 months post-angioplasty, the BA appears open, but the flow signal is heterogeneous, consistent with local large vessel disease.

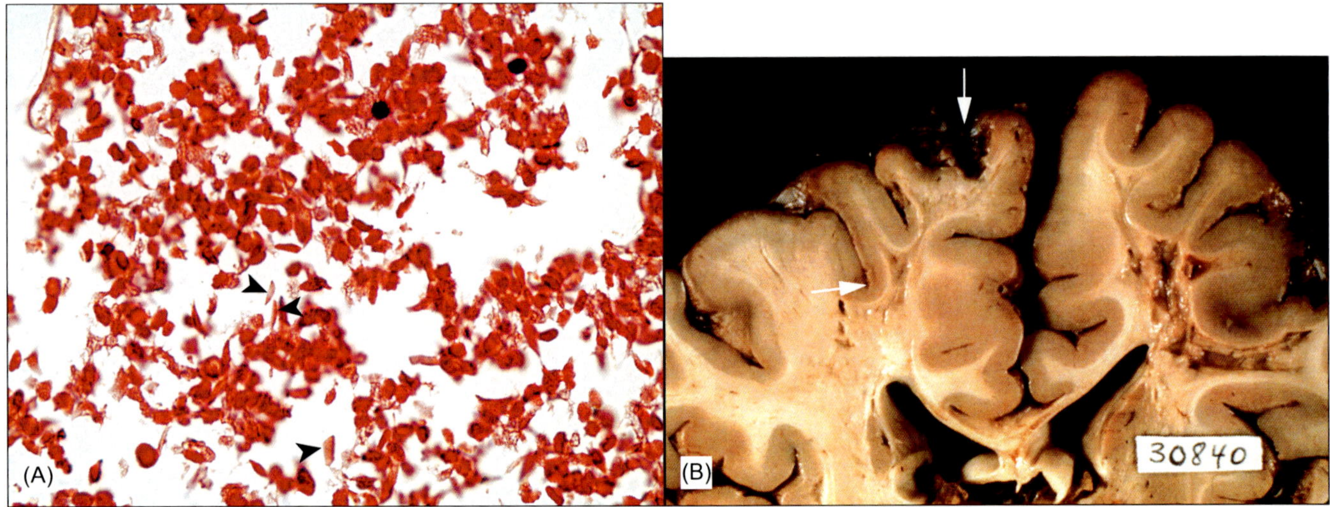

5.27 Sickle cell disease. A peripheral blood smear (A) shows individual sickle cells (arrowheads). Gross pathology (B) coronal section shows the brain of a patient with sickle cell disease who developed a border zone infarct (arrows), probably in the ACA–MCA territory, a common result of advanced moyamoya syndrome.

Spinal cord infarction and vascular malformations (5.28–5.30)

Neurovascular lesions in the spinal cord are rare. Most present with an acute and/or stepwise symptoms of cord dysfunction, specifically paraparesis or quadriparesis, and autonomic deficits, including sphincter flaccidity, atonic bladder, sexual dysfunction, and paralytic ileus.[24] True spinal transient ischemic attack (TIA) (e.g., from cardiac or aortic atheroembolism) is quite rare. Dural arteriovenous fistulae or malformations of the cord often cause fluctuating and subsequently progressive symptoms, with the potential for segmental pain due to increased venous pressure. The classification system of spinal cord vascular malformations is beyond the scope of this textbook[25] and other references delineate the complex vasculature of the spinal cord.[24]

The transverse size of the spinal cord is quite small such that even with magnetic resonance imaging (MRI) studies, individual lesions often may be difficult to discern. Similarly, delineating spinovascular lesions with conventional spinal angiography may be quite challenging. A few case examples of MRI studies are shown here.

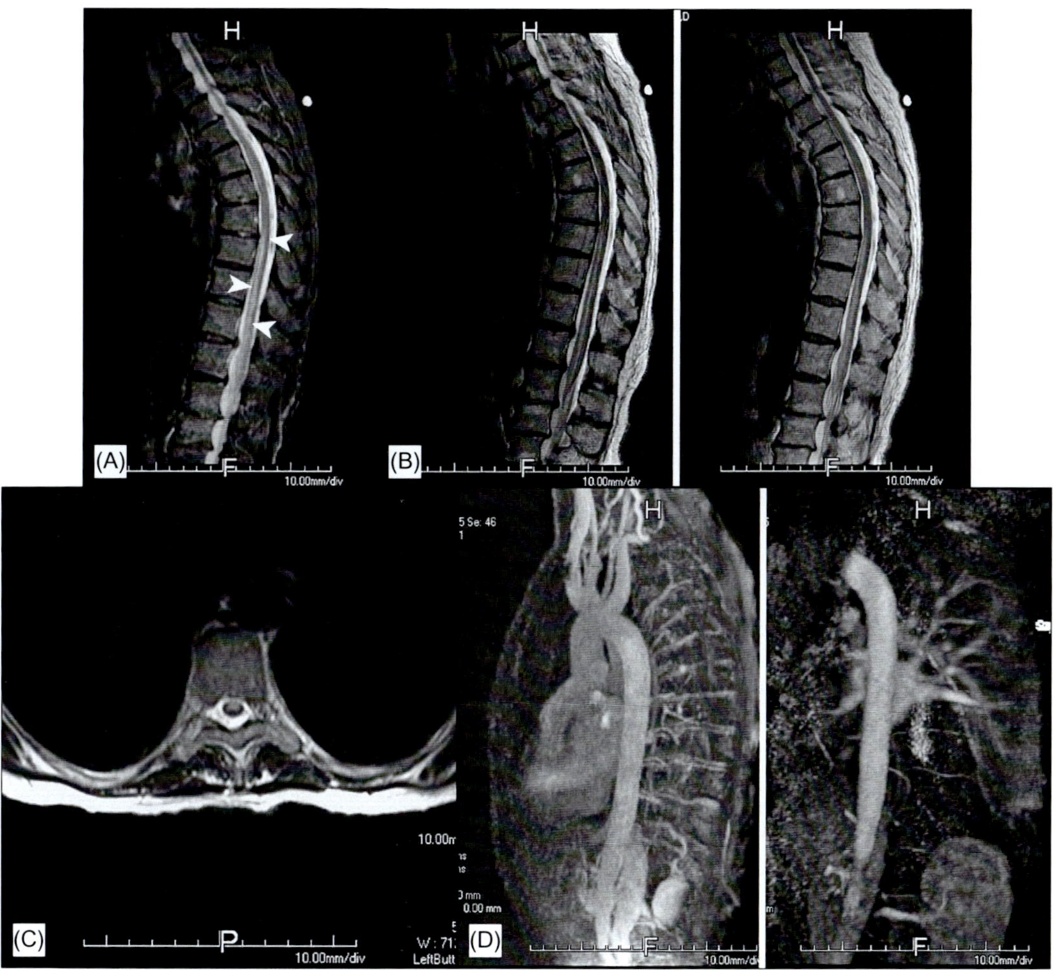

5.28 Spinal cord infarction (thoracic). The hallmark of this syndrome is the preservation of posterior column function (sensation to light touch, vibration, and position), due to an intact network of the posterior spinal arteries that spare the posterior third of the cord. This 64-year-old woman awoke with a dense paraparesis and a mid-thoracic sensory level. The spine MRI study shows abnormal signal through the anterior half of the spinal cord from the mid-thoracic level into much of the lumbar levels. The intramedullary lesion is shown on turbo spin echo (arrowheads) (A) as well as short tau inversion recovery (B, left) and T2-weighted (B, right) sequences. This lesion appears on a single transverse section in the thoracic region (C), demonstrating involvement of the anterior two-thirds of the cord. Arterial imaging of the aorta and its associated radicular arteries (D) are selected from sagittal maximum intensity projection (left) and MRA (right) studies. MRA will usually not provide adequate sensitivity (compared with conventional angiography) to delineate an occlusion of a single radicular artery.

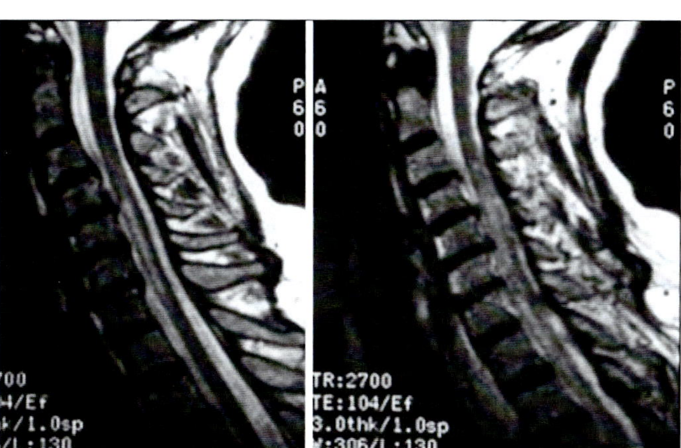

5.29 Spinal cord infarction (cervical). A sagittal cervical T2-weighted study shows a hyperintense signal (left image) in the anterior cord adjacent to the C5–C7 vertebral bodies, consistent with an anterior spinal artery–territory infarction.

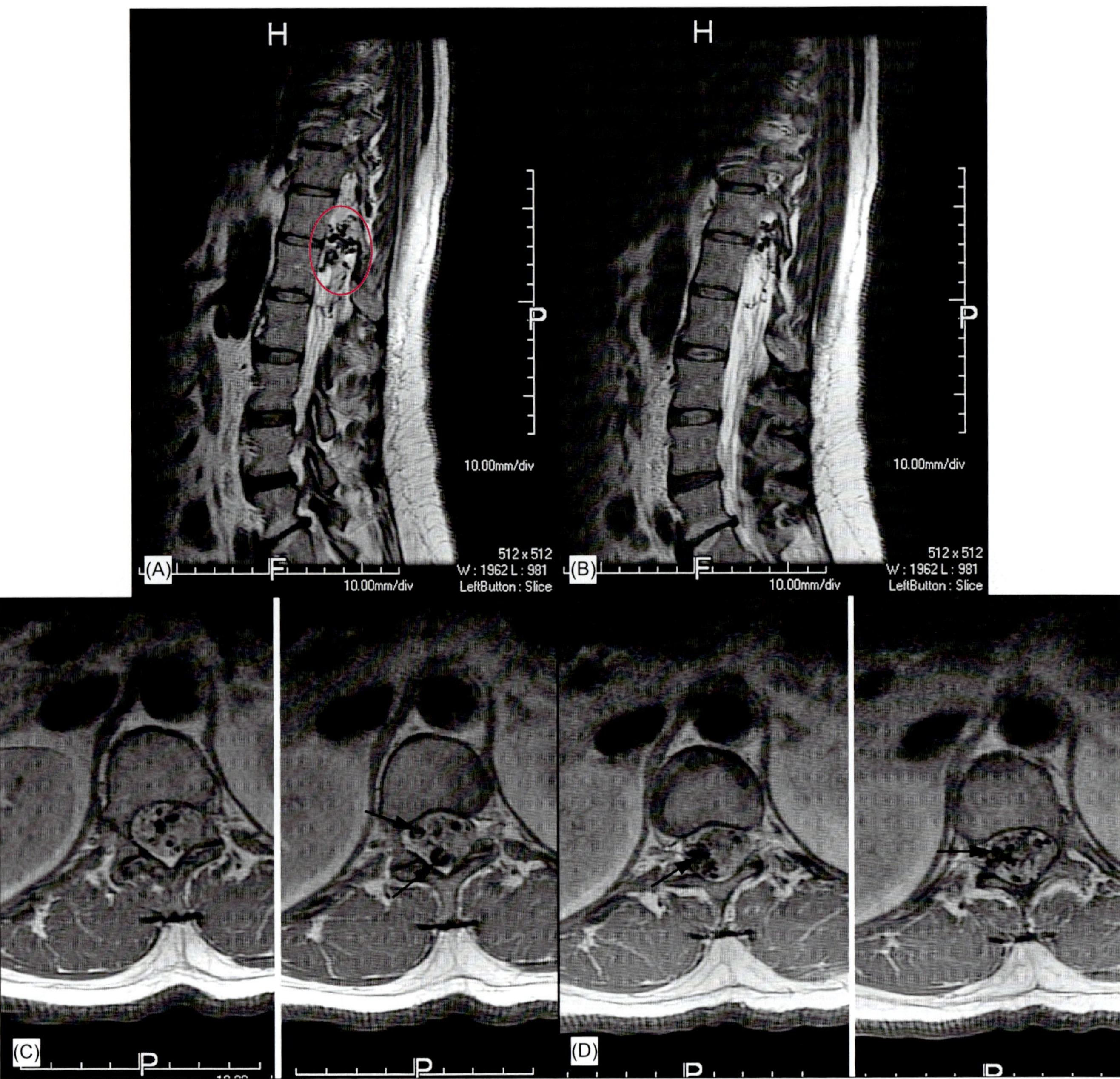

5.30 An AVM of the conus. This complex lesion is shown on sagittal T2WI (A,B; nidus encircled in A) and transaxial proton density images (C,D). In transaxial views, the lesion is appreciated as large, dark flow voids based in the right half of the spinal column (arrows), where nerve roots typically exit the spinal cord.

References

1. Bederson J. Pathophysiology and animal models of dural arteriovenous malformations. In: Awad I, Barrow D, eds. *Dural Arteriovenous Malformations*. Park Ridge, IL: American Association of Neurological Surgeons; 1993: 23–33.
2. Osborn A. Vascular malformations. In: *Diagnostic Cerebral Angiography*, 2nd ed. Philadelphia, PA: Lippincott Williams & Wilkins; 1999: 277–312.
3. Borden J, Wu J, Shucart W. A proposed classification for spinal and cranial dural arteriovenous fistulous malformations and implications for treatment. *J Neurosurg* 1995; **82**: 166–79.
4. Hinchey J, Chaves C, Appignani B, *et al*. A reversible posterior leukoencephalopathy syndrome. *N Engl J Med* 1996; **334**: 494–500.
5. Detsky M, Chiu L, Shandling M, Sproule M, Ursell M. Heading down the wrong path. *N Engl J Med* 2006; **355**: 67–74.
6. Duff J, Regli L. Von Hippel–Lindau disease. In: Bougousslavsky J, Caplan L, eds. *Uncommon Causes of Stroke*. New York: Cambridge University Press; 2001: 338–44.
7. Roach E. Sturge–Weber syndrome. In: Bougousslavsky J, Caplan L, eds. *Uncommon Causes of Stroke*. New York: Cambridge University Press; 2001: 330–7.
8. Moussouttas M, Fayad P, Rosenblatt M, *et al*. Pulmonary arteriovenous malformations: cerebral ischemia and neurologic manifestations. *Neurology* 2000; **55**: 959–64.
9. O'Sullivan M, Jarosz J, Martin R, Deasy N, Powell J, Markus H. MRI hyperintensities of the temporal lobe and external capsule in patients with CADASIL. *Neurology* 2001; **56**: 628–34.
10. Wityk RJ, Lapeyrolerie D, Stein BD. Rapid brain calcification after ischemic stroke. *Ann Intern Med* 1993; **119**: 490–1.
11. Manelfe C, Larrue V, von Kummer R, *et al*. Association of hyperdense middle cerebral artery sign with clinical outcome in patients treated with tissue plasminogen activator. *Stroke* 1999; **30**: 769–72.
12. Leary M, Kidwell C, Villablanca J, *et al*. Validation of computed tomographic middle cerebral artery 'dot' sign: an angiographic correlation study. *Stroke* 2003; **34**: 2636–40.
13. Yoon W, Seo J, Kim J, Cho K, Park J, Kang H. Contrast enhancement and contrast extravasation on computed tomography after intra-arterial thrombolysis in patients with acute ischemic stroke. *Stroke* 2004; **35**: 876–81.
14. Becker K, Baxter A, Bybee H, Tirschwell D, Abouelsaad T, Cohen W. Extravasation of radiographic contrast is an independent predictor of death in primary intracerebral hemorrhage. *Stroke* 1999; **30**: 2025–32.
15. Mayer S. Ultra-early hemostatic therapy for intracerebral hemorrhage. *Stroke* 2003; **34**: 224–9.
16. Johnson R, Leopold J, Loscalzo J. Vascular calcification: pathobiological mechanisms and clinical implications. *Circ Res* 2006; **99**: 1044–59.
17. Doherty T, Fitzpatrick L, Shaheen A, Rajavashisth T, Detrano R. Genetic determinants of arterial calcification associated with atherosclerosis. *Mayo Clin Proc* 2004; **79**: 197–210.
18. Passero S, Filosomi G. Posterior circulation infarcts in patients with vertebrobasilar dolichoectasia. *Stroke* 1998; **29**: 653–9.
19. Pico F, Labreuche J, Touboul P-J, Amarenco P. Intracranial arterial dolichoectasia and its relation with atherosclerosis and stroke subtype. *Neurology* 2003; **61**: 1736–42.
20. Blecic S, Bougousslavsky J. Other uncommon angiopathies. In: Bougousslavsky J, Caplan L, eds. *Uncommon Causes of Stroke*. New York: Cambridge University Press; 2001: 355–68.
21. Coull B, Skaff P. Disorders of coagulation. In: Bougousslavsky J, Caplan L, eds. *Uncommon Causes of Stroke*. New York: Cambridge University Press; 2001: 86–95.
22. Adams R, McKie V, Hsu L, *et al*. Prevention of a first stroke by transfusions in children with sickle cell anemia and abnormal results on transcranial Dopper ultrasonography. *N Engl J Med* 1998; **339**: 5–11.
23. Adams R, McKie V, Nichols F, *et al*. The use of transcranial ultrasonography to predict stroke in sickle cell disease. *N Engl J Med* 1992; **326**: 605–10.
24. Sturzenegger M. Spinal stroke syndromes. In: Bogousslavsky J, Caplan L, eds. *Stroke Syndromes*, 2nd edn. New York: Cambridge University Press; 2001: 691–704.
25. Chaloupka J, Huddle D. Classification of vascular malformations of the central nervous system. *Neuroimaging Clin North America* 1998; **8**: 295–321.

Further reading

Awad I, Barrow DL, eds. *Dural Arteriovenous Malformations*. Park Ridge, IL: American Association of Neurological Surgeons; 1993.

Bougousslavsky J, Caplan L, eds. *Uncommon Causes of Stroke*. New York: Cambridge University Press; 2001.

Digre K, Corbett J. Amaurosis fugax and not so fugax – vascular disorders of the eye. In: *Practical Viewing of the Optic Disc*. New York: Butterworth Heinemann; 2003: 269–344.

Osborn A. Vascular malformations. In: *Diagnostic Cerebral Angiography*, 2nd edn. Philadelphia: Lippincott Williams & Wilkins; 1999: 277–312.

Sturzenegger M. Spinal stroke syndromes. In: Bogousslavsky J, Caplan L, eds. *Stroke Syndromes*, 2nd edn. New York: Cambridge University; 2001: 691–704.

Index

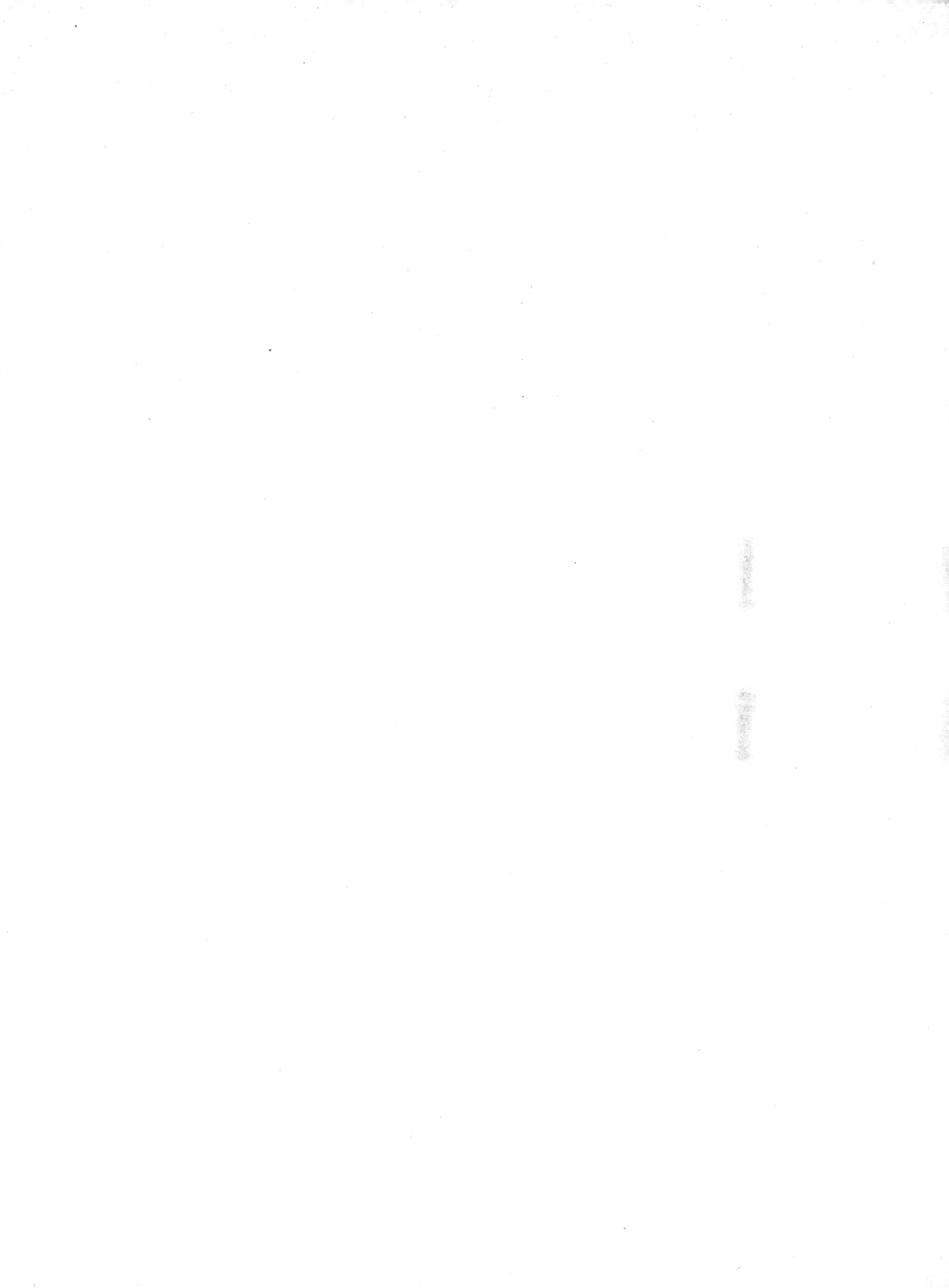